Pediatric Obesity

Prevention, Intervention, and Treatment Strategies for Primary Care

Sandra G. Hassink, MD, FAAP
Director, Pediatric Weight Management Clinic
AI duPont Hospital for Children
Wilmington, DE
Assistant Professor of Pediatrics
Thomas Jefferson University Medical School
Philadelphia, PA

American Academy of Pediatrics
141 Northwest Point Blvd
Elk Grove Village, IL 60007-1098

American Academy of Pediatrics Department of Marketing and Publications Staff

Maureen DeRosa, MPA
Director, Department of Marketing and Publications

Mark Grimes
Director, Division of Product Development

Jeff Mahony
Manager, Product Development

Eileen Glasstetter, MS
Manager, Consumer Publishing

Regina Moi Martinez
Manager, Patient Education

Sandi King, MS
Director, Division of Publishing and Production Services

Kate Larson
Manager, Editorial Services

Jason Crase
Editorial Specialist

Theresa Wiener
Manager, Editorial Production

Linda Diamond
Manager, Art Direction and Production

Jill Ferguson
Director, Division of Marketing and Sales

Linda Smessaert
Manager, Clinical and Professional Publications Marketing

Library of Congress Control Number: 2006928516
ISBN-10: 1-58110-221-6
ISBN-13: 978-1-58110-221-5

MA0355

1 2 3 4 5 6 7 8 9 10

....

To my husband Bill and my children Matthew, Stephen, and Alexa for your unfailing love and support.

Also to all my friends and colleagues along the way who have dedicated themselves to improving the lives of children.

Table of Contents

Foreword

Obesity is affecting more children than ever before. Up to one third of the childhood population has a body mass index (BMI) greater than 85% for age[1] and more than half of these children have a BMI greater than 95%.[2] These children are at risk for and are often already suffering from obesity-related comorbidities such as type 2 diabetes, nonalcoholic steatohepatitis, polycystic ovarian syndrome, sleep apnea, and Blount disease. They are also at risk for a lifetime of obesity with all its attendant medical and psychosocial consequences.

The evolution of obesity in childhood and adolescence is a complex interplay of gene-environment interactions, child temperament, parenting style, family dynamics, and home, school, and community environments. Children are influenced by parental role modeling, television advertising, and commercial food and entertainment offerings. Obesity and obesity-related comorbidities begin in childhood. Children in many ways are at the epicenter of the epidemic.

What does this mean for us as providers of pediatric health care? Not only can we not ignore the effects of obesity on the children we care for, we need to put ourselves in a position to take positive action in developing prevention, intervention, and treatment strategies for obesity.

This manual will help guide these efforts by providing information, strategies, and suggestions for approaches to prevention, intervention, and treatment at the primary care level. Starting with chapters on assessment and evaluation, each subsequent chapter focuses on a specific developmental stage with strategies for prevention of obesity in the normal weight population, intervention for children at risk for obesity, and treatment approaches for those children and adolescents whose BMIs are already greater than 95%. Families play a central role in modeling behavior, buffering the effects of an obesity-promoting environment and changing nutrition and activity habits to achieve a healthy energy balance for their children. Included in each chapter are questions for parents, self-assessment exercises, and points to touch on to enhance parenting information and skill in making family-based change. Additional information on practice-based changes and school interventions for primary care professionals can be used as a springboard for change in their own communities.

Patient handouts, American Academy of Pediatrics policy statements, a physician tracking form, and coding and reimbursement information are all collected in the appendices to aid the practitioner in implementing practice change aimed at obesity prevention, intervention, and treatment.

1. Ogden CL, Carroll MD, Curtin LR, McDowell MA, Tabak CJ, Flegal KM. Prevalence of overweight and obesity in the United States, 1999-2004. *JAMA.* 2006;295:1549–1555
2. Whitaker RC, Wright JA, Pepe MS, Seidel KD, Dietz WH. Predicting obesity in young adulthood from childhood and parental obesity. *N Engl J Med.* 1997; 337:869–873

Acknowledgments

Thanks for the thoughtful reviews of these chapters by the following members of the American Academy of Pediatrics Task Force on Obesity: Jamie Calabrese, MD, FAAP; Mark S. Jacobson, MD, FAAP; Nancy F. Krebs, MD, FAAP; Donald L. Shifrin, MD, FAAP; and Howard L. Taras, MD, FAAP.

Chapter 1

Childhood Obesity: An Overview

• •

1.1 The Rise in Obesity

Childhood obesity has risen to epidemic proportions. Pediatricians are faced with children at risk for obesity, obese children, and children suffering from the comorbidities of obesity every day. An overview of the problem will help us begin to create a strategy to respond to the needs of these patients and families.

What has happened to the population in the past 2 decades that has given rise to an increase of childhood and adult obesity of epidemic proportions?

There has been an inexorable shift in energy balance over the past 20 years. A combination of decreased activity, increased inactivity, and consumption of calories in excess of need have resulted in the steadily increasing prevalence rates of childhood and adolescent obesity. In 2003–2004, 33.6% of children between the ages of 2 and 19 years had body mass indexes (BMIs) greater than 85% (at risk for overweight/overweight) and 17.1% had BMI values greater than 95% (overweight/obese).[1]

This increase in obesity is occurring across the board and is alarmingly affecting our youngest patients. Of children aged 2 to 5 years, 26.2% had BMI values greater than 85%, while 13.9% were already obese with BMI values greater than 95%.[1]

Minority populations are being hit even harder. In 2003–2004, Mexican American and African American children aged 2 to 19 years who had BMI values greater than 85% made up 37% and 35.1% of these populations of children compared with non-Hispanic white children of the same age range with rates of 33.5%. These disparities are magnified by the number of children with BMI values greater than 95%, with 19.2% of Mexican American children and 20.0% of African American children 2 to 19 years of age obese compared with 16.3% of non-Hispanic white children aged 2 to 19 years.[1]

Genetic and Environmental Factors

What genetic and environmental interactions are involved?

There are hundreds of genes or gene markers associated in some way with obesity. Predisposition to energy imbalance, increased nutrient partitioning to adipose tissue, and susceptibility to intrauterine programming are among many proposed mechanisms involving gene-environment interaction. Families with one or both parents who are obese are at increased risk for having an obese child and adolescent.[2] Predisposition for obesity-related comorbidities may also be inherited. For example, it is common to see type 2 diabetes, hypertension, dyslipidemia, and insulin resistance clustered in families. In most cases of obesity, genetic susceptibility to the environment influences outcome.

The interaction between genetics and environment is complex. Nutritional components may influence gene regulation, the intrauterine environment may affect later susceptibility to an energy-abundant environment, and the environment may have a greater effect during periods of rapid growth.

Societal Effects of Obesity

How does this explosion of obesity and associated comorbidities involve the child, family, community, and society at large?

The societal costs of obesity are increasing. There will be a burden of illnesses in the young adult and adult population we have not seen before. More young parents will be chronically ill and this will affect their children. There will be increasing stress on the health care system in terms of economics, time, and personnel. The length of stay for discharges associated with obesity is longer than overall discharges. Costs associated with childhood obesity were calculated as $127 million per year in a recent review of hospital costs.[3] The overall health effects on the population and the cost to the larger economy are already threatening to become our biggest health expenditure.

1.2 The Medical Effects of Childhood Obesity

What are the medical effects of having an increasing population of obese children and adolescents?

Childhood obesity can be thought of as an accelerator of adult diseases. Obese children and adolescents are now experiencing comorbidities including type 2 diabetes, hypertension, dyslipidemia, obstructive sleep apnea, and nonalcoholic steatohepatitis (NASH) that had previously been seen predominantly in adults. In addition, obesity in childhood gives rise to serious orthopedic problems such as slipped capital femoral epiphysis (SCFE) and Blount disease and increases the incidence of less common but serious obesity-related conditions such as pseudotumor cerebri. These are diseases and complications few of us thought we would see in childhood or even adolescence; they give urgency to our need to institute prevention and early intervention as well as diagnosis and treatment.

Complications

Complications of obesity can be life threatening and even life ending. Some severe obesity-related emergencies include hyperglycemic hyperosmolar state (HHS), diabetic ketoacidosis, pulmonary embolism, and cardiomyopathy of obesity. All of these have been seen in obese children and adolescents.

Hyperglycemic hyperosmolar state can rarely be the first manifestation of type 2 diabetes. Patients may initially present with symptoms of vomiting, abdominal pain, dizziness, weakness, polyuria and polydipsia, weight loss, and diarrhea.[4] If unrecognized, patients may develop hyperosmolar nonketotic coma and death.[5] Diagnostic criteria for HHS include a plasma glucose level of greater that 600 mg/dL, serum carbon dioxide level of greater than 15 mmol/L, small ketonuria, absent to low ketonemia, an effective serum osmolality of greater than 320 mOsm/kg, and stupor or coma.[4,5]

Diabetic ketoacidosis can be an initial manifestation of type 2 diabetes. Insulin resistance often accompanies obesity and results in low baseline insulin sensitivity and relative insulin deficiency. This leads to increased lipolysis, increased free fatty acids in circulation, ketonemia, and ketonuria. Diabetic ketoacidosis should be treated as such, with the diagnosis of the type of diabetes made when the patient is stabilized.

Pulmonary embolism has been reported as a complication of gastric bypass in adolescence.[6] The risk factors for pulmonary embolism include obesity, obesity-hypoventilation syndrome, obstructive sleep apnea syndrome, and coagulation disorder. Symptoms include dyspnea, chest pain, decreased oxygen concentration, and hemoptysis.

Congestive heart failure resulting from obesity has been seen in morbidly obese adolescents. The effect of obesity on the heart is known as *cardiomyopathy of obesity* and is thought to result from high metabolic activity of excessive fat, which increases total blood volume and cardiac output and leads to left ventricular dysfunction. Dilation, increased left ventricular wall stress, and compensatory left ventricular hypertrophy then occur. Pulmonary hypertension caused by upper airway obstruction can also occur. Signs and symptoms of cardiac failure should point to this diagnosis.[7]

Comorbidities

Besides these frightening emergencies, there are a group of obesity-related comorbidities that require immediate attention. These include pseudotumor cerebri, SCFE, Blount disease, obstructive sleep apnea syndrome, NASH, cholelithiasis, metabolic syndrome, acanthosis nigricans, polycystic ovarian syndrome (PCOS), and type 2 diabetes.

Obesity occurs in 30% to 80% of children with *pseudotumor cerebri*.[8] Pseudotumor cerebri is defined as increased intracranial pressure with papilledema and normal cerebrospinal fluid in the absence of ventricular enlargement. Papilledema is part of the pathology of pseudotumor cerebri but may not occur initially. Presentation may range from an incidental finding on funduscopic examination to headaches, vomiting, blurred vision, or diplopia. Loss of peripheral visual fields and reduction in visual acuity may be present at diagnosis.[9] Neck, shoulder, and back pain have also been reported.[9] Treatment of pseudotumor cerebri includes acetazolamide, lumboperitoneal shunt in severe cases, and weight loss.[10] Pseudotumor cerebri is a diagnosis of exclusion after other causes of increased intracranial pressure are eliminated.

Slipped capital femoral epiphysis is a slipping of the femoral epiphysis through the zone of hypertrophic cartilage cells, which are under the influence of gonadal hormones and growth hormone.[11] Fifty percent to 70% of patients with SCFE are obese.[12] Patients can present with limp or complaints of groin, thigh, or knee pain. Hips should be examined and radiographs of both hips should be obtained because bilateral slips occur in 20% of cases. Medial and posterior displacement of the femoral epiphysis is seen through the growth plate relative to the femoral neck.[13] Treatment is surgical pinning of the hip.

The diagnosis of *Blount disease* involves the identification of bowing of the tibia and femur. This can affect one or both knees. This condition results from the overgrowth of the medial aspect of the proximal tibial metaphysis. Obesity has been reported in two thirds of patients with Blount disease.[14] Treatment requires surgical correction and weight loss.

Obstructive sleep apnea syndrome is a common diagnosis associated with obesity. This syndrome is defined as a disorder of breathing during sleep characterized by prolonged partial upper airway obstruction or intermittent complete obstruction that disrupts normal ventilation during sleep and normal sleep patterns.[15] Symptoms can include nighttime awakening, restless sleep, difficulty awakening in the morning, daytime sleepiness, napping, enuresis, decreased concentration and memory, and poor school performance.[16] Nighttime polysomnography is the diagnostic procedure of choice to make this diagnosis. If left untreated, children can have pulmonary hypertension, systemic hypertension, and right-sided heart failure.[15] Weight gain, hypertrophy of the tonsils and adenoids, and intercurrent upper respiratory infections can provoke symptoms.

Nonalcoholic steatohepatitis is suspected when elevated liver enzymes are found in the context of fatty liver discovered by ultrasound in the absence of other causes of liver disease. Twenty percent to 25% of obese children have been found to have evidence of steatohepatitis.[17] The definitive diagnosis is by liver biopsy in which evidence of inflammatory infiltrates and fibrosis can be seen. Nonalcoholic steatohepatitis can progress to cirrhosis and end-stage liver disease.[18] Weight loss reduces fatty infiltration and may decrease fibrosis.

Cholelithiasis symptoms in children include abdominal pain and tenderness with diagnosis made by ultrasound and appropriate laboratory studies. Fifty percent of cases in adolescents are associated with obesity.[19]

Metabolic syndrome is a condition characterized by insulin resistance. The components in childhood are obesity, elevated blood pressure, elevated triglyceride levels, decreased high-density lipoprotein (HDL) cholesterol, increased low-density lipoprotein cholesterol, and impaired glucose tolerance.

Acanthosis nigricans is often associated with metabolic syndrome, insulin resistance, and type 2 diabetes. This is a condition characterized by hyperpigmentation and velvety thickening that occurs in the neck, axillae, and groin.

Polycystic ovarian syndrome can occur in adolescence. It is characterized by insulin resistance in the presence of elevated androgens. Clinical signs and symptoms include oligomenorrhea or amenorrhea, hirsutism, acne, polycystic ovaries, and obesity. There is some evidence that girls with premature adrenarche are at risk for PCOS.[20]

Type 2 diabetes occurs when the diagnosis of hyperglycemia is made in the presence of insulin resistance and an elevated insulin level. Type 2 diabetes can present with HHS, diabetic ketoacidosis, or symptoms of polyuria, polydipsia, and weight loss. Diagnosis can also be made based on symptoms of hyperglycemia in an obese patient such as abdominal pain, vomiting, dizziness, and weakness.

1.3 The Pediatrician's Role in the Obesity Epidemic

Historical Perspective: From Malnutrition to Obesity

Pediatricians have always been focused on helping children maintain normal growth. One of the founding principles of pediatrics is that good nutrition is essential for health and growth. In 1897, L. Emmett Holt, Sr, MD, in *The Diseases of Infancy and Childhood* wrote, "Nutrition in its broadest sense is the most important branch of pediatrics." In the late 19th and early 20th centuries, cycles of gastroenteritis and resultant malnutrition and recurrent infections caused the death of countless infants. Efforts were made to promote breastfeeding, ensure a safe milk supply, and create formula tailored to infant needs. Vitamin deficiencies were identified and treated and the government created programs such as food stamps; the Special Supplemental Nutrition Program for Women, Infants, and Children (commonly referred to as WIC); and school lunch and breakfast programs to ensure that children's nutritional needs were met.

Pediatricians vigorously identified and treated children with failure to thrive and weight or height deceleration with the knowledge that growth disturbances were often the early signs of significant illness. Growth charts became tools used to assess overall health and there was always a feeling of reassurance when children were "staying on the growth chart." Attention to the optimum growth of premature infants, children with chronic disease, and children who are disadvantaged have all become integral parts of pediatric practice.

With a focus on optimum growth as a cornerstone to preventive care, pediatricians have

- Come to understand the importance of height and weight as measures of overall health
- Recognized the importance of breastfeeding in supporting healthy growth
- Given attention to environmental, social, and psychosocial factors as parameters that are crucial to healthy growth
- Recognized the importance of social supports in maintaining optimal nutrition and growth
- Recognized the effect of family life events on the growth of children
- Recognized the link between deviations in growth and disease

The obesity epidemic challenges us to use these same skills to examine our strategies for prevention, intervention, and treatment to help children stay on the growth curve. We have recognized that children with obesity are at risk for and suffer from diseases that we previously only saw in adults. Pediatricians have the opportunity to be involved with children and families from birth throughout adolescence. We have experience in taking a broad approach to growth and can use insights from our experiences to help our patients and families.

Today's Children at Risk

How does the obesity epidemic involve individual patients and our inter-action with them and their families?

As you end this chapter, ask yourself what as pediatricians do we want for our patients? A healthy start in life; a chance to participate in the normal activities of childhood; a childhood free of disease. The vignettes that close this chapter show us how close this problem is to our everyday practice. This manual will help you begin to address the prevention and treatment of obesity in your daily encounters with patients and families.

You are seeing newborns in the nursery and examine Marta, a 1-day-old little girl born of Hispanic parents. Her chances of developing type 2 diabetes over her lifetime are 50%.

The lifetime risk of developing diabetes for an average person born in the United States in 2000 until his or her death is

- Male—1 in 3 chance
- Female—2 in 5 chance
- Hispanic female—1 in 2 chance (high risk)

Progression to diabetes among those with prediabetes is not inevitable. Studies suggest that weight loss and increased physical activity among people with prediabetes prevent or delay diabetes and may return blood glucose levels to normal.[21]

You are seeing Tom, a 14-year-old who wants to play football, for a sports physical. His BMI is 35.

Adolescents who are obese have approximately an 80% likelihood of being obese adults.[22]

You are asked to speak at a preschool parents' meeting on nutrition and obesity.

The number of obese children has tripled in the past 3 decades.[23] One in 3 children are currently overweight or obese (BMI at 85% or higher).[1]

You meet Mr and Mrs Brown for a prenatal visit. Both the Browns are significantly obese.

There is a 75% chance that children will be overweight if both parents are obese; a 25% to 50% chance if just one parent is obese.[3]

Parents of an obese high school sophomore ask you if there is anything they can do to help him lose weight.

More than 90% of high schools have vending machines, stores, or snack bars, but only 21% sell low-fat yogurt, fruits, or vegetables.[23] Only 50% of schools offer intramural activity or clubs for students.[3] Only 6% to 8% of schoolchildren are in daily physical education.[23]

You are interviewed by your local newspaper and asked about the cost of the epidemic of childhood obesity.

Hospital costs of pediatric obesity in 1999 were $127 million per year.[1]

Parents of an overweight 8-year-old ask you about her health risks during a well examination.

Children with a BMI greater than 85% are more likely to have elevated cholesterol and triglycerides and lower HDL and higher blood pressure than children of normal weight.[24]

A mother of an overweight 4-year-old who is drinking 5 to 6 cups of juice a day feels that she is giving him a healthy drink.

Children increase their chances of becoming obese 1.6 times for each additional can or glass of sugared beverage they consume every day.[25]

Obesity prevention, intervention, and treatment will be integral to the practice of pediatrics in primary care practices, subspecialty pediatrics, and hospital-based care. Pediatricians are in a primary position to help children and families increase their knowledge and skills to combat obesity and obesity-related comorbidities.

References

1. Ogden CL, Carroll MD, Curtin LR, McDowell MA, Tabak CJ, Flegal KM. Prevalence of overweight and obesity in the United States, 1999-2004. *JAMA.* 2006;295:1549–1555

2. Whitaker RC, Wright JA, Pepe MS, Seidel KD, Dietz WH. Predicting obesity in young adulthood from childhood and parental obesity. *N Engl J Med.* 1997;337:869–873

3. Wang G, Dietz WH. Economic burden of obesity in youths aged 6 to 17 years: 1979-1999. *Pediatrics.* 2002;109:e81

4. Morales AE, Rosenbloom AL. Death caused by hyperglycemic hyperosmolar state at the onset of type 2 diabetes. *J Pediatr.* 2004;144:270–273

5. Rubin HM, Kramer R, Drash A. Hyperosmolality complicating diabetes mellitus in childhood. *J Pediatr.* 1969;74:177–186

6. Sugerman HJ, Sugerman EL, DeMaria EJ, et al. Bariatric surgery for severely obese adolescents. *J Gastrointest Surg.* 2003;7:102–108

7. Alpert MA. Obesity cardiomyopathy: pathophysiology and evolution of the clinical syndrome. *Am J Med Sci.* 2001;321:225–236

8. Scott IU, Siatkowski RM, Eneyni M, Brodsky MC, Lam BL. Idiopathic intracranial hypertension in children and adolescents. *Am J Ophthalmol.* 1997;124:253–255

9. Lessell S. Pediatric pseudotumor cerebri (idiopathic intracranial hypertension). *Surv Ophthalmol.* 1992;37:155–166

10. Distelmaier F, Sengler U, Messing-Juenger M, Assmann B, Mayatepek E, Rosenbaum T. Pseudotumor cerebri as an important differential diagnosis of papilledema in children. *Brain Dev.* 2006;28:190–195

11. Kempers MJ, Noordam C, Rouwe CW, Otten BJ. Can GnRH-agonist treatment cause slipped capital femoral epiphysis? *J Pediatr Endocrinol Metab.* 2001;14:729–734

12. Wilcox PG, Weiner DS, Leighley B. Maturation factors in slipped capital femoral epiphysis. *J Pediatr Orthop.* 1988;8:196–200

13. Busch MT, Morrissy RT. Slipped capital femoral epiphysis. *Orthop Clin North Am.* 1987;18:637–647

14. Dietz WH, Gross WL, Kirkpatrick JA. Blount disease (tibia vara): another skeletal disorder associated with childhood obesity. *J Pediatr.* 1982;101:735–737

15. Schechter MS, Section on Pediatric Pulmonology, Subcommittee on Obstructive Sleep Apnea Syndrome. Technical report: diagnosis and management of childhood obstructive sleep apnea syndrome. *Pediatrics.* 2002;109:e69

16. Gozal D. Sleep-disordered breathing and school performance in children. *Pediatrics.* 1998;102:616–620

17. Tazawa Y, Noguchi H, Nishinomiya F, Takada G. Serum alanine aminotransferases activity in obese children. *Acta Paediatr.* 1997;86:238–241

18. Harrison SA, Diehl AM. Fat and the liver—a molecular overview. *Semin Gastrointest Dis.* 2002;13:3–6

19. Crichlow RW, Seltzer MH, Jannetta PJ. Cholecystitis in adolescents. *Am J Dig Dis.* 1972;17:68–72

20. Ibanez L, Dimartino-Nardi J, Potau N, Saenger P. Premature adrenarche—normal variant or forerunner of adult disease? *Endocr Rev.* 2000;21:671–696

21. Diabetes Public Health Resource. Centers for Disease Control and Prevention Web site. Available at: www.cdc.gov/diabetes. Accessed May 25, 2006

22. Guo SS, Wu W, Chumlea WC, Roche AF. Predicting overweight and obesity in adulthood from body mass index values in childhood and adolescence. *Am J Clin Nutr.* 2002;76:653–658

23. Centers for Disease Control and Prevention Web site. Available at: www.cdc.gov. Accessed May 25, 2006

24. Freedman DS, Dietz WH, Srinivasan SR, Berenson GS. The relation of overweight to cardiovascular risk factors among children and adolescents: the Bogalusa Heart Study. *Pediatrics.* 1999;103:1175–1182

25. Ludwig DS, Peterson KE, Gortmaker SL. Relation between consumption of sugar-sweetened drinks and childhood obesity: a prospective, observational analysis. *Lancet.* 2001;357:505–508

Chapter 2

Assessment of Obesity

2.1 Introduction

Pediatricians' interest in assessing growth dates to the beginning of pediatrics when growth failure because of poor nutrition or chronic disease was a major focus of pediatric care. Now with the onset of the obesity epidemic, assessing the growth status of all children has never been more important. Preventive efforts, which focus on maintaining normal healthy weight gain, require that no opportunity is missed to measure height and weight and calculate body mass index (BMI). Frequent assessment of BMI also makes it possible to identify children who are overweight or obese and allows for early intervention to reinforce and reestablish good nutrition and activity habits. Children who have BMI values greater than 95% require screening for obesity-related comorbidities and intervention to manage obesity.

2.2 Assessing Obesity

Identifying excess adiposity in childhood is important for determining risk of obesity-associated comorbidities and future risk of obesity and obesity-related disease in adulthood. Direct measures of adiposity such as hydrodensitometry, dual-energy x-ray absorptiometry, and magnetic resonance imaging are used in research. Body mass index (weight/height^2) has been shown to correlate with direct measures of adiposity.[1] Because adipose tissue stores change as children grow and differ between boys and girls, BMI charts are specific for age and gender (figures 2.1 and 2.2).

Figure 2.1. Body mass index chart for boys.

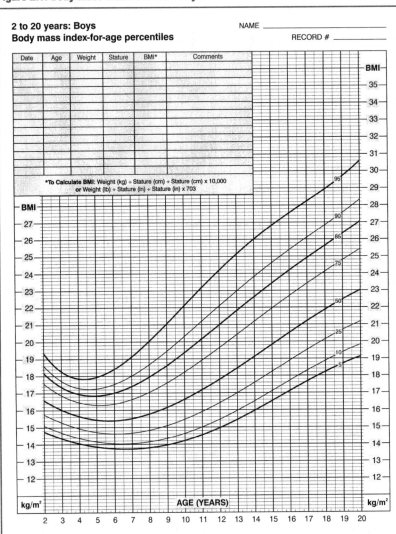

2 to 20 years: Boys
Body mass index-for-age percentiles

NAME _____

RECORD # _____

*To Calculate BMI: Weight (kg) ÷ Stature (cm) ÷ Stature (cm) x 10,000
or Weight (lb) ÷ Stature (in) ÷ Stature (in) x 703

SOURCE: Developed by the National Center for Health Statistics in collaboration with
the National Center for Chronic Disease Prevention and Health Promotion (2000).
http://www.cdc.gov/growthcharts

Figure 2.2. Body mass index chart for girls.

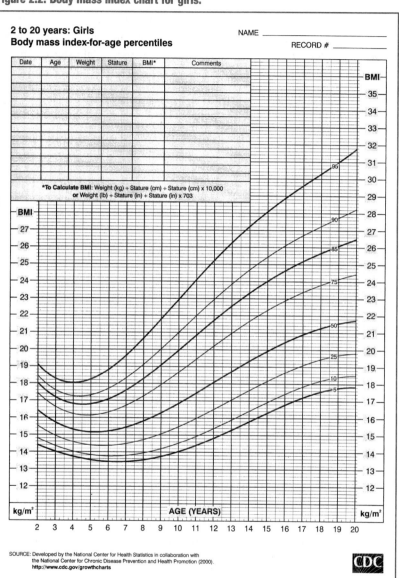

2 to 20 years: Girls
Body mass index-for-age percentiles

NAME _____

RECORD # _____

Date	Age	Weight	Stature	BMI*	Comments

*To Calculate BMI: Weight (kg) ÷ Stature (cm) ÷ Stature (cm) x 10,000
or Weight (lb) ÷ Stature (in) ÷ Stature (in) x 703

AGE (YEARS)

kg/m²

SOURCE: Developed by the National Center for Health Statistics in collaboration with
the National Center for Chronic Disease Prevention and Health Promotion (2000).
http://www.cdc.gov/growthcharts

CDC

Body mass index should be calculated at least once a year in all children and adolescents[2] and can be calculated as weight in kilograms divided by height in meters squared or weight in pounds multiplied by 703 and divided by (height in inches) squared. Once BMI is calculated, weight status can be assigned according to Table 2.1.

Table 2.1. Current Classification of Weight Status by Body Mass Index (BMI)

BMI <5%:	underweight
BMI 5%–85%:	normal weight
BMI 85%–95%:	overweight
BMI >95%:	obese

Body mass index measurements are important as a screening tool, but when they are applied to an individual patient they need to be used in the context of that individual. For example, a highly trained, muscular athlete may have an increased BMI but no excess adiposity. History and physical and anthropometric measurements such as skinfold thickness help to put BMI into proper focus for each individual.

For patients younger than 2 years, weight-for-length graphs should be used to characterize appropriate growth (figures 2.3 and 2.4). If weight is accelerating ahead of height, attention should be paid to identifying any underlying medical or metabolic cause of obesity and ensuring that optimal nutrition and activity habits are being fostered.

Rapid change in BMI can also be used to identify a rate of excessive weight gain relative to linear growth. Sequential BMI measurements should be plotted and compared to BMI charts for age and gender. Often the point at which excessive weight gain begins may allow an assessment of changes in risk factors for obesity that could be addressed.

Several states are now mandating BMI reporting by schools. If linked with communication with the child's pediatrician, this may provide additional opportunities to address risk for obesity and obesity in the school-age population.

Figure 2.3. Weight-for-length chart for boys.

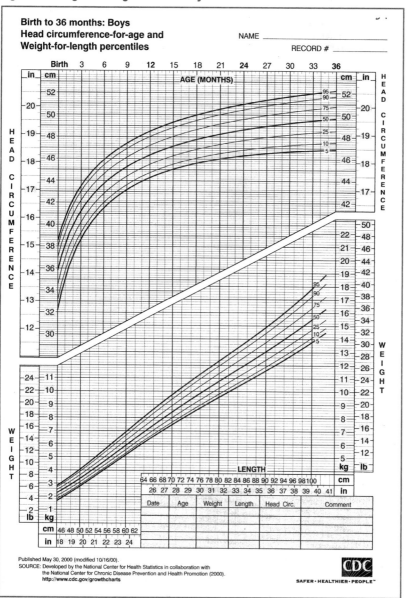

Birth to 36 months: Boys
Head circumference-for-age and
Weight-for-length percentiles

NAME _____

RECORD # _____

Published May 30, 2000 (modified 10/16/00).
SOURCE: Developed by the National Center for Health Statistics in collaboration with
the National Center for Chronic Disease Prevention and Health Promotion (2000).
http://www.cdc.gov/growthcharts

Figure 2.4. Weight-for-length chart for girls.

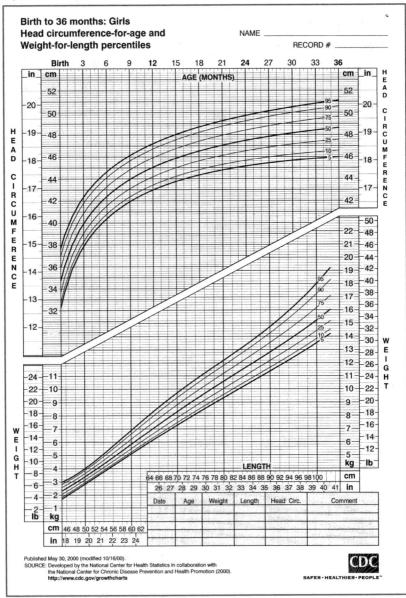

Birth to 36 months: Girls
Head circumference-for-age and
Weight-for-length percentiles

NAME _____

RECORD # _____

Published May 30, 2000 (modified 10/16/00).
SOURCE: Developed by the National Center for Health Statistics in collaboration with
the National Center for Chronic Disease Prevention and Health Promotion (2000).
http://www.cdc.gov/growthcharts

A Case in Point: CS

CS is an 11-year-old girl you are seeing for her yearly checkup. This year as you plot her height and weight and calculate her body mass index (BMI), you note that she has gained 20 lb (9.1 kg) since last year.

Over the past year she has been to your office several times for respiratory illnesses but has no other problems. She is not taking any medications. You ask about school and she and her mother report that her grades are good, but she is experiencing some teasing. When you ask CS about this she becomes upset and tells you that no one wants to play with her. Mom at this point says she has been worried about CS's self-esteem. You acknowledge the difficulty of getting teased and ask CS how she responds to this. She says she gets upset and usually says something back to the girls who tease her. You briefly discuss some responses to teasing and CS expresses some interest in trying to ignore their comments and walk away.

You then share the growth and BMI charts with Mom and CS and also share the thought that sometimes eating and activity habits change when someone is being teased and feeling bad. You let them know that staying healthy is important and you begin to ask specifically about her eating and activity. Mom notes that CS comes home from school and is starving and as soon as she finishes dinner she is asking for more food. CS says she is watching television or is on the computer a lot, which her mother translates as about 4 hours a day.

You then begin to explore CS's interest in out-of-school activities to give her another venue for physical activity and peer interaction. Mom says they have a YMCA membership; you ask CS and Mom to look into 2 or 3 possible activities she might join such as a dance class, karate, or swimming and then ask CS to choose one of them. You ask Mom if she would prepare an after-school snack for CS instead of having her daughter get her own, and Mom agrees.

You go over the laboratory studies that you want to order for CS based on her BMI, then ask CS and Mom to come back to check in with you in 3 to 4 weeks to review her laboratory studies and see how the changes in her eating and activity are going and most importantly, to see how she is doing with the kids at school.

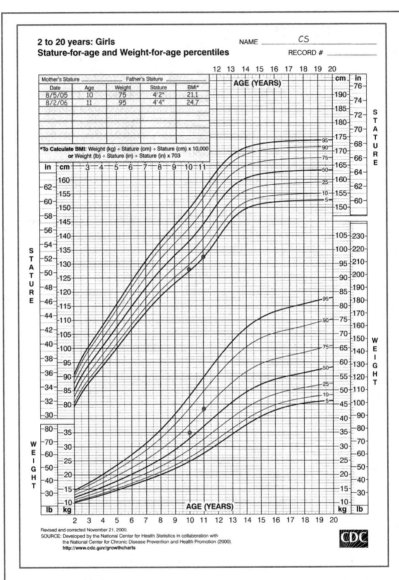

Second Visit

A month later CS returns to your office. You have reviewed the laboratory studies; she has a mild elevation of her triglycerides but no other abnormalities. This visit, her weight is 94 lb (42.6 kg), a decrease of 1 lb (0.5 kg), and she has joined a karate class at the YMCA and has

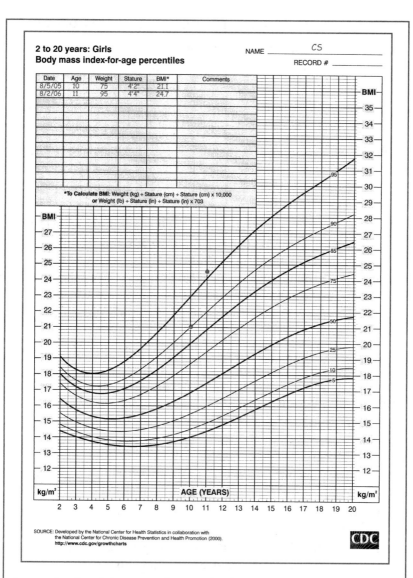

2 to 20 years: Girls
Body mass index-for-age percentiles

NAME _____ *CS* _____

RECORD # _____

Date	Age	Weight	Stature	BMI*	Comments
8/5/05	10	75	4'2"	21.1	
8/2/06	11	95	4'4"	24.7	

*To Calculate BMI: Weight (kg) ÷ Stature (cm) ÷ Stature (cm) x 10,000
or Weight (lb) ÷ Stature (in) ÷ Stature (in) x 703

AGE (YEARS)

SOURCE: Developed by the National Center for Health Statistics in collaboration with
the National Center for Chronic Disease Prevention and Health Promotion (2000).
http://www.cdc.gov/growthcharts

been going 2 to 3 times a week. Mom has been preparing an after-school snack and CS has not been asking for extra food. CS seems happier and says she has met some kids at karate that she likes. CS and Mom say they are willing to keep some diet records to address her elevated triglycerides at the next visit. You schedule the next visit and plan to continue to support CS and her family with the goal of normalizing her triglyceride levels and returning her to her previous growth trajectory.

2.3 Identifying Children and Families at Risk for Obesity

Risk factors for obesity can be identified in children and include

- Genetic and medical disorders associated with obesity
- Parental obesity
- Nutrition and activity patterns that have been associated with obesity
- Living in an at-risk environment

Obesity associated with genetic syndromes is a rare but important cause of childhood obesity.[3] Syndromes associated with obesity are frequently characterized by developmental delay, short stature, dysmorphic features, and involvement of specific organ systems.

Prader-Willi syndrome, which most commonly results from a deletion of 15q11q13, is the most common single gene obesity-associated syndrome, occurring in 1 of every 10,000 to 15,000 births. Primary features include infantile hypotonia, a poor sucking reflex, developmental delay, mental retardation, short stature, and skin picking. Obesity becomes apparent as early as 2 years of age along with hyperphagia, hypogonadism, and behavioral difficulties.[4] With early diagnosis and counseling, excessive weight gain can often be controlled. Additional obesity-associated genetic syndromes are listed in Table 2.2.

Medical conditions that may result in obesity include injury to the hypothalamus as a result of trauma or malignancy, surgery, or radiation treatment. Endocrinologic causes of obesity include Cushing syndrome, hypothyroidism, and growth hormone deficiency. Psychosocial conditions may also be associated with obesity. (See Table 2.3.)

Drug therapy can present a risk for weight gain. Table 2.4 shows commonly prescribed drugs that may be associated with obesity.

Children from pregnancies complicated by diabetes and children born small for gestational age have a greater incidence of obesity (see Chapter 3).

Parental obesity has been shown to be a strong predictor of childhood and adolescent obesity. By late adolescence a child who had at least one parent who was obese has an 80% chance of being obese.[7] The strong predictive value of parental obesity can allow early identification of children at risk for obesity and early intervention in helping families develop good nutrition and activity patterns. This is particularly important because activity and nutritional patterns are formed at a very early age. For example,

Table 2.2. Genetic Syndromes Associated With Obesity

Prader-Willi syndrome	Infantile hypotonia; poor feeding followed by hyperphagia and weight gain, developmental delay, mental retardation, short stature, skin picking, behavioral and psychosocial problems
Bardet-Biedl syndrome	Polydactyly, cognitive delay, short stature, retinitis pigmentosa, renal disease, hypogonadism
Alström syndrome	Nerve deafness, diabetes, pigmentary retinal degeneration, cataracts
Albright hereditary osteodystrophy	Short stature; may have pseudohypoparathyroidism, ectopic calcifications, hypocalcemia
Hereditary Cushing syndrome	Carney complex, an autosomal dominant syndrome of multiple neoplasia, spotty skin pigmentation, multiple endocrine neoplasia, testicular neoplasia, ovarian cysts[5]
Isolated growth hormone deficiency	Short stature, central obesity[5]
X-linked syndromic mental retardation	X-linked mental retardation with a high prevalence of obesity from mutations in the MECP2 gene[5]

studies have shown that preschool-aged children from obese or overweight families share food preferences with their parents and prefer sedentary activity.[8]

Nutritional patterns that may increase the risk of obesity include meals eaten at restaurants, increase in portion sizes, snacking, and meal skipping[9] as well as consumption of soda, sugar-sweetened beverages, and juice.[10,11] A major source of risk for obesity has been the increase in television watching and decrease in physical activity.[2] The importance of identifying nutritional and activity patterns that increase the risk of obesity is that many of these are directly influenced by parental and family behavior patterns and could be amenable to lifestyle change.

The school environment can increase the risk of obesity if soda, juice, and snack machines are available. Lack of physical education, longer

Table 2.3. Medical Conditions Associated With Obesity

Hypothalamic obesity	– Head injury; central nervous system malignancy, radiation, or surgery – Associated neurologic and endocrinologic deficits
Cushing syndrome	– Hypertension, centripetal obesity, striae – Elevated cortisol
Hypothyroidism	– Constipation, linear growth delay, myxedema, lethargy
Growth hormone deficiency	– Short stature
Depression or anxiety	– Change in eating and activity behavior or pharmacotherapy
Abuse	– Signs and symptoms consistent with physical, psychological, and/or sexual abuse[3]

Table 2.4. Drugs Associated With Obesity

– Glucocorticoids	– Carbamazepine
– Phenothiazines	– Beta-adrenergic blockers[6]
– Tricyclic antidepressants	– Insulin
– Valproic acid	– Selective serotonin-reuptake inhibitors[6]

school days, and decreases in recess also may contribute to a more obesity-promoting environment. Less walking to school has also been implicated in rising obesity trends.[9]

Once obesity is identified, screening for obesity-related comorbidities and intervention to normalize weight need to occur. These topics will be addressed at length in the following chapters.

References

1. Cole TJ, Bellizzi MC, Flegal KM, Dietz WH. Establishing a standard definition for child overweight and obesity worldwide: international survey. *BMJ.* 2000;320:1240–1243

2. Krebs NF, Jacobson MS, American Academy of Pediatrics Committee on Nutrition. Prevention of pediatric overweight and obesity. *Pediatrics.* 2003;112:424–430

3. Hassink S. Problems in childhood obesity. In: Bray GA. *Office Management of Obesity.* Philadelphia, PA: Elsevier; 2004:73–90

4. Cassidy SB. Prader-Willi syndrome. *Curr Probl Pediatr.* 1984;14:1–55

5. Perusse L, Rankinen T, Zuberi A, et al. The human obesity gene map: the 2004 update. *Obes Res.* 2005;13:381–490

6. Malone M, Alger-Mayer SA, Anderson DA. Medication associated with weight gain may influence outcome in a weight management program. *Ann Pharmacother.* 2005;39:1204–1208

7. Whitaker RC, Wright JA, Pepe MS, Seidel KD, Dietz WH. Predicting obesity in young adulthood from childhood and parental obesity. *N Engl J Med.* 1997;337:869–873

8. Wardle J, Guthrie C, Sanderson S, Birch L, Plomin R. Food and activity preferences in children of lean and obese parents. *Int J Obes Relat Metab Disord.* 2001;25:971–977

9. Nicklas TA, Baranowski T, Cullen KW, Berenson G. Eating patterns, dietary quality and obesity. *J Am Coll Nutr.* 2001;20:599–608

10. American Academy of Pediatrics Committee on School Health. Soft drinks in schools. *Pediatrics.* 2004;113:152–154

11. American Academy of Pediatrics Committee on Nutrition. The use and misuse of fruit juice in pediatrics. *Pediatrics.* 2001;107:1210–1213

Health Supervision Visits: Prevention, Early Intervention, and Treatment for the At-Risk Child

Chapter 3

Before Birth: The Prenatal Visit

·· ·

3.1 What Do We Know?

People often ask, "When should we begin to intervene in childhood obesity?" Surprisingly, the answer may be, "Before birth." Fetal life may be one of the critical times we can effectively focus a family's attention on genetic risk, parental influence, and environmental factors that will make it more or less likely that their unborn baby will develop childhood obesity.

The effect of genetics on obesity has been known for a long time. Stunkard et al determined that identical twins raised in different households had rates of obesity that correlated closely with each other and with their biological family independent of their adoptive families' weight status.[1] We know that there are a group of specific genetic deficits associated with obesity such as Prader-Willi syndrome, Bardet-Biedl syndrome, Alström syndrome, and leptin deficiency, to name a few. These disorders account for only a small fraction of childhood obesity and are usually associated with other systemic signs such as short stature and cognitive delay, but they have taught us a great deal about the fundamentals of energy regulation. The majority of our patients have an inherited predisposition toward obesity that is polygenic and in some way triggered by interaction with an obesity-promoting environment.

3.2 How Can This Help Us?

Clearly a child with obesity as part of a syndrome needs to be identified and genetic counseling is required. Table 3.1 shows a list of some of these syndromes associated with specific genetic defects.

In the case of most families, a clearer understanding of their own family history is in order when they are looking at obesity risk for their unborn

Table 3.1. Obesity-Related Syndromes

Single Gene Mutations Associated With Obesity	Clinical Findings
Leptin gene 7q31	Normal birth weight, hyperphagia, impaired satiety and rapid weight gain in infancy[2]
Leptin receptor gene 1p31	Normal birth weight, Prader-Willi–like eating behavior, severe infant obesity, central hypogonadism[3]
Proprotein convertase 1 deficiency (PCSK 1) 5q15-q21	Extreme childhood obesity, abnormal glucose homeostasis, low insulin and cortisol, hypogonadotropic hypogonadism, elevated plasma proinsulin[4]
Pro-opiomelanocortin (POMC) 2p23	Early-onset obesity, adrenal insufficiency, red hair[5]
Melanocortin 4 receptor (MC4R) 18q22	Severe childhood obesity, increased lean body mass, increase linear growth, hyperphagia, severe hyperinsulinemaia[6]
Obesity-Related Autosomal Disorders	**Clinical Findings**
Albright hereditary osteodystrophy 20q13.2	Short stature, obesity, brachydactyly, subcutaneous ossifications[7]
Familial partial lipodystrophy 1q21.2	Normal fat distribution in childhood, pubertal onset of adipose tissue accumulation in face and neck and decrease in upper and lower extremities; associated with insulin resistance and increased risk for diabetes in adulthood[8]
Prader-Willi syndrome 15q11-13	Diminished fetal activity, poor infantile weight gain with escalating hyperphagia and obesity, muscular hypotonia, mental retardation, short stature, hypogonadotropic hypogonadism, small hands and feet[9]
Insulin resistance syndrome type A	Younger females with signs of virilization, accelerated growth, and polycystic ovarian syndrome[10]

Obesity-Related Autosomal Recessive Disorders	Clinical Findings
Alstrom syndrome 2p13	Early childhood retinopathy, progressive sensorineural hearing loss, truncal obesity, advanced bone age, acanthosis nigricans with hyperinsulinemia and hypertriglyceridemia[11]
Bardet-Biedl syndrome 11q13, 16q21, 3p13p12, 15q22.3q23	Severe retinal dystrophy, dysmorphic extremities (polydactyly), obesity, variable developmental delay, renal abnormalities, small genitalia in males[12]
Obesity-Related X-linked Disorders	**Clinical Findings**
Mehmo syndrome Xp22.13p21.1	Mitochondrial disorder with mental retardation, epileptic seizures, hypogonadism and hypogenitalism, microcephaly, obesity, short life expectancy (<2 years)[13]
Fragile X syndrome with Prader-Willi–like phenotype Xq27.3	A Prader-Willi–like subphenotype of fragile X syndrome with obesity; full, round face; small, broad hands and feet; and regional skin hyperpigmentation; unlike Prader-Willi syndrome, patients lacked the neonatal hypotonia and feeding problems during infancy followed by hyperphagia during toddlerhood[14]
Wilson Turner syndrome Xp21.1q22	Obesity, gynecomastia, speech difficulties, emotional lability, tapering fingers, small feet[15]

baby. We know from work by Whitaker et al[16] that parental obesity is a large and significant risk for the development of obesity in the offspring. In this study children with one or both parents who are obese have an 80% chance of being obese by the time they are adolescents. Parents who are obese need to become aware of these risks and work with their pediatrician to develop a plan to address feeding, activity, and inactivity changes as a family, with the goal of preventing obesity in their child.

Taking a family history that focuses on obesity and obesity-related comorbidities could help the family understand the short- and long-term risks of obesity in their baby (Figure 3.1).

There is also growing evidence that "intrauterine life may be a critical period for the development of obesity."[17] It is known that infants of diabetic mothers have more adipose tissue than infants born to mothers without diabetes and are often large for gestational age. Even when macrosomia normalizes, these infants develop childhood obesity at higher rates than children born to mothers without diabetes.[18] Intrauterine exposure to hyperglycemia and resultant hyperinsulinemia may alter insulin receptor signaling in muscle and adipose tissue in utero.[19] There is evidence that intrauterine exposure to diabetes is associated with impaired glucose tolerance in adolescence[20] and a higher prevalence of type 2 diabetes.[21]

Alterations in the intrauterine environment during periods of maternal starvation may also play a role in later development of obesity. Male offspring of mothers subjected to famine in 1944 and 1945 during the first and second trimesters of pregnancy had higher than expected incidence of obesity.[22] A study in children born small for gestational age showed greater insulin resistance at ages 7 to 11 years than children born appropriate for gestational age with equivalent family history, gestational ages, and gender.[23] In an epidemiologic study of middle-aged adults, Barker showed that small birth size conferred a risk for hypertension, glucose intolerance, and dyslipidemia in adulthood.[24] Possibly related to the effects of impaired uterine growth on obesity risk is a report that maternal smoking during pregnancy had a close response relationship to obesity at school entry.[25]

Encouraging mothers to access health care before and during pregnancy is critical. Mothers who have diabetes, are at risk for a baby with growth impairment, or smoke need special focus when it comes to optimizing the intrauterine environment for their babies.

Pregnancy is also a time for planning for breastfeeding. Breastfeeding is recommended as the optimum source of nutrition for an infant. There are studies that show that breastfed babies have a reduced incidence of obesity.[26] The exact nature of this effect is not known, but breastfed babies may be able to regulate intake and satiety more precisely.[27] There are data showing increased difficulty initiating[28] and earlier cessation of breastfeeding in mothers who were obese prior to pregnancy.[29] Obesity mothers have a

Figure 3.1. Family history before birth.

	Mother	Father	Maternal Grandmother	Maternal Grandfather	Paternal Grandmother	Paternal Grandfather	Sibling 1	Sibling 2
Obesity	☐	☐	☐	☐	☐	☐	☐	☐
Cardiovascular disease	☐	☐	☐	☐	☐	☐	☐	☐
High blood pressure	☐	☐	☐	☐	☐	☐	☐	☐
Stroke	☐	☐	☐	☐	☐	☐	☐	☐
High cholesterol	☐	☐	☐	☐	☐	☐	☐	☐
High triglyceride	☐	☐	☐	☐	☐	☐	☐	☐
Type 1 or 2 diabetes	☐	☐	☐	☐	☐	☐	☐	☐
_____	☐	☐	☐	☐	☐	☐	☐	☐
_____	☐	☐	☐	☐	☐	☐	☐	☐
_____	☐	☐	☐	☐	☐	☐	☐	☐
_____	☐	☐	☐	☐	☐	☐	☐	☐
_____	☐	☐	☐	☐	☐	☐	☐	☐
_____	☐	☐	☐	☐	☐	☐	☐	☐

diminished prolactin response to suckling, which may explain their increased difficulty maintaining breastfeeding.[30] Obese mothers, therefore, may need increased help in initiating and maintaining breastfeeding. A lactation consultant may provide helpful information and support for these families.

References

1. Stunkard AJ, Sorensen TI, Hanis C, et al. An adoption study of human obesity. *N Engl J Med.* 1986;31:193–198
2. Montague CT, Farooqi IS, Whitehead JP, et al. Congenital leptin deficiency is associated with severe early-onset obesity in humans. *Nature.* 1997;387:903–908
3. Clement K, Vaisse C, Lahlou N, et al. A mutation in the human leptin receptor gene causes obesity and pituitary dysfunction. *Nature.* 1998;392:398–401
4. Jackson RS, Creemers JW, Ohagi S, et al. Obesity and impaired prohormone processing associated with mutations in the human prohormone convertase 1 gene. *Nat Genet.* 1997;16:303–306
5. Krude H, Biebermann H, Luck W, Horn R, Brabant G, Gruters A. Severe early-onset obesity, adrenal insufficiency and red hair pigmentation caused by POMC mutations in humans. *Nat Genet.* 1998;19:155–157
6. Farooqi IS, Keogh JM, Yeo GS, Lank EJ, Cheetham T, O'Rahilly S. Clinical spectrum of obesity and mutations in the melanocortin 4 receptor gene. *N Engl J Med.* 2003;348:1085–1095
7. Germain-Lee EL. Short stature, obesity, and growth hormone deficiency in pseudohypoaparathyroidism type 1a. *Pediatr Endocrinol Rev.* 2006;3(Suppl 2): 318–326
8. Kobberling J, Dunnigan MG. Familial partial lipodystrophy: two types of an X linked dominant syndrome, lethal in the hemizygous state. *J Med Genet.* 1986;23:120–127
9. Zipf WB. Prader-Willi syndrome: the care and treatment of infants, children and adults. *Adv Pediatr.* 2004;51:409–434
10. Kahn CR, Flier JS, Bar RS, et al. The syndromes of insulin resistance and acanthosis nigricans. Insulin receptor disorders in man. *N Engl J Med.* 1976;294:739–745
11. Marshall JD, Ludman MD, Shea SE, et al. Genealogy, natural history, and phenotype of Alstrom syndrome in a large Acadian kindred and three additional families. *Am J Med Genet.* 1997;73:150–161
12. Green JS, Parfrey PS, Harnett JD, et al. The cardinal manifestations of Bardet-Biedl syndrome, a form of Laurence-Moon-Biedl syndrome. *N Engl J Med.* 1989;321:1002–1009

13. Leshinsky-Silver E, Zinger A, Bibi CN, et al. MEHMO (mental retardation, epileptic seizures, hypogenitalism, microcephaly, obesity): a new X-linked mitochondrial disorder. *Euro J Hum Genet.* 2002;10:226–230

14. de Vries BB, Fryns JP, Butler MG, et al. Clinical and molecular studies in fragile X patients with a Prader-Willi-like phenotype. *J Med Genet.* 1993;30: 761–766

15. Wilson M, Mulley J, Gedeon A, Robinson H, Turner G. New X-linked syndrome of mental retardation, gynecomastia, and obesity is linked to DXS255. *Am J Med Genet.* 1991;40: 406–413

16. Whitaker RC, Wright JA, Pepe MS, Seidel KD, Dietz WH. Predicting obesity in young adulthood from childhood and parental obesity. *N Engl J Med.* 1997;337:869–873

17. Oken E, Gillman MW. Fetal origins of obesity. *Obes Res.* 2003;11:496–506

18. Plagemann A, Harder T, Kohlhoff R, Rhode W, Dorner G. Overweight and obesity in infants of mothers with long-term insulin-dependent diabetes or gestational diabetes. *Int J Obes Relat Metab Disord.* 1997;21:451–456

19. Freinkel N. Of pregnancy and progeny. *Diabetes.* 1980;29:1023–1035

20. Silverman BL, Metzger BE, Cho NH, Loeb CA. Impaired glucose tolerance in adolescent offspring of diabetic mothers. Relationship to fetal hyperinsulinism. *Diabetes Care.* 1995;18:611–617

21. Pettitt DJ, Aleck KA, Barrd H, Carraher MJ, Bennett PH, Knowler WC. Congenital susceptibility to NIDDM. Role of intrauterine environment. *Diabetes.* 1988;37:622–628

22. Ravelli GP, Stern ZA, Susser MW. Obesity in young men after famine exposure in utero and early infancy. *N Engl J Med.* 1976;295:349–353

23. Veening MA, Van Weissenbruch MM, Delemarre-Van De Waal HA. Glucose tolerance, insulin sensitivity, and insulin secretion in children born small for gestational age. *J Clin Endocrinol Metab.* 2002;87:4657–4661

24. Barker DJ. The intrauterine origins of cardiovascular disease. *Acta Paediatr Suppl.* 1993;82(Suppl 391):93–100

25. Von Kries R, Toschke AM, Koletzko B, Slikker W. Maternal smoking during pregnancy and childhood obesity. *Am J Epidemiol.* 2002;156:954–961

26. Arenz S, Ruckerl R, Koletzko B, von Kries R. Breast-feeding and childhood obesity—a systematic review. *Int J Obes Relat Metab Disord.* 2004;28:1247–1256

27. Agostoni C. Ghrelin leptin and the neurometabolic axis of breastfed and formula-fed infants. *Acta Paediatr.* 2005;94:523–525

28. Chapman DJ, Perez-Escamilla R. Identification of risk factors for delayed onset of lactation. *J Am Diet Assoc.* 1999;99:450–456

29. Li R, Jewell S, Grummer-Strawn L. Maternal obesity and breast-feeding practices. *Am J Clin Nutr.* 2003;77:931–936
30. Rasmussen KM, Hilson JA, Kjolhede CL. Obesity may impair lactogenesis II. *J Nutr.* 2001;131:3009S–3011S

Chapter 4

Newborn and Infant

4.1 Background

At birth, newborns need to be ready to transition to extrauterine sources of nutrition. Term neonates accumulate adipose tissue in the last trimester of pregnancy and the early postnatal months. Fat stores are mobilized during infections and transitions in sources of nutrition; this has been the explanation for the significant amount of adiposity in human neonates compared with other mammals.[1] Nutrient composition and intake may influence later obesity, especially in genetically susceptible babies. Evidence from multiple studies has shown a relationship between breastfeeding and reduced risk of obesity.[2] Mixed breastfeeding and formula feeding has been associated with higher weight- and length-for-age Z scores at 3 to 6 months, 6 to 9 months, and 9 to 12 months than exclusive breastfeeding.[3]

Breastfed newborns have slightly lower intake of energy and protein compared with formula-fed newborns[4] and gain more weight and lean body mass per gram of protein intake than formula-fed newborns.[5] Formula-fed newborns have increased fat mass deposition when compared with breastfed newborns.[6] This may indicate early differences in energy balance and body composition. Leptin, a cytokine integral to energy regulation, has been found in human milk[7] and is produced by mammary epithelial cells.[10] Human milk leptin has been found to vary with birth weight and rate of weight gain in small for gestational age, average for gestational age, and large for gestational age newborns during the first month of life.[9] At 2 months of age, leptin levels were found to be higher in breastfed than formula-fed infants independent of anthropometric measurements.[10]

Breastfeeding may be an indicator of maternal-child feeding interactions. Mothers who breastfed were found to have less restrictive patterns of child feeding at 1 year of age.[11] In formula-fed infants, rate of weight gain in the first 4 months of life has been associated with risk of overweight at age

7 years and may represent genetic influences on early energy balance or a vulnerable period of growth that affects later energy balance.[12] Total energy intake and sucking behavior during a test meal rather than energy expenditure were found to influence body weight of newborns over the first 2 years of life.[13]

Mothers who are overweight or obese before becoming pregnant have more difficulty initiating successful breastfeeding and stop breastfeeding earlier than normal-weight counterparts.[14] In one study, overweight or obese mothers had a decreased prolactin response to suckling, and this was hypothesized to compromise milk production and lead to premature cessation of lactation.[15] Maternal overweight and obesity may be an indication for additional lactation support to initiate and maintain breastfeeding. Health care professionals should anticipate this need and offer support at the onset of breastfeeding.

4.2 Prevention: Talking to Parents (BALANCE)

Prevention touch points for parents include **belief, assessment, lifestyle, activity, nutrition, child,** and **environment** (BALANCE).

Belief

- Bringing home a new baby is a time of change in every family. This may be a time when a family's childrearing beliefs are put to the test. This is a good time to help parents and families think about how their behavior and beliefs will affect the baby in terms of eating, activity, and the prevention of obesity.
- Parents who are obese often have a heightened concern about obesity prevention and are actively looking at ways to begin these preventive efforts as early as possible.
- Maintaining optimal growth requires managing eating and activity behavior and learning to interact with the baby around satiety (Table 4.1) and hunger. These interactions have particular importance for formula-fed babies.
- Learning to identify cues to hunger and satiety can help parents set the stage for an interactive approach to eating and feeding.
- Because feeding is an interactive process, it is important to remind parents to avoid propping a bottle.

Table 4.1. Signs of Satiety[16]

4 to 12 weeks	– Spontaneously releases nipple. – Moves head away from nipple. – Closes lips when nipple reinserted. – Slows sucking. – Falls asleep.
16 to 24 Weeks	– Bites nipple. – Blocks mouth with hands. – Turns away. – Cries or fusses if feeding persists. – Increases attention to surroundings. – Loses interest in feeding. – Releases nipple and withdraws head.
28 to 36 Weeks	– Changes posture. – Hands become more active. – Keeps mouth closed. – Plays with utensils. – Shakes head "no."
40 to 52 Weeks	– Does the above. – Hands bottle back to parent. – Spits.

Assessment

- Parents and grandparents have all kinds of ideas of what babies should look like and how much weight they should be gaining.
- Plotting the baby's height, weight, and weight for length and sharing this with parents is a good way to highlight the importance of following the growth chart.
- Parents can identify with the goal of "keeping the baby on the chart." This can focus discussion about the strategies to maintain energy balance, correct imbalances, and share strategies with other family members.

Lifestyle

- Helping new parents and families recognize the role of the family's lifestyle in supporting the proper nutrition and activity of the newborn is important.
- Encourage parents to communicate with the other members of the family about their plans and goals for feeding the baby and providing activity opportunities.
- Offering to have extended family members come to a doctor's visit if the parent wishes may also help to get everyone on the same page.

Activity

- Encouraging parents to spend time in face-to-face interaction with their baby making sounds, talking, and laughing lays the ground work for shared activity.
- Taking the baby for a daily walk in the stroller helps establish outdoor time as a part of the routine.
- Parents should make sure the baby has safe and soft toys to play with. Remind them that the toys should be small enough for the baby to pick up, but large enough so that they can't be put into the baby's mouth.
- Parents and family members should be discouraged from using television to "entertain" the baby.
- Parents need to know that television watching is associated with obesity and overweight in children.
- The American Academy of Pediatrics (AAP) currently recommends that TV should not be watched by children 2 years and younger.

Nutrition

- Every effort should be made to encourage and support breastfeeding for all newborns whenever possible. When breastfeeding is not possible, parents should be encouraged to hold their baby during formula feedings.
- Parents who are overweight or obese or who have obesity in their families should be acquainted with the benefits of breastfeeding with regard to obesity.

- Connections to lactation support may be especially helpful to overweight mothers.
- Parents who elect or need to formula feed should be encouraged to use hunger and satiety cues rather than feeding strictly by volume or a time schedule.

Child

- Parents often respond to crying by feeding their newborn. Help parents understand that crying is a baby's way of expressing its needs such as
  - Hunger
  - A diaper change
  - Gas pains
  - Help from a caregiver, eg, wanting to be wrapped in a blanket
  - Illness
  - To be held
- Remind parents that feeding will quiet babies even if they are not hungry because sucking is comforting, but if a baby learns to eat every time he or she has a problem, food may become an inappropriate source of comfort.
- Reassure parents that although they may be upset by their baby's crying, learning to interpret his or her particular cries is teaching the baby about communication.

Environment

- Work with parents on a safe home environment.
- Have parents find quiet spaces to play and read to their baby.
- Have families look in their neighborhood for safe and interesting places to walk with the baby.
- Remind parents that the AAP recommends that children younger than 2 years should not watch television. Watching television with the baby diverts people's attention away from each other, decreases face-to-face time, and can set up habits that contribute to obesity.

4.3 Intervention

Infancy is a time of feeding and eating transitions; paying careful attention to parent-child interactions can help to smooth the way for healthy eating. Patterns of activity and inactivity also emerge and families can be encouraged to take a close look at their own attitudes and behaviors toward eating, activity, and inactivity. Families with parental obesity are at risk for an obese child and may need to pay special attention to **energy balance, structure, and modeling healthy behavior.**

Energy Balance

Every visit is an opportunity to monitor growth, review feeding practices, and encourage activity. Attention to hunger and satiety cues need to be reinforced with families who choose to formula feed. Activity should be encouraged with safe and supervised floor time. Inactivity should be reduced by limiting time in infant seats. Reviewing the baby's intake and activity with parents at each visit will help reinforce their concept of the importance of energy balance.

Structure

By the end of the first year of life, families should be moving into a pattern of structured meals and activity. Parents may appreciate attention to time management and tips on balancing needs of the infant and other family members. Television time is not recommended for newborns or infants but may be the first thing parents think of when they need downtime. Active, supervised play may also get lost in the shuffle of child care, busy schedules, and siblings' activities and needs to be incorporated into families' overall plan.

Modeling Healthy Behavior

Parents may think that their baby is too young for the family to worry about their own habits affecting the baby, but family eating and activity patterns may sneak into the infant's routine. There is ample evidence that infants transition to foods that are already being consumed in the family. This is the time to review the family's diet and nutritional patterns with elimination of high-calorie snacks and excess sugared beverages the goal.

Use of desserts, sweets, and juice may be second nature to the family and roll right into the baby's diet. Other family members may have their own ideas of how and what to feed the baby, including larger-than-needed portion sizes and early solid foods. Parents need to begin to see themselves as in charge of the baby's environment at home and child care and with extended family. Families can use this time to get into a routine of outdoor activity, with stroller walks with the baby and reduction of screen time important aspects of that routine.

4.4 Treatment

Babies' weight trajectories can vary widely,[17] but if a newborn's or an infant's weight for length is above the normal curve, it is time to take a close look at the medical condition as well as the eating and activity patterns of the baby and family. Numerous studies have shown that babies who were classified as obese in infancy were more likely to be obese children,[12] adolescents,[18] and adults.[19] It is important to review the issues discussed in the preceding 2 sections because these are building blocks of good nutrition and activity habits. But you will also have to focus on the barriers to change that may have prevented parents and families from implementing these strategies.

Rate of weight gain in infancy as early as 4 months of age predicts obesity risk in children and adults.[20] Rate of sucking rather than energy expenditure was linked to infants' risk of later obesity.[13]

4.5 Family History

A useful way to begin is to obtain a family history (page 44) focused on obesity-related comorbidities. This can serve to emphasize the health risks involved and the necessity of taking early action before obesity has developed.

Family History, Newborn and Infant

Complete or update this family history targeted toward obesity and related comorbidities.

	Mother	Father	Maternal Grandmother	Maternal Grandfather	Paternal Grandmother	Paternal Grandfather	Sibling 1	Sibling 2
Obesity	☐	☐	☐	☐	☐	☐	☐	☐
Cardiovascular disease	☐	☐	☐	☐	☐	☐	☐	☐
High blood pressure	☐	☐	☐	☐	☐	☐	☐	☐
Stroke	☐	☐	☐	☐	☐	☐	☐	☐
High cholesterol	☐	☐	☐	☐	☐	☐	☐	☐
High triglyceride	☐	☐	☐	☐	☐	☐	☐	☐
Type 1 or 2 diabetes	☐	☐	☐	☐	☐	☐	☐	☐
_____	☐	☐	☐	☐	☐	☐	☐	☐
_____	☐	☐	☐	☐	☐	☐	☐	☐
_____	☐	☐	☐	☐	☐	☐	☐	☐
_____	☐	☐	☐	☐	☐	☐	☐	☐
_____	☐	☐	☐	☐	☐	☐	☐	☐
_____	☐	☐	☐	☐	☐	☐	☐	☐

4.6 Review of Systems

The review of systems can also serve as a point of departure to discuss obesity-related comorbidities, pointing out particular risk factors as they relate to increasing body mass index.

- Skin: Abnormal skin pigmentation
- Head, eyes, ears, nose, and throat (HEENT): Cataracts, deafness
- Cardiopulmonary:
- Gastrointestinal:
- Musculoskeletal: Infantile hypotonia and poor feeding, polydactyly
- Genitourinary: Hypogonadism
- Development: Delay in cognitive or motor development

4.7 Physical Examination

- Height
- Weight
- Weight for length

Note: For children younger than 2 years, the weight for length chart is useful to assess appropriateness of weight relative to length. The Centers for Disease Control and Prevention defines weight for length greater than 95% as overweight.[21]

- Blood pressure
- General: Dysmorphic features, poor linear growth, developmental delay
- Skin: Dermatitis in skin folds
- HEENT:
- Cardiopulmonary:
- Abdominal:
- Musculoskeletal/neurologic: Hypotonia
- Genitourinary: Hypogonadism

4.8 Family Constellation and Social History

Information about the family can provide a starting point to discuss how nutrition and activity decisions are made and how changes might take place.

- Who is living at home with the baby?
- Who else feeds and cares for the baby?
- Who decides what the baby will eat?
- Do family members agree on how to feed the baby?

4.9 Parenting Questions

Parenting styles and skills are important when families are trying to make changes in lifestyle. These questions may help you focus on family factors that may facilitate or hinder change.

	Never	Seldom	Sometimes	Often	Always
1. Parents agree on how to feed the baby.	☐	☐	☐	☐	☐
2. Parents set clear and simple expectations and limits.	☐	☐	☐	☐	☐
3. Parents understand the baby's developmental stage.	☐	☐	☐	☐	☐
4. Parents set boundaries and provide choices within them.	☐	☐	☐	☐	☐

4.10 Parenting Touch Points

Parenting touch points focus on helping families initiate and maintain change by helping them believe change can occur, identify the change needed, value the outcome of the change, know how to change, and have the energy to change and sustain the change.

- *Believe that change can occur.* Parents are the most important agents of change for the baby. Learning to assess the baby's nutrition and activity environment at child care and home and with other family members is a necessary skill if parents are to make the healthiest decisions for their baby.

- *Identify the change.* Parents base their feeding choices for their baby on their own knowledge of nutrition. This is the time to provide parents with information and an opportunity to explore and discuss their own choices and what they believe are the correct dietary choices for their baby. Juice is often seen as a healthy choice, but it should be virtually eliminated in the diet of a baby whose weight for length is greater than 95%. Parents may also see television time as educational or shared time with the family. Helping families to consider nutrition and activity as health behaviors may help them evaluate their habits in a different light.

- *Value the outcome.* Newborn and infant weight and feeding are important to parents and the measure of success may be the baby's weight gain and time or amount of feeding. Working with families to have the baby's weight stay on the growth curve is important. To accomplish this, parents may need to expand their ideas of successful feeding. Focusing families on the dynamics of satiety and cued feeding to allow value for the interaction between parent and baby to develop lays the groundwork for future eating behavior.

- *Know how to change.* Parents of a newborn may feel that their baby is driving the changes. Reassurance that they are offering an appropriate amount and type of nutrition can be helpful in allaying anxiety that their baby is still hungry. Changing the nutrition and activity environment for the baby begins with the parents' own behavior change.

- *Have energy to change and sustain.* Positive support at each physician visit for healthy nutrition and activity helps to sustain change. Involving the extended family members when appropriate in visits to discuss nutrition and activity may provide needed support for parents who are trying to effect family-based change.

4.11 Developmental Touch Point

Establishing communication is a critical step at this stage. Parents should be encouraged to have as much face-to-face interaction with their newborn as possible to notice the baby's unique responses and observe differences in cries. This interaction sets the stage for a responsive give and take.

4.12 Nutrition and Activity Questions and Interventions

Nutrition and activity questions (see page 49) can be answered by the
parents and provide a focal point for targeted intervention (see page 50)
in a brief encounter. Questions answered "Often" or "Always" can be targeted first for change. For example, if the parent answered questions 1, 7, 9,
and 13 on page 49 with "Often" or "Always," you would ask them
to rate the difficulty of change for questions 1, 7, 9, and 13 on page 50.

4.13 A Case in Point: SC

SC is a newborn girl you are seeing in the nursery. Her birth weight was
9 lb, 2 oz (41 kg), and she is a healthy full-term baby. You meet her parents
and note that both are significantly obese. SC is their first child and as you
ask about the family history, they note that SC's mother had gestational
diabetes and that 2 of the grandparents developed type 2 diabetes in midlife.
SC's mother wants to breastfeed but is having some difficulty and seems
somewhat discouraged. Both parents are anxious to do the right thing
for SC.

You note that SC's examination was normal and she seems to be a
healthy and vigorous baby. You support SC's mother's desire to breastfeed
and ask the nurse to support Mom in her efforts to breastfeed, showing her
how to best hold SC and help with latching on. You schedule an office visit
for 2 days later.

Second Visit

SC and Mom come to the office and Mom has had success initiating
breastfeeding. Mom wonders if SC is getting enough to eat and you reassure her after checking SC's weight and hydration. You offer Mom the
number of a lactation support group and encourage her to continue
breastfeeding. You mention SC's family history and the fact that Mom had
gestational diabetes. You note that these are risk factors for obesity and that
breastfeeding can help reduce the risk of obesity. You also ask mom to start
noticing SC's hunger and satiety cues.

Nutrition and Activity Questions, Newborn and Infant

These questions can be answered by the parents and provide a focal point for targeted intervention in a brief encounter. First have the parents answer these questions about the presence or absence of behaviors that promote weight gain, then refer to Nutrition and Activity Interventions, Newborn and Infant.

	Never	Seldom	Sometimes	Often	Always
1. Drinks juice between feedings.	☐	☐	☐	☐	☐
2. Seems hungry all the time.	☐	☐	☐	☐	☐
3. "Watches" television.	☐	☐	☐	☐	☐
4. Needs formula in bottle to go to sleep or awakens during the night and is fed.	☐	☐	☐	☐	☐
_____	☐	☐	☐	☐	☐
_____	☐	☐	☐	☐	☐
_____	☐	☐	☐	☐	☐
_____	☐	☐	☐	☐	☐
_____	☐	☐	☐	☐	☐
_____	☐	☐	☐	☐	☐

Nutrition and Activity Interventions, Newborn and Infant

Questions answered "Often" or "Always" in Nutrition and Activity Questions, Newborn and Infant, can be targeted first for change. Using these specific questions, ask the parent, "How difficult would it be for you to…?"

	Impossible	Could try	Could do sometimes	Could do most of the time	Easy
1. Change from juice to water between meals.	☐	☐	☐	☐	☐
2. Learn about and watch for satiety cues.	☐	☐	☐	☐	☐
3. Find alternatives to the television.	☐	☐	☐	☐	☐
4. Substitute water for formula.	☐	☐	☐	☐	☐
	☐	☐	☐	☐	☐
	☐	☐	☐	☐	☐
	☐	☐	☐	☐	☐
	☐	☐	☐	☐	☐
	☐	☐	☐	☐	☐
	☐	☐	☐	☐	☐
	☐	☐	☐	☐	☐
	☐	☐	☐	☐	☐

Ongoing Visits

As the visits progress, you plot SC's height, weight, and weight for length each time. You go over the growth charts with Mom with the goal of keeping SC "on the chart." You continue to support and encourage SC's parents in their efforts to provide healthy nutrition and activity for SC. You prepare Mom to start solid foods at 6 months, and encourage her and Dad to take stock of their own diet and activity habits, noting the importance of parental modeling of healthy behaviors. You remind SC's parents that television watching is not recommended for children younger than 2 years and encourage SC's parents to find family activities that they can do together besides watch television.

References

1. Kuzawa CW. Adipose tissue in human infancy and childhood: an evolutionary perspective. *Am J Phys Anthropol.* 1998;Suppl 27:177–209
2. Owen CG, Martin RM, Whincup PH, Smith GD, Cook DG. Effect of infant feeding on the risk of obesity across the life course: a quantitative review of published evidence. *Pediatrics.* 2005;115:1367–1377
3. Kramer MS, Guo T, Platt RW, et al. Feeding effects on growth during infancy. *J Pediatr.* 2004;145:600–605
4. Heinig MJ, Nommsen LA, Peerson JM, Lonnerdal B, Dewey KG. Energy and protein intakes of breast-fed and formula-fed infants during the first year of life and their association with growth velocity: the DARLING Study. *Am J Clin Nutr.* 1993;58:152–161
5. Butte NF, Wong WW, Hopkinson JM, Smith EO, Ellis KJ. Infant feeding mode affects early growth and body composition. *Pediatrics.* 2000;106:1355–1366
6. Pieltain C, De Curtis M, Gerard P, Rigo J. Weight gain composition in preterm infants with dual energy X-ray absorptiometry. *Pediatr Res.* 2001;49:120–124
7. Houseknecht KL, McGuire MK, Portocarrero CP, McGuire MA, Beerman K. Leptin is present in human milk and is related to maternal plasma leptin concentration and adiposity. *Biochem Biophys Res Commun.* 1997;240:742–747
8. Smith-Kirwin SM, O'Connor DM, De Johnston J, Lancey ED, Hassink SG, Funanage VL. Leptin expression in human mammary epithelial cells and breast milk. *J Clin Endocrinol Metab.* 1998;83:1810–1813
9. Dundar NO, Anal O, Dundar B, Ozkan H, Caliskan S, Buyukgebiz A. Longitudinal investigation of the relationship between breast milk leptin levels and growth in breast-fed infants. *J Pediatr Endocrinol Metab.* 2005;18:181–187

10. Savino F, Nanni GE, Maccario S, Costamagna M, Oggero R, Silvestro L. Breast-fed infants have higher leptin values than formula-fed infants in the first four months of life. *J Pediatr Endocrinol Metab.* 2004;17:1527–1532

11. Taveras EM, Scanlon KS, Birch L, Rifas-Shiman SL, Rich-Edwards JW, Gillman MW. Association of breastfeeding with maternal control of infant feeding at age 1 year. *Pediatrics.* 2004;114:e577–e583

12. Stettler N, Zemel BS, Kumanyika S, Stallings VA. Infant weight gain and child-hood overweight status in a multicenter, cohort study. *Pediatrics.* 2002;109: 194–199

13. Stunkard AJ, Berkowitz RI, Schoeller D, Maislin G, Stallings VA. Predictors of body size in the first 2 y of life: a high-risk study of human obesity. *Int J Obes Relat Metab Disord.* 2004;28:503–513

14. Hilson JA, Rasmussen KM, Kjolhede CL. Maternal obesity and breast-feeding success in a rural population of white women. *Am J Clin Nutr.* 1997;66:1371–1378

15. Rasmussen KM, Kjolhede CL. Prepregnant overweight and obesity diminish the prolactin response to suckling in the first week postpartum. *Pediatrics.* 2004;113:e465–e471

16. Trahms CM, Pipes PL, eds. *Nutrition in Infancy and Childhood.* 6th ed. New York, NY: WCB/McGraw Hill; 1997

17. Lovelady CA. Is maternal obesity a cause of poor lactation performance. *Nutr Rev.* 2005;63:352–355

18. Rolland-Cachera MF, Deheeger M, Guilloud-Bataille M, Avons P, Patois E, Sempe M. Tracking the development of adiposity from one month of age to adulthood. *Ann Hum Biol.* 1987;14:219–229

19. He Q, Karlberg J. Prediction of adult overweight during the pediatric years. *Pediatr Res.* 1999;46:697–703

20. Ekelund U, Ong K, Linne Y, et al. Upward weight percentile crossing in infancy and early childhood independently predicts fat mass in young adults: the Stockholm Weight Development Study (SWEDES). *Am J Clin Nutr.* 2006;83: 324–330

21. Skinner JD, Carruth BR, Wendy B, Ziegler PJ. Children's food preferences: a longitudinal analysis. *J Am Diet Assoc.* 2002;102:1638–1647

Chapter 5

Toddler

....

5.1 Background

Overweight is increasingly common in young children. The prevalence rate of overweight in 6- to 23-month-olds in a 1999–2000 survey was 11.6%.[1] One in 3 American babies born in 2000 will develop diabetes,[2] a trend driven by escalating rates of obesity and inactivity. Prevention of obesity has never been more important and the opportunity for prevention presents itself in the frequent contact these young children and their families have with their pediatricians.

Food preferences develop early[3] and may predict eating preferences through childhood.[4] By 1 year of age children will be eating an array of foods that usually reflects family preferences. A recent study of toddler diets found that the table foods they transitioned to reflected the same problem areas seen in the diets of older children and adults, namely high intake of sugar and fat.[5] For example, approximately 65% to 70% of 1- to 2-year-olds consumed dessert, ice cream, or candy once a day, while 30% to 50% consumed sweetened beverages daily.[6] Fruit and vegetable consumption did not fare much better, with fewer than 10% of 1- to 2-year-olds consuming a dark green vegetable a day, a general lack of fruits and vegetables, and potatoes and french fries accounting for the bulk of vegetable consumption.[5] Sugared beverage intake has been shown to be higher in obese children than non-obese children.[6] In essence, for good or ill, the toddler is a participant in the family's nutritional environment. Families have a tremendous influence on their children's food preferences and should be encouraged to provide the appropriate amount of nutritious foods at meals and snacks.

5.2 Prevention: Talking to Parents (BALANCE)

Prevention touch points for parents include **belief, assessment, lifestyle, activity, nutrition, child,** and **environment** (BALANCE).

Belief

- Parents need to feel comfortable that they are providing adequate nutrition for their toddler to make changes in the child's diet.
- The maxim "parents provide and the child decides" is important and can also be stated, "Your job (as a parent) is to provide optimal nutrition for your child. Your child's job is to decide how much of the correct portion to eat."
- Parents are the primary role models in developing good nutritional patterns for their child. "Good nutrition is a family affair."

Assessment

- Growth charts are essential tools for helping families understand the trajectory of normal growth.
- The goal of keeping the child on the chart is one that can capture the purpose of discussing nutrition, activity, and lifestyle change.
- Normal growth trajectories are also valuable reassurance to parents whose child is a picky eater, which makes the parents afraid the child is not getting enough to eat.

Lifestyle

- Children need structure, predictability, and limit-setting by parents for eating and activity. This fosters a sense of security for the child.
- Parents should make sure that toddlers do not get their own food or snacks, but that these are provided by parents and adult family members who can make healthy and appropriate choices.
- Parents may not realize that they carry over their own eating and activity patterns in interacting with their child and may need to reexamine their approach. For example,
  - Parents should exert control over meal timing, foods offered, and portion size, but not the amount of food consumed by the child.
  - Parents should decide on the location and activity at meals, such as "no television while eating."

Activity

- It is important for parents to know what age-appropriate physical skills develop to provide safe and appropriate activity opportunities for their child.
- When planning family activities, parents should think about making them as active as possible.
- Strollers should be used sparingly.
- Television watching is not a health-promoting activity for children. The American Academy of Pediatrics currently recommends that children 2 years and younger should not watch television.
- Children should not have televisions in their rooms or watch television during meals.
- For children older than 2 years, television watching (of educational, nonviolent programming) should be limited to no more than 1 to 2 hours a day.

Nutrition

- Providing good food choices is important for parents; it may be helpful for them to think of the nutritional requirement of the toddler in terms of daily servings. (The following information is taken from American Academy of Pediatrics. *Pediatric Nutrition Handbook.* Kleinman RE, ed. 5th ed. Elk Grove Village, IL: American Academy of Pediatrics; 2004.)
  - Daily servings for toddlers (2–3 years old)
    - ▾ Fruit: 2 servings a day
    - ▾ Vegetables: 3 servings a day
    - ▾ Dairy: 4 to 5 servings a day
    - ▾ Protein: 2 servings a day
    - ▾ Grain products: 3 to 4 servings a day
- Serving size (portion) may be one of the most confusing aspects of nutrition for parents. Even preschool-aged children eat more when large portions of highly palatable foods are offered. Providing parents with some guidelines for age-appropriate portions may be helpful.
  - Serving sizes for a 2- to 3-year-old
    - ▾ Fruit: Half to 1 small fruit, 2 to 4 tbsp canned fruit
    - ▾ Vegetables: 2 to 3 tbsp cooked vegetables
    - ▾ Dairy: ½ cup milk (whole milk for 2 years and younger) per serving or ½ cup yogurt

▼ Protein: 1 to 2 oz meat, 1 egg per serving, or 4 to 5 tbsp cooked
legumes

▼ Grain products: Half to 1 slice of bread; ¼ to ½ cups rice or pasta; or
½ to 1 cup dry cereal, quarter to half bagel, half to 1 tortilla

Child

● A child's behavior can often drive food consumption. It is important for
parents to understand and have support in changing these dynamics.
- Picky eaters
▼ Parents are often concerned about picky eaters. Providing reassur-
ance about normal growth using the growth and body mass index
(BMI) charts (or weight-for-height chart for children younger than
2 years) can help.
- Food refusal
▼ Children can gain control over their diets by refusing food.
▼ Parents will often say the child doesn't like certain types of food
and fall into a pattern of offering less nutritious alternative foods
just because the child cries or whines, thereby allowing the child
to direct the food selection.
▼ In this situation parents should provide nutritious meals and
appropriate snacks, let the child eat (or not eat) the amount of the
food offered, and redirect the focus away from food.
- Grazing
▼ One to 2 planned snacks a day should be part of a toddler's diet,
but grazing should be avoided.
▼ Parents' recognition of this pattern often is enough to promote
change, along with the reassurance that the child can get adequate
nutrition from the 3 meals and 2 snacks the parents provide.

Environment

● A safe and appropriate nutritional and activity environment is important.
- How to avoid choking should be part of nutritional counseling.
- Remind parents that children don't fully develop the grinding
motion involved in chewing until they are about 4 years old.
- Remind parents and family members to make sure to sit with their
child when they are eating to avoid choking.

- Parents can view providing a "safe" nutritional environment as they do childproofing the house for safety. If junk foods are not purchased, parents will not need to worry about limiting or refusing to serve them. It's easier to promote eating of healthy food if it's available in the home.

5.3 Intervention

When a toddler has a BMI greater than 85% and less than 95% or is crossing growth percentiles in an upward direction, this is the time for a more in-depth look at eating and activity, family health history, and parental obesity—all of which can contribute to the risk of becoming an obese older child and young adult. In addition to reemphasizing concepts covered previously, parents and families may need to give increased attention to their ability to provide and influence nutrition and activity by focusing on **energy balance, structure,** and **modeling healthy behavior.**

Energy Balance

Balancing energy intake for age and growth. Here is where many parents may need to be reminded of appropriate portion sizes for their toddler (see Nutrition under 5.2) and that balancing food groups and providing the variety of recommended food group servings provides balanced vitamin, mineral, fat, protein, and carbohydrate intake for growth and activity.

Balancing activity and inactivity. This means limiting television time, encouraging supervised playtime, and changing family activities from sedentary to active.

Diet and activity records from parents, child care providers, and other family members can contain valuable information and serve as a tool for monitoring desired changes in eating and activity.

Structure

Planning meals and mealtime, organizing snacks and limiting grazing, and eating meals together are all important factors in moving toward a healthier lifestyle. Parents need to find out what the child's day is really like. (What is he eating at child care? Is she going outdoors in nursery school? Is he watching television at grandmother's house?) Taking time to organize meals and activities is one of the most important factors in being able to stay with a health plan.

Modeling Healthy Behavior

Parents are the models for their children. Having parents reflect on their own eating and activity style and their hopes for their child and helping them recognize that they are the major influences on their toddler will help motivate them toward any changes that need to be made in the family's lifestyle.

Parents also will need to reflect on their own parenting style and ability to help their family and child make necessary changes.

5.4 Treatment

When a child's BMI is greater than 95% and you are usually dealing with excess adiposity or body fatness, it is time to initiate a focused treatment strategy. It is important to review the issues discussed in the preceding 2 sections because these are building blocks of good nutrition and activity habits. But you will also have to focus on the barriers to change that may have prevented parents and families from implementing these strategies.

Obtaining a family history focused on obesity-related comorbidities can serve to emphasize the health risks involved and the necessity of taking early action once obesity is identified.

5.5 Family History

The family history (page 59) provides information on obesity and obesity-related comorbidity risk as well as serves as a starting point to discuss the child's BMI.

If parents are obese or have a history of obesity, they may want to relate their personal struggles with their weight. Often the desire to avoid these same struggles in their child motivates parents to make family changes in nutrition and activity.

5.6 Review of Systems

The review of systems can also serve as a point of departure to discuss obesity-related comorbidities, pointing out particular risk factors as they relate to increasing BMI.

- Skin: Acanthosis nigricans
- Head, eyes, ears, nose, and throat (HEENT): Headache, snoring, sleep disturbance

Family History, Toddler

Complete or update this family history targeted toward obesity and related comorbidities.

	Mother	Father	Maternal Grandmother	Maternal Grandfather	Paternal Grandmother	Paternal Grandfather	Sibling 1	Sibling 2
Obesity	☐	☐	☐	☐	☐	☐	☐	☐
Cardiovascular disease	☐	☐	☐	☐	☐	☐	☐	☐
High blood pressure	☐	☐	☐	☐	☐	☐	☐	☐
Stroke	☐	☐	☐	☐	☐	☐	☐	☐
High cholesterol	☐	☐	☐	☐	☐	☐	☐	☐
High triglyceride	☐	☐	☐	☐	☐	☐	☐	☐
Type 1 or 2 diabetes	☐	☐	☐	☐	☐	☐	☐	☐
_____	☐	☐	☐	☐	☐	☐	☐	☐
_____	☐	☐	☐	☐	☐	☐	☐	☐
_____	☐	☐	☐	☐	☐	☐	☐	☐
_____	☐	☐	☐	☐	☐	☐	☐	☐
_____	☐	☐	☐	☐	☐	☐	☐	☐
_____	☐	☐	☐	☐	☐	☐	☐	☐

- Lungs: Asthma, shortness of breath during activity, cough at end of activity, decreased ability to keep up with other children at play
- Cardiac: History of congenital heart disease
- Abdomen: Gastroesophageal reflux, stomach pain before or after eating, chronic diarrhea or constipation, rapid eating
- Musculoskeletal: Limping, hip pain, knee pain
- Development: Delay, hypotonia, coordination difficulties, social interaction, poor height growth

5.7 Physical Examination

- Height
- Weight
- Weight for length or BMI

Note: For children younger than 2 years, length should be measured. The weight-for-length chart is useful to assess appropriateness of weight relative to length. The Centers for Disease Control and Prevention defines weight for length above 95% as overweight.[5]

- General: Dysmorphic features, poor linear growth, developmental delay
- Skin: Dermatitis in skinfolds
- HEENT: Funduscopic examination for papilledema, tonsillar hypertrophy
- Cardiopulmonary: Wheezing, poor ventilation, heart murmur
- Abdominal: Hepatomegaly
- Musculoskeletal: Range of motion, genu varum, limp, hip or knee pain
- Genitourinary: Undescended testicles

5.8 Family Constellation and Social History

Information about the family can provide a starting point to discuss how nutrition and activity decisions are made and how changes might take place.

- Who is living at home with the child?
- Who else feeds and cares for the child?
- Who decides what the child will eat?
- Who is in charge of the child's daily schedule?

5.9 Parenting Questions

Parenting styles and skills are important when families are trying to make changes in lifestyle. These questions may help you focus on family factors that may facilitate or hinder change.

	Never	Seldom	Sometimes	Often	Always
1. Parents agree on how to feed the child.	☐	☐	☐	☐	☐
2. Child and parents fight about food.	☐	☐	☐	☐	☐
3. Parents set clear and simple expectations and limits.	☐	☐	☐	☐	☐
4. Parents understand the child's developmental stage.	☐	☐	☐	☐	☐
5. Parents set boundaries and give child choice within them.	☐	☐	☐	☐	☐

5.10 Parenting Touch Points

Parenting touch points focus on helping families initiate and maintain change by helping them believe change can occur, identify the change needed, value the outcome of the change, know how to change, and have the energy to change and sustain the change.

- *Believe that change can occur.* Parents need to feel that change is possible. Setting realistic goals is important. For example, in the toddler age group, weight stability to allow the height to catch up is a realistic and healthy goal. Goals can be behavioral, keying on the attainment of a desired behavior change (ie, sitting at the table for meals and snacks), or incremental, starting with making diet records. It is important to demonstrate early on that realistic goals can be achieved.

- *Identify the change.* Parents need to have the necessary information to understand what change needs to occur.
  - This is often the area in which pediatricians feel most comfortable. However, it is important to offer the family an array of possible changes and have a discussion about what might be possible in their situation rather than simply tell them what to do.

– For example, a toddler may be drinking too much juice, grazing,
and getting snacks by refusing food at mealtimes. Parents may be
ready to make a change in juice drinking as a first step because
changing grazing and food refusal depends on speaking to grandparents. It is best to start where the family is and continue to work
over time on other changes that need to be made.

● *Value the outcome.* Parents need to believe that a healthy weight is
important for their child. Each parent and family is unique in their
perspective about obesity. Reasons for managing a toddler's weight may
range from "Doesn't look like his friends" to "I don't want her to have
to suffer like I did being overweight as a child." It is important that
parents are able to identify what they value and why because this provides energy and motivation for change.

● *Know how to change.* Parents often need help to devise concrete steps
to make the desired change. This is a key step in the process of helping
families change nutrition and activity patterns. Your knowledge of the
family's circumstances, parenting attitudes and skills, and the child can
all come into play as you help families implement the desired change.
For example, in one family, eliminating sugared beverages may simply
require a decision on the part of the parent not to buy them and the rest
of the family will go along. In another family, a parent may feel that the
thinner sibling "needs" juice and the decision to limit juice may require
more extensive discussion about good family nutrition and parenting
children with different body types.

● *Have energy to change and sustain.* Parents need to have resources
and support not only to make the initial change, but also to sustain the
change. Maintenance of any behavioral change is difficult. Engaging
family support, making small incremental changes, and allowing the
family to adjust to and feel good about the changes they have made
is important. Difficult behavior can also get in the way of sustaining
change. For example, a 2-year-old throwing a tantrum can make even
the most committed parent give in if a strategy is not in place to deal
with the tantrums.

5.11 Developmental Touch Point

At this stage of development children need confirmation of trust, to know that a parent is nearby while they explore the world. They are ambivalent, testing limits of authority. Food selection and inactivity (ie, television) may be a battleground for self-control. The child at this stage has an egocentric view of the world.

5.12 Nutrition and Activity Questions and Interventions

Nutrition and activity questions (see pages 64–65) can be answered by the parents and provide a focal point for targeted intervention (see pages 66–67) in a brief encounter. Questions answered "Often" or "Always" can be targeted first for change. For example, if the parent answered questions 1, 7, 9, and 13 on pages 64 and 65 with "Often" or "Always," you would ask them to rate the difficulty of change for questions 1, 7, 9, and 13 on pages 66 and 67.

These questions and answers may give you some targeted starting points that the parents feel they can tackle. For example, if the parents answered questions 1 with "often" drinks juice and then answered that they thought they could change juice to water "most of the time" this would be a good starting point for change. Even if the family feels that a change will be doable, it is a good idea to explore with them exactly how they will make the change, what might make the desired change easier to make, and what would make it harder. For example, if the mother thinks she would like to eliminate juice, she might also say that getting grandmother to do this when the child is visiting might be hard or that the child's older brother would object. Given this information you can help her troubleshoot a solution.

You should aim in general for weight stability with continued height growth in a toddler unless there is a medical morbidity, which has to be resolved quickly. Frequent visits to facilitate change are important, as is monitoring for nutritional adequacy and developmentally appropriate activity.

Nutrition and Activity Questions, Toddler

These questions can be answered by the parents and provide a focal point for targeted intervention in a brief encounter. First have the parents answer these questions about the presence or absence of behaviors that promote weight gain, then refer to Nutrition and Activity Interventions, Toddler.

	Never	Seldom	Sometimes	Often	Always
1. Drinks milk, juice, or sugared beverages between meals.	☐	☐	☐	☐	☐
2. Eats junk food.	☐	☐	☐	☐	☐
3. Eats more than 2 snacks between meals a day.	☐	☐	☐	☐	☐
4. Eats as much as an adult.	☐	☐	☐	☐	☐
5. Eats at fast-food restaurants.	☐	☐	☐	☐	☐
6. Eats in the car.	☐	☐	☐	☐	☐
7. People other than parents feed the child snacks.	☐	☐	☐	☐	☐
8. Eats snacks at child care.	☐	☐	☐	☐	☐
9. Demands food or snacks.	☐	☐	☐	☐	☐
10. Refuses fruit products.	☐	☐	☐	☐	☐

	Never	Seldom	Sometimes	Often	Always
11. Refuses vegetable products.	☐	☐	☐	☐	☐
12. Refuses dairy products.	☐	☐	☐	☐	☐
13. Parents or grandparents disagree on what child should eat.	☐	☐	☐	☐	☐
14. Eats in front of the television.	☐	☐	☐	☐	☐
15. Skips meals.	☐	☐	☐	☐	☐
16. Eats alone.	☐	☐	☐	☐	☐
17. Watches more than 1 hour of television each day.	☐	☐	☐	☐	☐
18. Plays outside.	☐	☐	☐	☐	☐
19. Rides in a stroller.	☐	☐	☐	☐	☐
20. Has a scheduled active playtime.	☐	☐	☐	☐	☐

Nutrition and Activity Interventions, Toddler

Questions answered "Often" or "Always" in Nutrition and Activity Questions, Toddler, can be targeted first for change. Using these specific questions, ask the parent, "How difficult would it be for you to…?"

	Impossible	Could try	Could do sometimes	Could do most of the time	Easy
1. Change from juice to water between meals.	☐	☐	☐	☐	☐
2. Eliminate junk food.	☐	☐	☐	☐	☐
3. Eliminate extra snacks.	☐	☐	☐	☐	☐
4. Decrease portion sizes.	☐	☐	☐	☐	☐
5. Decrease fast food.	☐	☐	☐	☐	☐
6. Stop eating in the car.	☐	☐	☐	☐	☐
7. Find out what other people are feeding your child.	☐	☐	☐	☐	☐
8. Provide healthy snacks for your child to take to child care.	☐	☐	☐	☐	☐
9. Distract your child when he or she is hungry between meals or snacks.	☐	☐	☐	☐	☐
10. Offer fruit at meals.	☐	☐	☐	☐	☐

	Impossible	Could try	Could do sometimes	Could do most of the time	Easy
11. Offer vegetables at meals.	☐	☐	☐	☐	☐
12. Offer dairy products at meals.	☐	☐	☐	☐	☐
13. Have family agree on what child should eat.	☐	☐	☐	☐	☐
14. Turn off the television during meals and snacks.	☐	☐	☐	☐	☐
15. Schedule regular meals and snacks.	☐	☐	☐	☐	☐
16. Eat meals together.	☐	☐	☐	☐	☐
17. Reduce television time.	☐	☐	☐	☐	☐
18. Increase supervised outdoor play.	☐	☐	☐	☐	☐
19. Put away the stroller.	☐	☐	☐	☐	☐
20. Schedule supervised indoor play time.	☐	☐	☐	☐	☐

5.13 A Case in Point: LQ

LQ comes to your office at 2 years and 9 months of age for an upper respiratory infection. You note her height is 37" (94 cm) (90% for age) and weight is 58 lb (26.4 kg) (>95% for age). You calculate her BMI at 30, which is well above 95% for age. You look back in her chart and note that she gained 15 lb (6.8 kg) in the past 6 months. When you mention this to her parents they note, "We're not concerned about her weight." They explain that her father's family was large and that he was chunky until 5 years of age. They also note that LQ is very active, even in the house.

You ask about family history and they note that a paternal grandfather had bypass surgery and a maternal grandmother has diabetes.

Your physical examination is unremarkable except for tibial torsion. You ask them to fill out the first set of questions (pages 64–65) and they answer "Often" or "Always" to

1. Drinks milk, juice, or sugared beverages between meals.
   They think they could change juice to water most of the time.

3. Eats more than 2 snacks between meals a day.
   Parents think they could set times for meals and 2 snacks most of the time.

4. Eats as much as an adult.
   They think it would be difficult to limit portions.

9. Demands food or snacks.
   Mom thinks Dad is more likely to give in to the child's demands but could try, and Mom thinks that she could distract her when she demanded food "most of the time."

16. Eats alone.
    Because Mom works at night, Dad says he will eat his dinner with LQ.

You ask them to try to change her juice to water and wean her from the bottle to a cup at night. You go over a schedule of meals and snacks and the father agrees to eat dinner with her. You briefly discuss limiting portions as something to try and report back on.

In addition you order laboratory work, which shows elevated cholesterol of 194 mg/dL with normal triglyceride, glucose, insulin, thyroid, and liver function studies.

You ask the family to return in 3 weeks.

Second Visit

LQ's weight on return is 57 lb (26.0 kg), a decrease of 1 lb (0.4 kg). The parents report that they followed the previous instructions exactly. She is now drinking water between meals, her father is no longer giving her junk food for dinner, and mealtimes are now regular. You reinforce the changes and ask them to come back in 1 month.

Third Visit

Now LQ's weight has gone up to 60 lb (27.0 kg). Mom notes that Dad has changed his work schedule and is taking her outside less. Mom is also in the last part of her pregnancy and is less active with LQ. Review of the diet records you have asked them to keep shows a slight increase in her portions. You raise the issue of activity. Mother says that in their area there are no particular playgroups or outlets for her. Dad said he would look into building a fenced-in area of the yard so she can play outdoors. When she goes out now with Mom, she bolts and runs away, so outdoor safety is a priority.

Fourth Visit

You wanted to see LQ in 1 month, but because of the new baby, she comes back 3 months later. Her weight is still 60 lb (27.0 kg) and she has grown to 40" (100.4 cm), lowering her BMI from 30 to 26.78. On dietary review you note she is eating 3 meals and 2 snacks per day. Unfortunately you notice her bowing is worse and you send her to orthopedics where the diagnosis of Blount disease is made and she is prescribed a brace.

Fifth Visit

Two months later you see LQ again. Her weight is 55 lb (25.1 kg). Mom attributes this to increased activity ("She is running all the time"). Parents are still structuring her meals and snacks; the quality of her diet is improved with no junk or snack food. You repeat her cholesterol and it is still elevated at 204 mg/dL. You give them specific dietary advice on lowering cholesterol.

Sixth Visit

LQ returns to your office 4 months later in midsummer with a weight of 50 lb (22.5 kg). Her height is 40" (101.4 cm) and her BMI is 21.9. Her parents have maintained her dietary changes.

References

1. Ogden CL, Flegal KM, Carroll MD, Johnson CL. Prevalence and trends in overweight among US children and adolescents 1999-2000. *JAMA.* 2002;288: 1728–1732

2. Narayan KM, Boyle JP, Thompson TJ, Sorensen SW, Williamson DF. Lifetime risk for diabetes mellitus in the United States. *JAMA.* 2003;290:1884–1890

3. Birch LL. Development of food acceptance patterns in the first years of life. *Proc Nutr Soc.* 1998;57:617–624

4. Skinner JD, Carruth BR, Wendy B, Ziegler PJ. Children's food preferences: a longitudinal analysis. *J Am Diet Assoc.* 2002;102:1638–1647

5. Fox MK, Pac S, Devaney B, Jankowski L. Feeding infants and toddlers study: what foods are infants and toddlers eating? *J Am Diet Assoc.* 2004;104 (1 Suppl 1):S22–S30

6. Ludwig DS, Peterson KE, Gortmaker SL. Relation between consumption of sugar-sweetened drinks and childhood obesity: a prospective, observational analysis. *Lancet.* 2001;357:505–508

Chapter 6

Preschool Age

··

6.1 Background

The preschool period is a time when children transition from a period of relative slowing in weight gain to a time when many children accelerate their weight. Children who are overweight or obese at this age are at significant risk for becoming obese as adults. In one study more than 50% of 3- to 6-year-olds with a body mass index (BMI) at or above 95% became obese adults.[1] The point when BMI reaches its nadir in early childhood normally occurs around 5 to 6 years of age (adiposity rebound).[2,3] Children who cross BMI percentiles at younger than 4.8 years (early adiposity rebound) have a greater likelihood of becoming obese adults.[2,3]

Parental obesity is still a major risk factor for overweight and obesity in this age group; parents also exercise a tremendous influence over their preschooler's nutrition and activity environment. A dietary factor that contributes to disorders in energy balance is increased consumption of sweetened beverages.[4] For children aged 2 to 3 years between 85% and 95% for BMI, as little as 1 extra sweetened drink a day (eg, juice, soda, fruit drink) doubled their risk of having a BMI greater than 95% in the following year.[4]

Accelerated weight gain in preschool children has been associated with higher baseline fat intakes[5] and inappropriately large portion sizes[6] that can negatively affect daily energy balance.

A low level of physical activity in preschoolers has been reported to be associated with an increased amount of subcutaneous fat in children by first grade.[7] The same study showed that preschool children with active parents were more likely to be active than those with sedentary parents.[7] The increase in stroller use and highly structured activity may also be limiting physical activity in this age group.

Time spent outdoors strongly correlates with physical activity in young children.[8] Between 1981 and 1997, time for free play dropped by 25%. Free play in the preschool age group is composed of brief bouts of varied activity interspersed with frequent rest periods.[9] Time spent watching television has a direct relationship to overweight and obesity.[10] A recent study found that 40% of low-income children aged 1 to 5 years have a television in their room.[10]

Child temperament and behavior has also been associated with a risk for overweight. In one study, young children with persistent tantrums over food and highly emotional temperament were at increased risk for overweight.[11] Parenting skills that help deal with their child's anger, temper tantrums, and emotions around boundary settings are crucial if parents are to guide their preschoolers through challenges to healthy eating and activity.

Parents of a preschool-aged child are challenged to achieve consistency between spouses, family members, and caregivers in the nutritional choices offered to their child. Recognizing the importance of appropriate portion sizes, limiting sweetened beverages, and encouraging outdoor play need to become common themes among the adults who care for the overweight or obese child. Communication about the child's daily activities and eating is essential as the preschooler moves into environments outside the home. Small exceptions in portion sizes, treats, and snacks can add up to weight gain over time—as little as 150 kcal extra intake per day can become a 15-lb (6.8-kg) weight gain over the next year.

Because food and activity choices often become emotional for parents and children, it is important to have parents set the initial boundaries such as what kinds of food will be in the house, how much television time the family will have, and what kind of activities are available to the child. Within these boundaries parents should provide the child with choices such as a variety of possible healthy snacks and options for what they will do during outside play. This not only prevents every decision from becoming a battle, but also encourages healthy decision making and avoids over-restriction.

6.2 Prevention: Talking to Parents (BALANCE)

Prevention touch points for parents include **belief, assessment, lifestyle, activity, nutrition, child,** and **environment** (BALANCE).

Belief

- Because preschool children are becoming more independent, parents and families may believe that they can make good food and activity decisions independently as well.
- At this point it is important to remind parents that they still need to be in charge of the nutrition and activity environment, allowing children to choose food and activity within the boundaries set by parents.

Assessment

- As eating patterns, eating venues, and caregivers change, it is important to review growth charts with parents and families. This helps them remain in charge of the knowledge of the child's daily activity and nutrition with the goal of staying on the chart.

Lifestyle

- Busy families frequently eat out, often leaving the decision about what to eat up to the preschool child. Remind parents it is important to limit eating out and to maintain oversight of their child's food choices when they do so.
- Parents are important role models for physical activity and inactivity and need to take stock of their own behavior to set up healthy patterns for their child.

Activity

- During a child's preschool years, parents should encourage free play as much as possible to help develop motor skills.
- Outdoor time is the best way to encourage free play. Parents need to be reminded to avoid micromanaging their child's play. Providing appropriate supervision, however, is their job.
- It's appropriate for parents to provide their child with age-appropriate play equipment, from balls to plastic bats, to make exercise fun, but they should let the child choose exactly what to play with at any given time.
- The television should be off when the family is eating. This not only encourages conversation but also allows parents to model good eating behavior.

- If the child has a television in the bedroom, recommend that it be removed.
- The American Academy of Pediatrics advises a daily limit not to exceed 1 to 2 hours of television viewing, including time spent playing computer and video games.

Nutrition

- Younger children should be served smaller portions than older siblings and parents.
- Parents and families still need to be reminded of the appropriate portion size and number of servings appropriate for the preschooler. Sometimes referring to a sample menu can help them calibrate the right amount of food to offer their child (Table 6.1).
- Sugar-sweetened beverages and juice creep in again at child care, pre-schools, relatives, and friends and parents may want to provide milk or water or the occasional diet beverage as alternatives.

Child

- Parents need to understand that children as young as preschool age are a major target of food advertising.
- Parents may give in to requests for energy-dense or highly sugared foods when food shopping or out to eat with their child.
- Dealing with a child's complaints of hunger between meals and snacks is often difficult for parents.
- Information about what constitutes an adequate diet and reassurance about other drivers for hunger such as visual cues, boredom, situational cues, and television advertising can help parents respond appropriately.
- Parents should observe the food advertising their child is exposed to with a critical eye and discuss with their child the untruths and exaggerations that are often present.

Environment

- Maintaining a structured eating environment is important. Predictable times for meals and snacks help children manage hunger and families deliver good nutrition instead of relying on filling in the gaps with snack food.

Table 6.1. Sample Menu and Serving Sizes for a 4-year-old Who Weighs About 36 lb (16.3 kg)

Breakfast	– One-half cup of 2% milk
	– One-half cup of cereal
	– Four to 6 oz of 100% citrus or tomato juice or ½ cup of cantaloupe or strawberries
Snack	– One-half cup of 2% milk
	– One-half cup of banana
	– One slice of whole wheat bread
	– One teaspoon of margarine (or butter)
	– One teaspoon of jelly
Lunch	– One-half cup of 2% milk
	– One sandwich—2 slices of whole wheat bread, 1 teaspoon of margarine (or butter) or 2 teaspoons of salad dressing, and 1 oz of meat or cheese
	– One-fourth cup of dark-yellow or dark-green vegetable
Snack	– One teaspoon of peanut butter or 1 slice of low-fat cheese
	– One slice of whole wheat bread or 5 crackers
Dinner	– One-half cup of 2% milk
	– Two oz (slightly less than a deck of cards) or about ¼ cup of meat, fish, or chicken
	– One-half cup of pasta, rice, or potato
	– One-half cup of vegetables
	– One teaspoon of margarine (or butter) or 2 teaspoons of salad dressing

From American Academy of Pediatrics. The preschool years. In: Hassink SG, ed. *A Parent's Guide to Childhood Obesity: A Road Map to Health.* Elk Grove Village, IL: American Academy of Pediatrics; 2006:179

- Many parents assume that child care, preschool, and other caregivers are providing good nutrition and activity options for their child. It is important for families to ask about these options and provide healthy alternatives if needed.

6.3 Intervention

When a preschool-aged child has a BMI greater than 85% and less than 95% or is crossing growth percentiles in an upward direction, this is the time for a more in-depth look at eating and activity, family health history, and parental obesity—all of which can contribute to the risk of becoming an obese older child and young adult. In addition to reemphasizing concepts covered previously, parents and families may need to give increased attention to their ability to provide and influence nutrition and activity by focusing on **energy balance, structure,** and **modeling healthy behavior.**

Energy Balance

There are many factors that can alter energy balance by disrupting nutrition or activity and begin an upward trend in a child's weight gain. Many of these have to do with increased family or child stress, including

- Parental divorce or separation
- Illness or death of a close family member
- Family move
- Birth of a sibling
- Physical illness or injury in child
- Parental depression

If the causes of altered energy balance can be understood, many times a more effective intervention can be designed.

Parents of preschoolers can gradually reduce the energy imbalance by

- Switching from whole milk to skim, 1%, or 2% milk
- Selecting grilled or broiled fish or lean meats
- Serving cheese only in modest portions
- Serving whole fruit to meet recommended fruit intake
- Limiting fruit juice consumption to no more than 4 to 6 oz per day (from ages 1 to 6 years)—and this should be 100% juice, not juice drinks
- Relying on low-fat snack choices such as pretzels, fresh fruit, and fat-free yogurt
- Using cooking methods like steaming, broiling, and roasting that do not require fat during cooking, or using only a small amount of olive oil or nonstick spray

Structure

Structured meals, snacks, and time for activity become more important as the time the family has together decreases. Parents need to become acutely aware of what their preschooler is eating and what kind of activity is taking place at child care, preschool, or time with extended family. A change in scheduling or the environment (eg, switch of child care, grandparents watching the child over vacation) can affect weight gain. It is equally important to review scheduling of television, computer, and outdoor time so these activities become part of the family's health plan.

Modeling Healthy Behavior

Parents will need to work together and with other family members to help their preschooler. At this point a family meeting may be helpful to get all family members on the same page. At this meeting, it can be helpful to review growth rate, family history, age-appropriate activity, eating, and access to food. The family can also discuss ways to make sure other family members are on board with the strategy of offering healthy food choices to the child.

6.4 Treatment

When a child's BMI is greater than 95% and you are dealing with excess adiposity, it is time to initiate a focused treatment strategy. It is important to review the issues discussed in the previous 2 sections because these are building blocks of good nutrition and activity habits. But you will also have to focus on the barriers to change that may have prevented parents and families from implementing these strategies.

A useful way to begin is to obtain a family history focused on obesity-related comorbidities. This can serve to emphasize the health risks involved and the necessity of taking early action once obesity is identified.

6.5 Family History

The family history (page 79) provides information on obesity and obesity-related comorbidity risk as well as serves as a starting point to discuss the child's BMI.

If parents are obese or have a history of obesity, they may want to relate their personal struggles with their weight. Often the desire to avoid these same struggles in their child motivates parents to make family changes in nutrition and activity.

6.6 Review of Systems

The review of systems can also serve as a point of departure to discuss obesity-related comorbidities, pointing out particular risk factors as they relate to increasing BMI.

- Skin: Acanthosis nigricans, striae, cervical fat pad, skin picking
- Head, eyes, ears, nose, and throat (HEENT): Headache, blurred vision
- Lungs: Snoring, sleep disturbance, sleep apnea, restless sleep, sleep position, daytime tiredness, napping, asthma, shortness of breath or subjective chest tightness on exercise, cough after exercise
- Cardiac: Murmur
- Abdomen: Gastroesophageal reflux, stomach pain, nausea or vomiting after eating
- Musculoskeletal: Limping, hip pain, knee pain, bowing
- Development: School problems, learning difficulties, attention problems
- Psychosocial: Depression, anxiety, behavior problems

6.7 Physical Examination

- Height
- Weight
- BMI + previous BMI measurements
- Blood pressure

- General: Dysmorphic features, poor linear growth, developmental delay
- Skin: Skin picking, acanthosis nigricans, dermatitis in skinfolds, striae, cervical fat pad
- HEENT: Funduscopic examination for papilledema, tonsillar hypertrophy
- Cardiopulmonary: Murmur, wheezing
- Abdominal: Hepatomegaly
- Musculoskeletal: Range of motion, genu varum, limp, hip or knee pain
- Genitourinary: Tanner stage

Family History, Preschool Age

Complete or update this family history targeted toward obesity and related comorbidities.

	Mother	Father	Maternal Grandmother	Maternal Grandfather	Paternal Grandmother	Paternal Grandfather	Sibling 1	Sibling 2
Obesity	☐	☐	☐	☐	☐	☐	☐	☐
Cardiovascular disease	☐	☐	☐	☐	☐	☐	☐	☐
High blood pressure	☐	☐	☐	☐	☐	☐	☐	☐
Stroke	☐	☐	☐	☐	☐	☐	☐	☐
High cholesterol	☐	☐	☐	☐	☐	☐	☐	☐
High triglyceride	☐	☐	☐	☐	☐	☐	☐	☐
Type 1 or 2 diabetes	☐	☐	☐	☐	☐	☐	☐	☐
_____	☐	☐	☐	☐	☐	☐	☐	☐
_____	☐	☐	☐	☐	☐	☐	☐	☐
_____	☐	☐	☐	☐	☐	☐	☐	☐
_____	☐	☐	☐	☐	☐	☐	☐	☐
_____	☐	☐	☐	☐	☐	☐	☐	☐
_____	☐	☐	☐	☐	☐	☐	☐	☐

6.8 Family Constellation and Social History

Information about the family can provide a starting point to discuss how nutrition and activity decisions are made and how changes might take place.

- Who is living at home with the child?
- Who is with the child before school?
- Who is with the child after school?
- Who else besides parents is responsible for the child's meals or snacks?

6.9 Parenting Questions

Parenting styles and skills are important when families are trying to make changes in lifestyle. These questions may help you focus on family factors that may facilitate or hamper change.

	Never	Seldom	Sometimes	Often	Always
1. Parents set clear and simple expectations and limits.	☐	☐	☐	☐	☐
2. Parents set boundaries and give the child choice within them.	☐	☐	☐	☐	☐
3. Parents have developmentally appropriate goals for the child.	☐	☐	☐	☐	☐
4. Parents model healthy nutrition, activity, and inactivity behavior.	☐	☐	☐	☐	☐

6.10 Parenting Touch Points

Parenting touch points focus on helping families initiate and maintain change by helping them believe change can occur, identify the change needed, value the outcome of the change, know how to change, and have the energy to change and sustain the change.

- *Believe that change can occur.* Parents need to feel that change is possible. Parents may start with the thought that "We are just a big family," or "My child isn't eating anything the other kids aren't eating." This is a good time to reinforce the individual factors that affect weight gain.

- Family history
- Parental obesity
- Child's temperament
- Family and cultural eating patterns

  Parents may need to be encouraged that they can take charge of the nutrition and activity environment of their child and that this will make a difference if done consistently.

- *Identify the change.* Families may be concerned but not aware of what factors need to be changed. Asking families to go through their child's day often turns up unexpected problems such as a child eating breakfast at home and again at preschool, not going outside at child care, or other caregivers rewarding the child with food. Families seeing this will often spontaneously change; other families will need help identifying possible changes to choose from.

- *Value the outcome.* Parents at this point may begin to worry about the child's constant hunger or the fact that he or she is being teased. Getting in touch with the family's worries and what they value (eg, good eating behavior, acceptance by other children, not fighting about food) is the first step toward helping them make necessary change. Each family will have a slightly different concern and time spent on articulating these concerns is well worth the effort.

- *Know how to change.* Parents often need to be helped to devise concrete steps to make the desired change. Watchwords for parents of the preschooler are consistency, appropriate choices, a calm approach to change, and patience. Change is often best accomplished in small, measurable increments.

- *Have energy to change and sustain.* Parents need to have resources and support not only to make the initial change, but also to sustain the change. Often strong emotions are at play and parents need to be able to have a strategy to deal with anger and tantrums, whining, and pouting when the preschooler cannot get his or her way. Encouraging parents to discuss ways they will manage these situations, suggestions for time-outs, distracting the child, and remaining calm are all part of helping the family to be able to implement the changes important to the child's health.

6.11 Developmental Touch Point

Children begin to develop impulse control, which leads to self-esteem. Social awareness of events outside home and cultural norms leads to approval-seeking behavior. This is a good age to initiate time-outs to deal with inappropriate behavior.

6.12 Nutrition and Activity Questions and Interventions

Nutrition and activity questions (see pages 84–85) can be answered by the parents and provide a focal point for targeted intervention (see pages 86–87) in a brief encounter. Questions answered "Often" or "Always" can be targeted first for change. For example, if the parent answered questions 1, 7, 9, and 13 on pages 84 and 85 with "Often" or "Always," you would ask them to rate the difficulty of change for questions 1, 7, 9, and 13 on pages 86 and 87.

6.13 A Case in Point: OG

OG is a 5-year, 4-month-old boy who comes into your office because his mother is concerned about his constant hunger. She notes he is constantly bugging her for something to eat, even when he has just finished a meal. You look at his growth chart and note that he has gained 3 pounds in the past 6 weeks since he had come in for an upper respiratory infection. His current height is 48" (121.9 cm) and weight is 65 lb (29.5 kg), giving him a BMI of 19.8 (>97% for age and gender). Mom also notes that she is worried about his weight because she and her husband have weight problems and she doesn't want OG to go through the teasing they did as children.

Mom filled out the family history questionnaire (page 79) in the waiting room and you note that 3 of the 4 grandparents have hypertension, 2 are overweight, and 1 has type 2 diabetes. Dad has elevated blood pressure and sleep apnea as well as being overweight.

OG's review of systems reveals that he snores and is restless during sleep. Mom thinks he may have pauses in his breathing but is not sure. His physical examination shows a very active, overweight boy with no other abnormal physical findings except somewhat enlarged tonsils.

You review his family constellation and note that OG lives with his mother, father, older brother (age 10 years), and maternal grandparents. He attends half-day preschool and his grandmother and grandfather look after him before and after school until his parents get home from work. Mom and Grandmother share the cooking and shopping.

Mom answers "Always" or "Often" to questions 1 (Drinks juice or sugared beverages between meals), 8 (Sneaks or hides food), 13 (Constantly complains of being hungry), 14 (Becomes angry when demands for food are not met), and 16 (Watches more than 2 hours of television or the computer each day).

On the second questionnaire she doesn't indicate that anything would be easy, but she could do a change from juice to water between meals most of the time, sometimes reduce television time, and use time-outs to help OG calm down.

Problem #1: Obesity

You order laboratory studies to screen for obesity-related metabolic abnormalities and explain these to Mom.

Problem #2: Possible Sleep Apnea

Based on his obesity, enlarged tonsils, positive family history, snoring, restless sleep, and possible apnea, you arrange a sleep study.

Problem #3: Excess Consumption of Sweetened Beverages

From his diet history you estimate he is drinking 4 to 6 8-oz glasses of juice or soda a day.

- *Parenting dilemma*
  Mom agrees that she would like to get the juice and soda out of the house; she is worried because her husband "needs his soda." She suggests she just ask Dad to hide it.

- *Strategy*
  You ask Mom to talk to Dad and try a soda- and juice-free house for 3 to 4 weeks, then come back to the office to recheck OG's weight and see how the family managed without these beverages in the house.

Nutrition and Activity Questions, Preschool Age

These questions can be answered by the parents and provide a focal point for targeted intervention in a brief encounter. First have the parents answer these questions about the presence or absence of behaviors that promote weight gain, then refer to Nutrition and Activity Interventions, Preschool Age.

	Never	Seldom	Sometimes	Often	Always
1. Drinks juice or sugared beverages between meals.	☐	☐	☐	☐	☐
2. Eats junk food.	☐	☐	☐	☐	☐
3. Eats more than 2 snacks between meals a day.	☐	☐	☐	☐	☐
4. Requests second helpings or eats more than an older sibling.	☐	☐	☐	☐	☐
5. Is a fast eater.	☐	☐	☐	☐	☐
6. Eats at fast-food restaurants on a regular basis.	☐	☐	☐	☐	☐
7. Gets own snacks.	☐	☐	☐	☐	☐
8. Sneaks or hides food.	☐	☐	☐	☐	☐
9. Demands certain food or snacks.	☐	☐	☐	☐	☐
10. Refuses to eat fruit or vegetables.	☐	☐	☐	☐	☐

	Never	Seldom	Sometimes	Often	Always
11. Refuses to eat dairy products.	☐	☐	☐	☐	☐
12. Eats in front of the television.	☐	☐	☐	☐	☐
13. Constantly complains of being hungry.	☐	☐	☐	☐	☐
14. Becomes angry when demands for food are not met.	☐	☐	☐	☐	☐
15. Still wants to ride in the stroller.	☐	☐	☐	☐	☐
16. Watches more than 2 hours of television or the computer each day.	☐	☐	☐	☐	☐
17. Does not want to go outside to play.	☐	☐	☐	☐	☐
18. Prefers quiet activities.	☐	☐	☐	☐	☐
19. Has a television or computer in the bedroom.	☐	☐	☐	☐	☐
20. Parents and family members disagree on what, when, where, and how much the child should eat.	☐	☐	☐	☐	☐

Nutrition and Activity Interventions, Preschool Age

Questions answered "Often" or "Always" in Nutrition and Activity Questions, Preschool Age, can be targeted first for change. Using these specific questions, ask the parent, "How difficult would it be for you to…?"

	Impossible	Could try	Could do sometimes	Could do most of the time	Easy
1. Change from juice to water between meals.	☐	☐	☐	☐	☐
2. Eliminate or cut down on junk food.	☐	☐	☐	☐	☐
3. Eliminate unnecessary snacks.	☐	☐	☐	☐	☐
4. Offer vegetables instead of second helpings.	☐	☐	☐	☐	☐
5. Work on a plan to slow down eating.	☐	☐	☐	☐	☐
6. Decrease fast food.	☐	☐	☐	☐	☐
7. Pack healthier school snacks.	☐	☐	☐	☐	☐
8. Work with your child on a plan to stop sneaking.	☐	☐	☐	☐	☐
9. Keep only healthy snacks in the house.	☐	☐	☐	☐	☐
10. Offer fruit and vegetables at meals.	☐	☐	☐	☐	☐

	Impossible	Could try	Could do sometimes	Could do most of the time	Easy
11. Offer dairy products at meals.	☐	☐		☐	☐
12. Turn off the television during meals and snacks.	☐	☐		☐	☐
13. Distract child.	☐	☐	☐	☐	☐
14. Use a time-out to help child calm down.	☐	☐	☐	☐	☐
15. Put the stroller away.	☐	☐	☐	☐	☐
16. Reduce television and computer time.	☐	☐	☐	☐	☐
17. Schedule time for you and your child to go outside.	☐	☐	☐	☐	☐
18. Come up with some suggestions that involve physical activities for your child.	☐	☐	☐	☐	☐
19. Take the television or computer out of the bedroom.	☐	☐	☐	☐	☐
20. Work with family members on getting agreement and setting boundaries on snacks, sweetened drinks, and portion sizes.	☐	☐	☐	☐	☐

Problem #4: Too Much Screen Time

- *Parenting dilemma*
  Mom notes that the television is on all the time and OG is often watching.

- *Strategy*
  You ask if Mom can work with Dad and the grandparents to get OG
  on a schedule in the afternoon after kindergarten. You ask if he could
  combine outdoor play with some small chores to reduce television time,
  only turning on the television when he is scheduled for a show. Mom
  is nervous about turning off the television, so you and she decide to try
  30 minutes a day without television and move up from there to 30 more
  minutes each week. You suggest that the family fill out a chart to detail
  its progress.

Problem #5: Constant Hunger

- *Parenting dilemma*
  Mother feels constant hunger is OG's biggest problem, but she doesn't
  know what to do about it because he becomes very angry if she denies
  him food.

- *Strategy*
  You introduce the concept of distracting him. You ask OG, "What could
  you do besides eat when you are hungry?" Surprisingly to Mom, he
  answers, "Go out and play." You encourage her to work with OG to
  think about things he could do instead of eating, such as play with toys.

  You schedule a return appointment for OG, Mom, and Dad in 3 to 4
  weeks to check on OG's progress and see how the family has done with
  beginning to make changes

Second Visit

One month later, OG, Mom, and Dad return. His weight is 64 lb (29.0 kg),
a decrease of 1 lb (0.5 kg).

- *Problem #1: Obesity.* You review his laboratory studies, all of which were
  within the normal range.

- *Problem #2: Possible sleep apnea.* Mom reports that his sleep study is
  scheduled for next week.

- *Problem #3: Excess consumption of sweetened beverages.* Mom and Dad report that except for a few times when they ate out, they were able to limit OG and the family's beverage consumption to milk with meals and diet beverages or water between meals. OG has accepted this fairly well, especially because Dad is doing the same thing.

- *Problem #4: Too much screen time.* Reducing screen time has been more difficult, especially because all family members are big television watchers. They were able to turn the television off during dinner and keep it off for about an hour every day. Mom noted that they frequently played a board game after dinner to accomplish this. They feel they can keep trying to reduce television time and note that as the weather gets nicer, it will be easier because OG likes being outside.

- *Problem #5: Constant hunger.* Mom wants to work on OG's complaints of constant hunger; she notes that it is very hard distracting him but has tried it a few times.
  - *Strategy*
    Mom says she thinks OG sometimes eats because he is bored. You and Mom talk about enrolling him in an after-school activity 1 to 2 days a week and she thinks this is a good idea, possibly a karate class or swimming at the Y. You reinforce her attempts to distract him, rewarding him with a sticker if he can transition to another activity. You also give her a list of healthy snacks to use if she can't distract him (Table 6.2).

You schedule OG for a return appointment in 1 month to check his progress and the results of the sleep study.

Table 6.2. Examples of Healthy Snacks

– Fruit	– Bran muffins	– Sugar-free cereals
– Low-fat/frozen yogurt	– Fresh strawberries	– Unsalted pretzels
– Celery stalks	– Air-popped popcorn	– Dried raisins or apricots
– Low-fat oatmeal cookies	– Low-fat cheeses	
– Cucumber slices	– Frozen juice bars	
– Frozen bananas	(without added sugar)	
– Baked potato chips	– Crackers	

Adapted from American Academy of Pediatrics. *A Parent's Guide to Childhood Obesity: A Road Map to Health.* Hassink SG, ed. Elk Grove Village, IL: American Academy of Pediatrics; 2006:39

Third Visit

This time Grandmother brings him in because of Mom and Dad's work schedule. You note that you received the results of his sleep study; he is having some apneic episodes and you recommend that he see the pediatric otolaryngologist to inquire about a tonsillectomy.

His weight on this visit is 62 lb (28.1 kg) and height is 49" (124.5 cm). His BMI is 18.2, just at 95% (down 1.6% since his first visit). You show Grandmother the plot and praise the efforts the family has been making.

- *Problem #3: Excess consumption of sweetened beverages.* The family is now used to drinking water or diet drinks between meals and has adjusted very well to this. Grandmother notes that parties and extended family get-togethers are still a problem, and you suggest they may want to offer to bring along a diet drink.

- *Problem #4: Too much screen time.* Grandmother notes that he is watching about 2 hours of television a day and going outside more, and the family is getting better at helping him think of other things to do instead of watching television. For example, they bought a basketball hoop for outside.

- *Problem #5: Constant hunger.* OG seems less hungry; he is enjoying his karate class and spends some time at home practicing his moves. They have substituted the low-calorie snacks for the chips and ice cream he used to have and he doesn't seem to mind.

You reschedule him for a 2-month visit.

References

1. Whitaker RC, Wright JA, Pepe MS, Seidel KD, Dietz WH. Predicting obesity in young adulthood from childhood and parental obesity. *N Engl J Med.* 1997;337:869–873

2. Rolland-Cachera MF, Deheeger M, Bellisle F, Sempe M, Guillound-Bataille M, Patois E. Adiposity rebound in children: a simple indicator for predicting obesity. *Am J Clin Nutr.* 1984;39:129–135

3. Whitaker RC, Pepe MS, Wright JA, Seidel KD, Dietz WH. Early adiposity rebound and the risk of adult obesity. *Pediatrics.* 1998;101:e5

4. Welsh JA, Cogswell ME, Rogers S, Rockett H, Mei Z, Grummer-Strawn LM. Overweight among low-income preschool children associated with the consumption of soft drinks: Missouri, 1999-2002. *Pediatrics.* 2005;115:e223–e229

5. Klesges RC, Klesges LM, Eck LH, Shelton ML. A longitudinal analysis of accelerated weight gain in preschool children. *Pediatrics.* 1995;95:126–130

6. Orlet Fisher J, Rolls BJ, Birch LL. Children's bite size and intake of an entrée are greater with large portions than with age-appropriate or self-selected portions. *Am J Clin Nutr.* 2003;77:1164–1170

7. Moore LL, Lombardi DA, White MJ, Campbell JL, Oliveria SA, Ellison RC. Influence of parents' physical activity levels on activity levels of young children. *J Pediatr.* 1991;118:215–219

8. Burdette HL, Whitaker RC, Daniels SR. Parental report of outdoor playtime as a measure of physical activity in preschool-aged children. *Arch Pediatr Adolesc Med.* 2004;158:353–357

9. Burdette HL, Whitaker RC. Resurrecting free play in young children: looking beyond fitness and fatness to attention, affiliation, and affect. *Arch Pediatr Adolesc Med.* 2005;159:46–50

10. Dennison BA, Erb TA, Jenkins PL. Television viewing and television in bedroom associated with overweight risk among low-income preschool children. *Pediatrics.* 2002;109:1028–1035

11. Agras WS, Hammer LD, McNicholas F, Kraemer HC. Risk factors for childhood overweight: a prospective study from birth to 9.5 years. *J Pediatr.* 2004;145:20–25

Chapter 7

School Age

....

7.1 Background

Over the past 3 decades the percentage of 6- to 11-year-olds with weight greater than 95% for age has more than tripled, from 6% to 18.8%.[1,2] Eleven percent of children entering kindergarten are already overweight.[3] A study of predictors of overweight in children found that 20% of obese boys younger than 8 years became obese adults.[4]

Elementary school enrollment characterizes this age group and factors in the school environment add to family and environmental factors in promoting obesity. Families need skills and information to assess and structure their children's nutrition and activity as time demands shift on school entry.

Physical activity tends to decrease with age. In one meta-analysis, 6- to 7-year-olds engaged in 46 minutes per day of moderate to vigorous activity, compared with 10- to 16-year-olds who had only 16 to 45 minutes per day. Mean activity levels decreased with age by 2.7% per year in boys and 7.4% per year in girls.[5]

Physical education (PE) time is not uniform across schools. In a national study of 1,000 schools, approximately 65% of first graders had PE 1 to 2 times a week, 16.2% had PE 2 to 3 times a week, and only 12.5% had daily PE.[6]

Time that had previously been spent on physical activity is often taken up with academic subjects in school and homework after school. Parents are increasingly challenged to create activity opportunities for their children at home, find opportunities in the community, and encourage schools to increase PE and recess. It is important to remember that incremental increases or decreases in regular activity can have a major effect over time. It has been predicted that adding 30 minutes a week to PE time could decrease the prevalence of obesity among girls by 5% and the prevalence of overweight among girls by 10%.[7]

Schools can also be the site of exposure to increased amounts of sweetened beverages and snack foods. These beverages can add to total energy consumption and enhance weight gain.[8] A 12-oz sugar-sweetened drink consumed daily has been associated with an 0.18% increase in a child's body mass index (BMI).[9] In 2000 the Centers for Disease Control and Prevention found that 50% of all school districts have a soft drink contract. Of these schools, almost 80% received a percentage of sales and almost two thirds were given a financial incentive for meeting target sales. In addition, one third of schools allowed soft drink advertising in their buildings.[10] Juice consumption of more than 12 oz per day has also been linked to overweight.[11] The American Academy of Pediatrics recommends that children 7 to 18 years of age should limit their juice consumption to 8 to 12 oz per day, while children 6 years and younger should limit juice to 4 to 6 oz per day.[12]

Pediatricians are encouraged to work to eliminate sweetened drinks in schools. This involves educating parents, families, and patients as well as school authorities about the health effects of soft drink consumption.[13]

Parents may be unaware of exactly what kind of food their children are purchasing at school. In addition to sweetened beverages, many children are exposed to snack food offered in vending machines, school stores, and the cafeteria. These items are available and often purchased with a food credit card funded by monthly allotments from parents.

Many children are also eating breakfast and lunch at school. School breakfast and lunch choices may be limited in elementary school to one high-calorie offering. Mid-morning snacks are often encouraged and after-school programs usually provide a snack. This means that the bulk of the child's caloric intake may occur outside the home without parents being aware of the quality or quantity of the food consumed. Parents need to be knowledgeable about what is being offered at each meal so they can adjust eating patterns at home if needed. In a study of 8- to 10-year-old African American girls, greater low-fat food preparation at home was related to lower consumption of total fat.[14] Children may occasionally eat breakfast at home or child care and again at school, or add on to a packed lunch from home with lunch or snacks at school.

Parents need to assess their child's level of daily physical activity. Most PE occurs only 1 to 2 times a week and children may not be active for the entire class. Recess may or may not be outside and after-school programs or child care may not offer extended periods of free play.

After-school time can be problematic for many overweight children. This is a time where hunger and access to food at home combined with unstructured time and boredom can give rise to excess caloric intake. Parents often view after-school time, once homework is complete, as time for their child to wind down. While true, this may take the form of television or computer use that can take up all of the child's free time. In a study of 5- to 9-year-old girls, those who watched more television consumed more snacks in front of the television and those from families in which one or both parents were overweight had more frequent higher fat snacks.[15] Parents need to be encouraged to structure after-school and evening time to include a regular mealtime, screen time limited to less than 2 hours a day, homework time, and time for free play. Parents and families may feel that structure precludes free or playtime, but the message these days is clear that unless parents create an opportunity for activity, screen time tends to take over.

Planning skills for parents have become increasingly important as they help their child juggle the increased time demands of school. Planning ahead for school events, visits to friends, and parties at which children will be exposed to different nutritional environments become important for the overweight children.

Elementary school entry provides an opportunity to discuss with parents their role in planning, assessing, and structuring their child's activity and nutritional environment.

7.2 Prevention: Talking to Parents (BALANCE)

Prevention touch points for parents include **belief, assessment, lifestyle, activity, nutrition, child,** and **environment** (BALANCE).

Belief

- Parents may believe that a child's weight will take care of itself as the child grows. While this may be true in an environment of optimal activity and nutrition, it is clear that parents and families will have to participate in the effort to achieve energy balance and optimal weight.
- Parents may also assume, without checking, that school, after-school care, and extracurricular activities are providing healthy snacks and time for activity.

- It may help to alert parents to the fact that their role in helping to oversee their child's nutrition and activity environment outside of the home is part of helping their child achieve optimal energy balance.

Assessment

- It is important to help keep parents focused on assessing their child's dietary and exercise habits while health professionals are attending to ongoing changes in energy balance and BMI.
- As the child begins school, assessing the school's nutrition and activity environment and advocating for needed change are important skills for parents.
- Helping parents and families monitor shifts in the nutrition and activity environment over time is also important. Weekends, vacations, summers, and seasonal changes in activity may require different decisions to balance nutrition and activity and do not necessarily happen automatically.

Lifestyle

- These are very important years for helping a child adopt healthy eating and activity habits that last a lifetime.
- Parents should continue to focus on a wholesome lifestyle for everyone in the family.
  - Develop a structured family meal and snack schedule (3 well-thought-out meals and 2 snacks a day).
  - Minimize junk food consumption.
  - Eliminate sugared beverages like soft drinks.
  - Pay attention to portion sizes.
  - Add some physical activity to the mix.
- A reasonable approach for parents at this age is to frame the changes in eating and nutrition in terms of "health decisions" for the family.

Activity

- Free play is still important at this age.
- Parents will need to start striking a balance between unstructured outdoor time and entry-level sports such as baseball and soccer.
- Children still have short attention spans and are improving their reaction times and directionality. Fundamental skill development is the main task with minimal competitions and flexible rules.

- Organized and spontaneous activity should focus on fun and participation.
- Television and computer use may start to increase and parents need to keep in mind that no more than 2 hours of screen time daily is recommended. Limiting television and computer time is usually best accomplished by
  - Not having a television or computer in a child's bedroom
  - Not watching television during meals
  - Having the whole family limit television use
  - Not being outnumbered by the number of televisions in the house
  - Helping the child and other family members find other indoor activity options

Nutrition

- Nutritional choices begin at the grocery store. Parents who buy a few pieces of fruit and a selection of high-fat or high-sugar snacks have inadvertently set their families up for difficult choices. Providing larger amounts of fruits and vegetables than had previously been the case and avoiding purchases of other snack foods paves the way for easier choices for all family members.
- Family meals are important and can be planned around selections like
  - Fresh fruits and vegetables
  - Whole-grain cereals and breads
  - Low-fat or nonfat dairy products like milk, yogurt, and cheeses
  - Lean and skinless meats including chicken, turkey, fish, and lean hamburger
- Portion sizes at this age should be less than that of an adult-sized serving.
- If the school cafeteria doesn't offer many healthy choices, parents can pack a healthy lunch each day. Some ideas include
  - Prepare a turkey sandwich on multigrain or pita bread (a peanut butter and jelly sandwich is fine, too).
  - Add a piece of fruit or perhaps a bag of pretzels.
  - Pack a small water bottle or encourage the child to buy low-fat milk in the cafeteria.
  - Avoid pastrami, salami, and other high-fat lunch meats.
- Parents may also need to pack a healthy snack for after-school care or activities if one is not offered.

Child

- Although children at this age are becoming increasingly independent, they still need structure and support of nutrition and activity by the family.
- After-school time can be problematic for children and parents.
  - Children tend to come home hungry, ready for a snack and downtime, and are not in a position to make good nutritional choices.
  - Parents can help by preparing a snack to have ready for the child.
  - Children may not automatically ask to go outside after school. Parents may need to plan this time into the after-school schedule, reserving television and computer time for later in the evening.

Environment

- Managing the child's nutrition and activity environment takes on an expanded dimension at this age with home, school, after-school care, and activities all having their own balance of activity, inactivity, and eating.
- Parents may need to have an active role in promoting change. For example, parents can advocate for more PE in school, promote healthier snacking in after-school care, and ask if teachers can use healthier snacks for class rewards and parties.
- Extended family members may need to be reminded about healthy after-school snacks, encouraging activity, and helping to limit television and computer time.

7.3 Intervention

When a school-aged child has a BMI greater than 85% and less than 95% or is crossing growth percentiles in an upward direction, this is the time for a more in-depth look at eating and activity, family health history, and parental obesity—all of which can contribute to the risk of becoming an obese older child and young adult. In addition to reemphasizing concepts covered previously, parents and families may need to give increased attention to their ability to provide and influence nutrition and activity by focusing on **energy balance, structure,** and **modeling healthy behavior.**

Energy Balance

As children move out into the environment the challenges to staying in optimal energy balance increase. When a child starts to cross percentiles or is in the at-risk range of BMI between 85% and 95%, an examination of the daily nutrition and activity routine is in order. In an otherwise reasonable diet, an increase in snacks and portion sizes are ways energy balance can shift, often without parents noticing. Once recognized, parents could initiate changes by preparing healthy snacks for their child and eliminating the child walking in the front door after school right to the refrigerator or cabinets. Parents can also continue to serve meals restaurant style (portioning out food onto plates) instead of family style (everyone helping themselves from the food on the table).

Structure

Planning and time management become increasingly important, particularly when the actual time the family has to manage homework, dinner, bedtime routines, and free time shrinks because of school and work. A reasonable look at the flow of after-school time is in order and often parents can restructure this to include a snack, outdoor time, dinner, homework, and free time, in that order. When a child is in after-school care, time for activity may be squeezed out and parents have to be creative in finding indoor activities and limiting television and computer time. Weekends can also be a challenge because unless parents plan the time, children may go to the television or computer as the activity that is most available.

Modeling Healthy Behavior

Children at this age are quick to detect and point out discrepancies in what a parent is asking them to do and what the parent is actually doing for them. They are also sensitive to what other children are doing and fairness issues in relation to siblings and friends. This may cycle into resistance to change and cause parents to give in to demands for snacking and television time more than they realize. This is a good time to establish positive lifestyle changes as a household with boundaries set by parents and input from the child on how to limit television watching, get the family more active, and eliminate junk food. Parents, however, need to stay in the role of setting overall boundaries for healthy eating and activity.

7.4 Treatment

When a child's BMI is greater than 95% and you are dealing with excess adiposity, it is time to initiate a focused treatment strategy. It is important to review the issues discussed in the previous 2 sections because these are building blocks of good nutrition and activity habits. But you will also have to focus on the barriers to change that may have prevented parents and families from implementing these strategies.

A useful way to begin is to obtain a family history focused on obesity-related comorbidities. This can serve to emphasize the health risks involved and the necessity of taking early action once obesity is identified.

7.5 Family History

The family history (page 101) provides information on obesity and obesity-related comorbidity risk as well as serves as a starting point to discuss the child's BMI.

If parents are obese or have a history of obesity, they may want to relate their personal struggles with their weight. Often the desire to avoid these same struggles in their child motivates parents to make family changes in nutrition and activity.

7.6 Review of Systems

The review of systems can also serve as a point of departure to discuss obesity-related comorbidities, pointing out particular risk factors as they relate to increasing BMI.

- Skin: Acanthosis nigricans, striae, cervical fat pad, skin picking
- Head, eyes, ears, nose, and throat (HEENT): Headache, blurred vision
- Lungs: Snoring, sleep disturbance, sleep apnea, restless sleep, sleep position, daytime tiredness, napping, asthma, shortness of breath or subjective chest tightness on exercise, cough after exercise
- Cardiac: Murmur
- Abdomen: Gastroesophageal reflux, stomach pain, nausea or vomiting after eating
- Musculoskeletal: Limping, hip pain, knee pain
- Development: School problems, learning difficulties, attention problems
- Psychosocial: Depression, anxiety, behavior problems

Family History, School Age

Complete or update this family history targeted toward obesity and related comorbidities.

	Mother	Father	Maternal Grandmother	Maternal Grandfather	Paternal Grandmother	Paternal Grandfather	Sibling 1	Sibling 2
Obesity	☐	☐	☐	☐	☐	☐	☐	☐
Cardiovascular disease	☐	☐	☐	☐	☐	☐	☐	☐
High blood pressure	☐	☐	☐	☐	☐	☐	☐	☐
Stroke	☐	☐	☐	☐	☐	☐	☐	☐
High cholesterol	☐	☐	☐	☐	☐	☐	☐	☐
High triglyceride	☐	☐	☐	☐	☐	☐	☐	☐
Type 1 or 2 diabetes	☐	☐	☐	☐	☐	☐	☐	☐
_____	☐	☐	☐	☐	☐	☐	☐	☐
_____	☐	☐	☐	☐	☐	☐	☐	☐
_____	☐	☐	☐	☐	☐	☐	☐	☐
_____	☐	☐	☐	☐	☐	☐	☐	☐
_____	☐	☐	☐	☐	☐	☐	☐	☐
_____	☐	☐	☐	☐	☐	☐	☐	☐

7.7 Physical Examination

- Height
- Weight
- BMI + previous BMI measurements
- Blood pressure
- General: Dysmorphic features, poor linear growth, developmental delay
- Skin: Skin picking, acanthosis nigricans, dermatitis in skinfolds, striae, cervical fat pad, evidence of skin picking
- HEENT: Funduscopic examination for papilledema, tonsillar hypertrophy
- Cardiopulmonary: Murmur, wheezing
- Abdominal: Hepatomegaly
- Musculoskeletal: Range of motion, genu varum, limp, hip or knee pain
- Genitourinary: Tanner stage

7.8 Family Constellation and Social History

Information about the family can provide a starting point to discuss how nutrition and activity decisions are made and how changes might take place.

- Who is living at home with the child?
- Who is with the child before school?
- Who is with the child after school?
- Who else besides parents is responsible for the child's meals or snacks?

7.9 Parenting Questions

Parenting styles and skills are important when families are trying to make changes in lifestyle. These questions may help you focus on family factors that may facilitate or hinder change.

	Never	Seldom	Sometimes	Often	Always
1. Parents set clear and simple expectations and limits.	☐	☐	☐	☐	☐
2. Parents set boundaries and give the child choice within them.	☐	☐	☐	☐	☐
3. Parents have developmentally appropriate goals for the child.	☐	☐	☐	☐	☐
4. Parents model healthy nutrition, activity, and inactivity behavior.	☐	☐	☐	☐	☐
5. Parents limit the availability of high-sugar or high-fat snacks in the home.	☐	☐	☐	☐	☐
6. Parents maintain an abundant supply of fruits and vegetables in the home.	☐	☐	☐	☐	☐

7.10 Parenting Touch Points

Parenting touch points focus on helping families initiate and maintain change by helping them believe change can occur, identify the change needed, value the outcome of the change, know how to change, and have the energy to change and sustain the change.

- *Believe that change can occur.* Parents may feel that the pressure of school, homework, and activity, as well as parents' jobs and responsibilities, do not allow for any changes. The idea of incremental changes being effective and important is crucial to allowing families to attempt to change behavior. Helping parents pick a doable, feasible, and measur-able change to tackle, such as packing a lunch, taking a daily walk, or enrolling the child in an activity, will help encourage parents that change is possible.

- *Identify the change.* After-school time is a major area of focus when it comes to looking at ways to improve nutrition and activity. Helping parents identify alternatives to the television, computer, and snacking will be useful. Some options might be
    - Create a time schedule for after-school time, allowing for snack, outdoor, dinner, homework, and television or computer time.
    - Sign the child up for an after-school program or activity.

– Extracurricular activities should be chosen to emphasize participation and skill building.
– Children who are reluctant to participate may benefit by picking an activity such as karate or dance rather than a team sport at first.
– Activities that require involvement with peers and participation such as scouts, church groups, or school clubs can be very important in structuring time, relieving boredom, decreasing screen time, and enhancing social skills.
– For a reluctant child, parents can provide 2 or 3 activity options and have the child choose among these rather than requiring a "yes" or "no" to a specific activity.

● *Value the outcome.* Screening for obesity-related comorbidities is always important and becomes increasingly more so as children get older. Health outcomes of obesity in childhood and the future can be powerful motivators for families. The family history and laboratory and physical assessments of the child can be focused on obesity-related outcomes. For many families the link between health, weight, and behavior will be enough to help them begin to initiate change. Psychosocial issues such as teasing and lowered self-esteem may also motivate families to change.

When a family seems unable to initiate change, it may be useful to explore barriers to change with them such as
– Parents may have had a history of failed attempts to change their own weight and feel discouraged.
– Other family issues may be overwhelming and prevent the family from focusing their energy on making change.
– Parents may feel that it is up to the child to make change.
– External factors such as an unsafe community, other caregivers, or lack of money may be operative.
– Families that have been able to change lifestyle but have had little improvement in BMI may become discouraged. It is important to point out that healthier diet and physical activity habits are predictors of longer lives, independent of weight or BMI.

● *Know how to change.* It is important for the family to work together to make change. It's equally important for parents to be on the same page for the changes they want to make. Extended families and parents who are separated or divorced face special challenges that make communication even more important. Talking over family goals and ways to implement them are an integral part of moving forward. For example, asking a child, "How many hours of TV or computer time do you need?" will be enlightening and can start the discussion of how to decrease television time. Another question worth asking the child is, "What can you do when you're not watching TV?" Frequently it is evident that the child doesn't have any alternate plans in mind and the family can then help design some activities to fill the time.

- *Have energy to change and sustain.* As families get busier and busier, it is important for parents to take time to be with their child—take time for just hanging out together. These special times can energize the parent-child relationship and fuel the changes in nutrition and activity the family is trying to make. Parents and extended family members, if appropriate, need to communicate frequently about how things are going and support each other in their efforts to sustain the desired changes.

7.11 Developmental Touch Point

School-aged children are balanced between tuning into their parents and peer group. Structure and negotiation are effective tools in modifying behaviors. This may be a good time to have families initiate family meetings to establish house rules, vent feelings and thoughts, and make positive lifestyle changes. Input from the children gives them a sense of control and engages them in following through on changes discussed. Topics can include how to limit television watching, getting the family more active, and eliminating junk food from the house.

7.12 Nutrition and Activity Questions and Interventions

Nutrition and activity questions (see pages 106–107) can be answered by the parents and provide a focal point for targeted intervention (see pages 108–109) in a brief encounter. Questions answered "Often" or "Always" can be targeted first for change. For example, if the parent answered questions 1, 7, 9, and 13 on pages 106 and 107 with "Often" or "Always," you would ask them to rate the difficulty of change for questions 1, 7, 9, and 13 on pages 108 and 109.

Nutrition and Activity Questions, School Age

These questions can be answered by the parents and provide a focal point for targeted intervention in a brief encounter. First have the parents answer these questions about the presence or absence of behaviors that promote weight gain, then refer to Nutrition and Activity Interventions, School Age.

	Never	Seldom	Sometimes	Often	Always
1. Drinks juice or sugared beverages between meals.	☐	☐	☐	☐	☐
2. Eats junk food.	☐	☐	☐	☐	☐
3. Eats more than 1 snack between meals each day.	☐	☐	☐	☐	☐
4. Requests second helpings.	☐	☐	☐	☐	☐
5. Is a fast eater.	☐	☐	☐	☐	☐
6. Eats at fast-food restaurants.	☐	☐	☐	☐	☐
7. Gets own snacks.	☐	☐	☐	☐	☐
8. Sneaks or hides food.	☐	☐	☐	☐	☐
9. Demands certain food or snacks.	☐	☐	☐	☐	☐
10. Refuses to eat fruits or vegetables.	☐	☐	☐	☐	☐

	Never	Seldom	Sometimes	Often	Always
11. Refuses to eat dairy products.	☐	☐	☐	☐	☐
12. Eats in front of the television.	☐	☐	☐	☐	☐
13. Skips meals.	☐	☐	☐	☐	☐
14. Eats alone.	☐	☐	☐	☐	☐
15. Eats when bored.	☐	☐	☐	☐	☐
16. Watches more than 2 hours of television or the computer each day.	☐	☐	☐	☐	☐
17. Stays indoors after school.	☐	☐	☐	☐	☐
18. Prefers quiet activities.	☐	☐	☐	☐	☐
19. Seems unmotivated to get active.	☐	☐	☐	☐	☐
20. Lacks interest in peer activities.	☐	☐	☐	☐	☐

Nutrition and Activity Interventions, School Age

Questions answered "Often" or "Always" in Nutrition and Activity Questions, School Age, can be targeted first for change. Using these specific questions, ask the parent, "How difficult would it be for you to…?"

	Impossible	Could try	Could do sometimes	Could do most of the time	Easy
1. Change from juice to water between meals.	☐	☐	☐	☐	☐
2. Eliminate junk food.	☐	☐	☐	☐	☐
3. Eliminate extra snacks.	☐	☐	☐	☐	☐
4. Offer vegetables instead of second helpings.	☐	☐	☐	☐	☐
5. Work on a plan to slow down eating.	☐	☐	☐	☐	☐
6. Decrease fast food.	☐	☐	☐	☐	☐
7. Pack healthier school snacks.	☐	☐	☐	☐	☐
8. Work with your child on a plan to stop sneaking.	☐	☐	☐	☐	☐
9. Keep only healthy snacks in the house.	☐	☐	☐	☐	☐
10. Offer fruit and vegetables at meals.	☐	☐	☐	☐	☐

	Impossible	Could try	Could do sometimes	Could do most of the time	Easy
11. Offer dairy products at meals.	☐	☐	☐	☐	☐
12. Turn off the television during meals and snacks.	☐	☐	☐	☐	☐
13. Schedule regular meals and snacks.	☐	☐	☐	☐	☐
14. Eat meals together.	☐	☐	☐	☐	☐
15. Help your child find activities to do instead of munching.	☐	☐	☐	☐	☐
16. Reduce television time.	☐	☐	☐	☐	☐
17. Schedule time for your child to go outside after school.	☐	☐	☐	☐	☐
18. Come up with some suggestions that involve physical activities for your child.	☐	☐	☐	☐	☐
19. Partner with your child in a physical activity.	☐	☐		☐	☐
20. Make a peer group activity part of after-school time.	☐	☐		☐	☐

7.13 A Case in Point: SB

SB is a 6-year, 10-month-old boy who has been followed in your practice for several years. On his recent checkup you ordered a lipid panel because of a family history of hyperlipidemia. SB's cholesterol was elevated at 200 mg/dL and his low-density lipoprotein (LDL) cholesterol was 143 mg/dL. You note that his weight gain has been steadily accelerating and his parents are concerned because of his preoccupation with food.

They note that he tends to argue with them a lot, especially about food, and they are worried about his self-esteem. They answer "Always" to questions 3 (Eats more than 1 snack between meals each day), 4 (Requests second helpings), and 5 (Is a fast eater). They also answer "Often" to question 19 (Seems unmotivated to get active). The family has already made numerous dietary changes and answer "Never" to questions 1 (Drinks juice or sugared beverages between meals), 2 (Eats junk food), and 7 (Eats at fast-food restaurants), having eliminated juice, junk food, and fast food from their diet.

SB is in good health with no problems except for an occasional ear infection and complaints of stomach pain after eating on the review of systems. He is in first grade and doing well.

Family history is positive for high cholesterol (in 3 of 4 grandparents) and negative for diabetes, hypertension, and obesity.

The results of the physical examination are that his height is 50" (125.9 cm) and weight is 91 lb (41.4 kg), with a BMI of 26.2 (>97% for age and gender). Blood pressure is 111/67 mm Hg with systolic and diastolic pressure at 90%. Physical examination is essentially normal with no positive findings.

All laboratory values are normal with the exception of the total and LDL cholesterol.

Problem #1: Snacking

Based on the answers to your questionnaire and the family's responses, you ask the family how they view his snacking. They say they know he is eating too many snacks between meals and would like to change this but have found it difficult to do in the past.

- *Parenting dilemma: Fairness*
  The parents want to be fair and avoid SB's angry outbursts if they limit snacks. They are concerned because his 13-year-old (thin) brother "needs" snacks and SB always wants whatever he sees his brother eating. SB becomes upset if he can't eat too.

- *Strategy: Family-based change*
  You take care of their older son and note that he is growing along his weight and height curves and is not underweight. You ask about his eating and parents note that he is picky eater, often eating very little at meals and then asking for snacks.

  You note that fairness is not necessarily equality. Meeting each child's needs is the goal and each child's nutritional and activity needs may vary.

  You also note that grazing or frequent snacking is not a recommended eating behavior at any weight because snacks tend to be less nutritious than food offered at a well-balanced family meal and that eating 3 meals and 1 snack is a goal for the whole family.

  The parents feel somewhat encouraged and are ready to try to structure eating times to 3 meals and 1 snack per day for everyone.

Problem #2: Rapid Eating

The parents note that SB eats rapidly, gets done eating before anyone else, and always asks for seconds.

- *Parenting dilemma: Need for a new approach*
  Parents have tried telling SB to slow down but that hasn't worked. They tell you that they are not sure what to do next.

- *Strategy: Splitting portions*
  You ask them to offer salad or vegetables as an appetizer for the meal with a small glass of water. You then ask them to portion out his dinner on a plate, divide the portion, and place half on another plate. They will give the first plate with a half portion and offer the second plate. If SB is still hungry he can have extra salad or vegetables.

Problem #3: Unmotivated to Get Active

The parents are very aware that SB needs to increase his activity; in fact, they are active themselves.

- *Parenting dilemma: Dealing with resistance*
  When they ask him if he wants to join a sport he always says "no," and when they try to get him outside he resists and they get worn out.

- *Strategy: Partnering*
  One-to-one time with parents can be an important motivator for children. SB's father offers to walk with him after dinner. He says they could take a ball along and toss it, and this would be their special time together. Hearing this, SB brightens and says he thinks this would be OK.

Problem #4: Hypercholesterolemia

To address his hypercholesterolemia you ask the parents to keep detailed diet records for a few days for review during SB's next visit.

Second Visit

For his second visit 1 month later, his weight decreased by 4 lb (1.9 kg).

- *Problem #1: Snacking.* SB's parents feel that the diet records they were asked to keep actually helped them to keep on track with the scheduled snacking. After a few weeks SB and his brother seemed to adjust to the new routine and the parents feel things are going OK except for a few complaints.

- *Problem #2: Rapid eating.* The parents think the technique of splitting portions has worked; SB now seems to feel full after the meal.

- *Problem #3: Unmotivated to get active.* SB has been walking every day, rain or shine, and he and his father are now up to 25 minutes a day. They take a football with them and toss it during their walk and SB seems to enjoy this.

- *Problem #4: Hypercholesterolemia.* You review his diet and ask the family to pack a lunch to lower total fat. His review of systems and physical examination are normal.

- *New Problem #5: Eating at parties.* The parents have questions about parties and you ask them to talk to SB before parties and ask him to take only one helping of food, praising him for making good decisions.

Third Visit

Six weeks later, his weight is down 4 lb (1.7 kg) from the previous visit. The family is now taking walks together. They say it is harder to get him outside when the weather is not so good, but they are persevering. They are concerned that he will not eat the carrots or other vegetables they pack in his lunch.

His repeated cholesterol is now 159 mg/dL; you reinforce the positive changes the family has made.

Fourth Visit

SB returns with a weight loss of 5 lb (2.2 kg) over the 11 weeks since his last visit. His BMI has been reduced from 26.2 to 22.2, which places his BMI just at 97%. He is eating a well-balanced diet and is walking daily. His family notes he has been increasingly more active and that his endurance is increasing.

His review of systems and physical examination continue to be normal. The family has now established a solid family-based approach to eating and activity. SB is more positive about himself and is willing to try new activities. You ask the family to return in 6 months and to feel free to check in with you if they have any difficulties.

References

1. Ogden CL, Flegal KM, Carroll MD, Johnson CL. Prevalence and trends in overweight among US children and adolescents, 1999-2000. *JAMA*. 2002;288: 1728-1732

2. Ogden CL, Carroll MD, Curtin LR, McDowell MA, Tabak CJ, Flegal KM. Prevalence of overweight and obesity in the United States, 1999-2004. *JAMA*. 2006;295:1549–1555

3. Datar A, Sturm R, Magnabosco JL. Childhood overweight and academic performance: national study of kindergartners and first-graders. *Obes Res*. 2004;12:58–68

4. Guo SS, Wu W, Chumlea WC, Roche AF. Predicting overweight and obesity in adulthood from body mass index values in childhood and adolescence. *Am J Clin Nutr*. 2002;76:653–658

5. Sallis JF. Epidemiology of physical activity and fitness in children and adolescents. *Crit Rev Food Sci Nutr*. 1993;33:403–408

6. Datar A, Sturm R. Physical education in elementary schools and body mass index: evidence from the early childhood longitudinal study. *Am J Public Health*. 2004;94:1501–1506

7. National Institute for Health Care Management. Obesity in young children: impact and intervention. Research brief. August 2004. Available at: www.nihcm.org/OYCbrief.pdf. Accessed May 25, 2006

8. Berkey CS, Rockett HR, Field AE, Gillman MW, Colditz GA. Sugar-added beverages and adolescent weight change. *Obes Res*. 2004;12:778–788

9. Ludwig DS, Peterson KE, Gortmaker SL. Relation between consumption of sugar-sweetened drinks and childhood obesity: a prospective, observational analysis. *Lancet*. 2001;357:505–508

10. Wechsler H, Brener ND, Kuester S, Miller C. Food service and foods and beverages available at school: results from the School Health Policies and Programs Study 2000. *J Sch Health*. 2001;71:313–324

11. Dennison BA, Rockwell HL, Baker SL. Excess fruit juice consumption by preschool-aged children is associated with short stature and obesity. *Pediatrics*. 1997;99:15–22

12. American Academy of Pediatrics Committee on Nutrition. The use and misuse of fruit juice in pediatrics. *Pediatrics*. 2001;107:1210–1213

13. American Academy of Pediatrics Committee on School Health. Soft drinks in schools. *Pediatrics*. 2004;113:152–154

14. Cullen KW, Baranowski T, Klesges LM, et al. Anthropometric, parental, and psychosocial correlates of dietary intake of African-American girls. *Obes Res*. 2004;12:20S–31S

15. Francis LA, Lee Y, Birsch LL. Parental weight status and girls' television viewing, snacking, and body mass indexes. *Obes Res*. 2003;11:143–151

Chapter 8

Early Adolescent

··

8.1 Background

Body size, shape, and composition change dramatically during puberty. Adolescent females increase deposition of body fat; regional deposition of adipose tissue changes in boys and girls; and concerns about body image may heighten. At the hormonal level, gonadotropins, leptin, sex steroids, and growth hormone interact to produce and complete the pubertal transition.[1]

The increase in insulin resistance that occurs with the onset of puberty may accentuate the risk for obesity and obesity-related comorbidities. This increase is born out in a study of an urban population of African American and non-Hispanic urban children in which it was found that carbohydrate intolerance or near-diabetes was more likely to develop in pubertal than post-pubertal children.[2] Pubertal transition from Tanner stage 1 to Tanner stage 3 has been associated with a 32% reduction in insulin sensitivity and increases in fasting glucose, insulin, and insulin resistance. These changes were similar across gender, ethnicity, and obesity and were not associated with changes in body fat, visceral fat, insulin-like growth factor,[1] androgens, or estradiol.[3]

Timing of menarche can also affect factors such as insulin, glucose, blood pressure, fat-free mass, and peripheral body fat levels. Girls with early menarche were found to have higher glucose, insulin, and blood pressure measurements than girls who had average or late onset of menses. These changes were independent of age and changes in fat-free mass or peripheral body fat.[4] Early maturity differs in effect between boys and girls. In one study, body mass index (BMI) and skinfold thickness were associated with early sexual maturity stages in boys and girls, but early maturing boys were leaner than their counterparts while early maturing girls had increased adiposity when compared with girls maturing at average ages or later.[5]

Physical activity in children is important for the maintenance of metabolic control. In a study of 589 Danish children with an average age of 9.7 years, a strong relationship was found between insulin resistance and physical activity.[6] In boys and girls there has been found to be an inverse relationship between physical activity and increasing age.[7] Decreases in physical education classes and participation in extracurricular activities may play a role. Only 6.4% of middle schools have daily physical education, and 62% of children aged 9 to 13 years do not spend any time outside of school hours in organized physical activities such as sports.[8] A study of children examining the link between childhood obesity, activity, and screen time found that heavier children spend more time in sedentary activities than those with lower BMI.[9] Physical activity behaviors track from early to middle childhood[10] and from adolescence to adulthood.[11]

Insulin resistance is more common in obese children and is important in the etiology of cardiovascular disease and development of metabolic syndrome.[12] Risk factors for metabolic syndrome include[13,14]

1. Abdominal obesity
2. Elevated triglyceride levels (>150 mg/dL)
3. Low high-density lipoprotein (HDL) cholesterol levels (<40 mg/dL)
4. Increased low-density lipoprotein cholesterol (>130 mg/dL)
5. Increased blood pressure (systolic or diastolic blood pressure >90%)
6. Impaired fasting glucose[15] (fasting glucose >100 mg/dL, random glucose >200 mg/dL)

The diagnosis of metabolic syndrome is made when 3 of the 6 criteria are met.

Other components of metabolic syndrome include a pro-thrombotic and proinflammatory state and hyperuricemia.[13] Indicators of metabolic syndrome have been demonstrated to be stable from childhood and adolescence to young adulthood.[16]

Hyperinsulinemia and insulin resistance are already present in prepubertal obese children. Because hyperinsulinemia is a potentially reversible condition and the complications related to it may be prevented, early assessment should be undertaken so that obese children lose body weight before the onset of puberty, which may enhance the problem of insulin insensitivity.[3]

8.2 Prevention: Talking to Parents and Teens (BALANCE)

Prevention touch points for parents and teens include **belief, assessment, lifestyle, activity, nutrition, child/young adolescent,** and **environment** (BALANCE).

Belief

- Parents may see the middle school child as being able to negotiate food and activity choices independently. While it is true that the child will push to have choices, decision support is still needed and desired by the child.
- As the peer group becomes more of an influence on the middle school child, the drive to fit in may become more important in determining nutrition and activity choices.
- Food choices, packing a lunch, and family activities that were taken for granted by the younger child may become areas of conflict.
- Early adolescents may feel that it's not fair that they have to follow a nutrition and activity plan while their friends do not.
- This is a time when parents need to be encouraged to maintain a calm, supportive, and communicative environment when encouraging change to avoid going negative.

Assessment

- Self-assessment is still important, but this can be shared. For example, talking over situations such as food choices that an early adolescent made at a recent family gathering sets the stage for two-way communication and avoids the potential power struggle when parents try for complete control.
- Parents and their child can participate in setting goals together by jointly setting the goal (eg, getting outside every day) and communicating about exactly how the goal will be achieved.

Lifestyle

- Caregivers can be reminded that modeling the behavior they desire is a powerful way to stay believable.
- Family meals continue to be important anchors of the day for providing good nutrition and enhancing communication.

- It is tempting for parents to have televisions and computers in their child's room, but they may need to be reminded that this not only increases sedentary time, but also decreases parent-child communication.

Activity

- Unfortunately, middle school can be a time of dramatic decrease in activity for many children. Demands of schoolwork and increased competitiveness of sports teams as well as elimination of recess can dramatically shift energy balance.
- Parents can emphasize the value of participation versus competition in activities. Clubs, volunteer groups, and church groups can all be valuable activities for this age group, getting them away from "screen and snack" mode after school.
- Total screen time should continue to have a 2-hour limit.
- Parents and children are often surprised at the energy cost of snacks and drinks. For example, 12 oz of a fruit drink can be 180 kcal (>1 hour of outdoor activity) and large fast-food french fries 430 kcal (1 hour of karate).
- Helping parents and children understand the energy output required to balance snacks, fast food, and sugared beverages can affect their motivation to change.
- In addition, the time it takes to consume 250 kcal can be very short (5–10 minutes), while the time it takes to expend 250 kcal can be up to 1 hour of activity. A child can literally run out of time in the day to exercise (Table 8.1).

Table 8.1. One Hour of Activity for a 100-lb Child

Outdoor cycling, exercise of moderate intensity	160 kcal
Basketball	270 kcal
Dancing	216 kcal
Martial arts	450 kcal
Soccer	325 kcal

Nutrition

- Many children come home from school "starving"; if they have unlimited access to food, they will often eat a high-calorie snack or even small meal.
- Although young adolescents have greater freedom to purchase foods of their choice outside of the home, the home is still where good nutrition habits are formed. Parents establish the food choices a child has at home when they shop at the grocery store. Growing appetites should be satisfied with fruits and vegetables instead of snack food. It's unfair to expect children at this age to resist temptation when they are hungry at home if the parent purchasing the products cannot resist those temptations when shopping.
- Early lunch periods, eating to unwind, or boredom if there is nothing to do after school can all contribute to over-snacking. Parents still need to oversee the young adolescent's selections of snacks.
- Packing a snack eliminates the child's decision making at a time when the child is feeling too hungry to choose well.
- Stopping at a neighborhood store after school may also be an issue. Limiting snack money and discussing choices may help.

Child/Young Adolescent

- The physical changes of puberty may lead young adolescents to feel unsure and critical about their bodies.
- Parents need to educate their child about the normal diversity of body types at this age and discuss individual differences.
- Puberty may also trigger increased expectations from parents and disappointment if these expectations are not met.[17]
- Parents need to be encouraged to continue to support their child in terms of nutrition and activity while encouraging the development of independent decision making.

Environment

- Finding venues for activity may be more challenging at this age.
- Safety issues that are important for parents may cause early adolescents to complain about undue restriction.
- Parents continue to need to provide transportation and financing for extracurricular activities.

- Computer and television time can creep upward rapidly at this age. Parents need to continue to limit screen time and explore alternatives for activity with their child.
- It is probably not enough to assume that the child will automatically find something to replace screen time without ideas and opportunities offered by the parents and family.

8.3 Intervention

When an early adolescent has a BMI greater than 85% and less than 95% or is crossing growth percentiles in an upward direction, this is the time for a more in-depth look at eating and activity, especially related to emotional eating, increase in sedentary time, and poor food choices—all of which can contribute to the risk of becoming an obese young adult. In addition to reemphasizing concepts covered previously, parents and families may need to give increased attention to their ability to provide and influence nutrition and activity by focusing on **energy balance, structure,** and **modeling healthy behavior.**

Energy Balance

- "How has the energy balance shifted?" is the question to ask (eg, increased snacking after school, more screen time, late-night eating).
- "Why has it shifted?" may be even more important.
- After-school eating may become an increasing problem when young adolescents are not participating in after-school activities.
- Sports participation may fall off because of increased competitiveness of teams or the youngster's self-consciousness about level of skill or body image.
- Increased eating linked to boredom, stress, anxiety, or depression may also occur.
- Shifts in meal patterns, with breakfast skipping and late-night eating, may have altered calorie balance.
- Activity may be harder to sustain with increased demands of homework and less spontaneous activity opportunities.
- Identifying the reasons for the shift in energy balance can help parents and families target areas for change.

Structure

- Meal timing and structure can become more difficult at this age because of breakfast skipping, early school lunches, and late-night eating.
- Because of a shift in sleep schedule, adolescents may find it difficult to get up, get ready for school, and eat a meal. Simplifying breakfast may help. Pre-filling a bowl with cereal or putting cereal in a plastic bag for eating on the go may make eating breakfast easy enough for the young adolescent to accomplish.
- It is important to have a plan for the after-school snack. Preparing a snack in advance that the child and parents agree on may limit the foraging that can take place.
- Predictable family meals are still important; it is hard for the teen to manage hunger if dinner can occur unpredictably, for example, between 5:00 and 8:00 pm.
- It is important to carry meal and activity structure through the weekend and vacations. These times are often seen as downtimes when the rigor of school schedules can be loosened; however, meal and activity structure often become disorganized and can lead to overeating and underactivity.

Modeling Healthy Behavior

- Modeling healthy behavior takes on a new twist—parents are still major influences on their adolescents, but peer groups and media are also giving these children messages about eating and activity that may be unhealthy.
- Fad diets are appealing to young teens concerned about their weight. Parents need to be on the lookout for these and emphasize healthy approaches to weight control.
- It is important for parents to stay positive and supportive as they try to help their teen with weight issues and continue to take a family-based approach to healthy nutrition and activity without targeting the teen as the only one who has to change.
- Parents can also help with some media education for teens concerning food advertisements and how eating and activity are portrayed in the media.
- Helping teens look their best and strengthening their competencies, whether academic achievement, club participation, individual hobbies, or positive personality traits, are important buffers for the negative self-image that can develop when a young teen is struggling with weight.

8.4 Treatment

When an early adolescent's BMI is greater than 95% and you are dealing with excess adiposity, it is time to initiate a focused treatment strategy. It is important to review the issues discussed in the previous 2 sections because these are building blocks of good nutrition and activity habits. But you will also have to focus on the barriers to change that may have prevented parents, families, and teens from implementing these strategies.

A useful way to begin is to obtain a family history focused on obesity-related comorbidities. This can serve to emphasize the health risks involved and the necessity of taking early action once obesity is identified.

8.5 Family History

The family history (page 123) provides information on obesity and obesity-related comorbidity risk as well as serves as a starting point to discuss the child's BMI.

If parents are obese or have a history of obesity, they may want to relate their personal struggles with their weight. Often the desire to avoid these same struggles in their child motivates parents to make family changes in nutrition and activity.

8.6 Review of Systems

The review of systems can also serve as a point of departure to discuss obesity-related comorbidities, pointing out particular risk factors as they relate to increasing BMI.

- Skin: Acanthosis nigricans, striae, cervical fat pad
- Head, eyes, ears, nose, and throat (HEENT): Headache, blurred vision
- Lungs: Snoring, sleep disturbance, sleep apnea, restless sleep, sleep position, daytime tiredness, napping, asthma, shortness of breath or subjective chest tightness on exercise, cough after exercise
- Cardiac: Murmur
- Abdomen: Gastroesophageal reflux, stomach pain, nausea or vomiting after eating
- Musculoskeletal: Limping, hip pain, knee pain
- Development: School problems, learning difficulties, attention problems
- Psychosocial: Depression, anxiety, behavior problems

Family History, Early Adolescent

Complete or update this family history targeted toward obesity and related comorbidities.

	Mother	Father	Maternal Grandmother	Maternal Grandfather	Paternal Grandmother	Paternal Grandfather	Sibling 1	Sibling 2
Obesity	☐	☐	☐	☐	☐	☐	☐	☐
Cardiovascular disease	☐	☐	☐	☐	☐	☐	☐	☐
High blood pressure	☐	☐	☐	☐	☐	☐	☐	☐
Stroke	☐	☐	☐	☐	☐	☐	☐	☐
High cholesterol	☐	☐	☐	☐	☐	☐	☐	☐
High triglyceride	☐	☐	☐	☐	☐	☐	☐	☐
Type 1 or 2 diabetes	☐	☐	☐	☐	☐	☐	☐	☐
_____	☐	☐	☐	☐	☐	☐	☐	☐
_____	☐	☐	☐	☐	☐	☐	☐	☐
_____	☐	☐	☐	☐	☐	☐	☐	☐
_____	☐	☐	☐	☐	☐	☐	☐	☐
_____	☐	☐	☐	☐	☐	☐	☐	☐

8.7 Physical Examination

- Height
- Weight
- BMI + previous BMI measurements
- Blood pressure

- General: Dysmorphic features, poor linear growth, developmental delay
- Skin: Skin picking, acanthosis nigricans, dermatitis in skinfolds, striae, cervical fat pad
- HEENT: Funduscopic examination for papilledema, tonsillar hypertrophy
- Cardiopulmonary: Murmur, wheezing
- Abdominal: Hepatomegaly
- Musculoskeletal: Range of motion, genu varum, limp, hip or knee pain
- Genitourinary: Tanner stage

8.8 Family Constellation and Social History

Information about the family can provide a starting point to discuss how nutrition and activity decisions are made and how changes might take place.

- Who is living at home with the early adolescent?
- How is the early adolescent spending time before and after school?
- Is someone other than the early adolescent responsible for meal or snack preparation?

8.9 Parenting Questions

Parenting styles and skills are important when families are trying to make changes in lifestyle. These questions may help you focus on family factors that may facilitate or hinder change.

	Never	Seldom	Sometimes	Often	Always
1. Parents set clear and simple expectations and limits.	☐	☐	☐	☐	☐
2. Parents set boundaries and give their young teen choices within those boundaries.	☐	☐	☐	☐	☐
3. Parents have developmentally appropriate goals for the young teen.	☐	☐	☐	☐	☐
4. Parents model healthy nutrition and activity.	☐	☐	☐	☐	☐
5. Parents limit the availability of high-sugar or high-fat snacks in the home.	☐	☐	☐	☐	☐
6. Parents maintain an abundant supply of fruits and vegetables in the home.	☐	☐	☐	☐	☐

8.10 Parenting and Teen Touch Points

Parenting touch points focus on helping families initiate and maintain change by helping them believe change can occur, identify the change needed, value the outcome of the change, know how to change, and have the energy to change and sustain the change.

- *Believe that change can occur.* Early teens may feel that change is too hard and be very aware that not everyone in their peer group needs to focus so acutely on eating and activity patterns. Acknowledging the difficulties and staying positive about what change can accomplish is important for parents. Bringing up areas in the teen's life where they have been successful, such as academic work, having a musical talent, or being a good friend, can help the teen focus on what he or she can do.

- *Identify the change.* Parents may be concerned and very explicit about eating behaviors and attitudes they want to see their young teens change. It is important to provide background and education to parents and young teens about the etiology of obesity and factors that effect energy balance. Identifying needed changes can lead to a discussion of what is possible in the current family setting. Parents and teens frequently want to attempt to change everything at once and it is worth emphasizing the incremental nature of lifestyle change and the importance of choosing achievable goals.

- *Value the outcome.* Issues of health, family history of obesity-related comorbidities, and their teen's declining self-esteem are often uppermost in parents' minds. Young teens may be much more concerned about fitting in with their peers in terms of body type, eating style, and clothing selections. It is important to take some time and let the parents and teens share each others' concerns. Parents can be reassured that they have legitimate interests in and responsibility for the teen's health. However, the teen's concerns also need to be validated and seen as developmentally appropriate.

- *Know how to change.* The techniques of establishing structure such as helping the teen organize after-school time, planning ahead for family and social events, and helping create activity opportunities are important. At this age parents can provide the structure and encouragement for change. Communicating about how to make the desired change and troubleshooting when things don't go as expected are keys to supporting the young teen. Structured times for parents and the teen to touch base can be important. This is a good time to initiate family meetings to establish house rules, express feelings and thoughts, and make positive lifestyle changes. Parents need to maintain and help teenagers follow through on a schedule of meals, activity, homework, and chores. Input from the teen gives him or her a sense of control and engages the teen in following through on discussed changes.

- *Have energy to change and sustain.* Time with parents is still important and shared activities, family meals, and car rides can be venues for sharing thoughts and feelings on how things are going. Parents need to be alert for the times when teens want to talk as well. When setbacks occur (eg, eating more than intended at a party), it helps parents to discuss these calmly and ask what different choices the young teen might have made, how the parent could help, and what to do next time.

8.11 Developmental Touch Point

In this age group, children strive to fit in with defined peer groups through cooperation and competition. They are absorbed with their bodily changes as they approach puberty. Concern about being different from their peers can be a painful topic and parents need to help the early adolescent understand the concept of individual nutrition and activity needs.

During early to mid-adolescence, more formal thought processes with the ability to evaluate logic with deductive reasoning appear. Teens grow more emancipated from the adults in their lives and follow their peer groups.

8.12 Nutrition and Activity Questions and Interventions

Nutrition and activity questions (see pages 128–129) can be answered by the parents and provide a focal point for targeted intervention (see pages 130–131) in a brief encounter. Questions answered "Often" or "Always" can be targeted first for change. For example, if the parent answered questions 1, 7, 9, and 13 on pages 128 and 129 with "Often" or "Always," you would ask them to rate the difficulty of change for questions 1, 7, 9, and 13 on pages 130 and 131.

8.13 A Case in Point: AN

AN is an 11-year-old African American boy who comes to you for his yearly school physical. He is being raised by his maternal grandparents, and his grandmother says she has no specific health concerns about AN currently but notes that his grandfather has diabetes and hypertension, as do several of his great aunts and uncles.

Grandmother answers 5 (Feels bad about self) as "Often," 7 (Gets own snacks) as "Always," 12 (Eats in front of the television) as "Often" or "Always," and 18 and 19 (Prefers quiet activities; Seems unmotivated to get active) as "Often."

During review of systems, AN notes that he cannot keep up with his peers when playing, but other than that he has no physical complaints. He had a tonsillectomy and adenoidectomy at 8 years and no longer snores. He has been having some difficulty in the sixth grade with math and reading. He also has been getting teased and occasionally bullied by classmates.

Nutrition and Activity Questions, Early Adolescent

These questions can be answered by the parents and provide a focal point for targeted intervention in a brief encounter. First have the parents answer these questions about the presence or absence of behaviors that promote weight gain, then refer to Nutrition and Activity Interventions, Early Adolescent.

	Never	Seldom	Sometimes	Often	Always
1. Drinks juice or sugared beverages between meals.	☐	☐	☐	☐	☐
2. Eats junk food.	☐	☐	☐	☐	☐
3. Eats more than 1 snack between meals each day.	☐	☐	☐	☐	☐
4. Eats a school lunch and snacks at school.	☐	☐	☐	☐	☐
5. Feels bad about self.	☐	☐	☐	☐	☐
6. Eats at fast-food restaurants.	☐	☐	☐	☐	☐
7. Gets own snacks.	☐	☐	☐	☐	☐
8. Sneaks or hides food.	☐	☐	☐	☐	☐
9. Demands certain food and snacks.	☐	☐	☐	☐	☐
10. Does not eat any vegetables.	☐	☐	☐	☐	☐

	Never	Seldom	Sometimes	Often	Always
11. Overeats after school.	☐	☐	☐	☐	☐
12. Eats in front of the television.	☐	☐	☐	☐	☐
13. Skips breakfast.	☐	☐	☐	☐	☐
14. Eats alone.	☐	☐	☐	☐	☐
15. Eats when bored.	☐	☐	☐	☐	☐
16. Watches more than 2 hours of television or the computer each day.	☐	☐	☐	☐	☐
17. Stays indoors after school.	☐	☐	☐	☐	☐
18. Prefers quiet activities.	☐	☐	☐	☐	☐
19. Seems unmotivated to get active.	☐	☐	☐	☐	☐
20. Lacks interest in peer activities.	☐	☐	☐	☐	☐

Nutrition and Activity Interventions, Early Adolescent

Questions answered "Often" or "Always" in Nutrition and Activity Questions, Early Adolescent, can be targeted first for change. Using these specific questions, ask the parent, "How difficult would it be for you to…?"

	Impossible	Could try	Could do sometimes	Could do most of the time	Easy
1. Change from juice to water between meals.	☐	☐	☐	☐	☐
2. Eliminate junk food.	☐	☐	☐	☐	☐
3. Pack a school lunch and snacks; limit extra money.	☐	☐	☐	☐	☐
4. Pack healthier school snacks.	☐	☐	☐	☐	☐
5. Help teens find areas of competence.	☐	☐	☐	☐	☐
6. Decrease fast food.	☐	☐	☐	☐	☐
7. Help teen prepare healthy snacks ahead of time	☐	☐	☐	☐	☐
8. Work with your teen on a plan to stop sneaking.	☐	☐	☐	☐	☐
9. Keep only healthy snacks in the house.	☐	☐	☐	☐	☐
10. Offer vegetables at meals.	☐	☐	☐	☐	☐

	Impossible	Could try	Could do sometimes	Could do most of the time	Easy
11. Pack a snack for after school; limit purchase of snack foods.	☐	☐	☐	☐	☐
12. Turn off the television during meals and snacks.	☐	☐	☐	☐	☐
13. Allow simple on-the-run breakfast choices.	☐	☐	☐	☐	☐
14. Eat meals together.	☐	☐	☐	☐	☐
15. Help your teen find activities to do instead of munching.	☐	☐	☐	☐	☐
16. Reduce television and computer time.	☐	☐	☐	☐	☐
17. Schedule time for your child to go outside after school.	☐	☐	☐	☐	☐
18. Come up with some suggestions that involve physical activities for your teen.	☐	☐	☐	☐	☐
19. Have your teen partner with a family member or friend in a physical activity.	☐	☐	☐	☐	☐
20. Make a peer group activity part of after-school time.	☐	☐	☐	☐	☐

His weight is 145 lb (65.8 kg). His height is 4'10" (147.3 cm), giving him a BMI of 30.3. His blood pressure is elevated at 124/78 mm Hg. On physical examination you note mild acanthosis nigricans of his neck and axilla. His Tanner stage is 2. His waist circumference is 30" (76.2 cm).

His laboratory studies show that his triglyceride level is elevated at 185 mg/dL, his insulin level is 2.5 times the laboratory normal at 45 µU/L, and his HDL cholesterol is decreased (30 mg/dL).

His combination of abdominal obesity, elevated triglyceride levels, low HDL cholesterol levels, and increased blood pressure meet the criteria for metabolic syndrome. His elevated insulin and family history of type 2 diabetes and acanthosis nigricans further raise your concerns about associated abnormalities such as impaired glucose tolerance or diabetes and nonalcoholic steatohepatitis.

You order a 2-hour glucose tolerance test (GTT) and find that his glucose at 2 hours is 155 mg/dL, which indicates impaired glucose tolerance. His liver function studies are within normal limits.

Problem #1: Metabolic Syndrome, Increased Risk for Type 2 Diabetes

This increases the emphasis that needs to be placed on diet and activity management for weight loss and will intensify your behavioral intervention.

Problem #2: Inactivity

- *Parenting dilemma: Lack of motivation*
  Grandmother understands that AN needs to increase his activity but worries about the safety of the neighborhood. She also notes that although he seems to love basketball, he refuses to try out for the community center basketball team.

- *Strategy: Create boundaries and allow choice*
  You explore community and family resources with Grandmother to evaluate activity options. Grandmother notes that a Boys & Girls Club is close by. She is willing to take him there after school and pick him up. She also says that his 13-year-old cousin lives nearby and he could come over and shoot baskets with AN. There is also a Boy Scout troop at their church that has activities every weekend. You encourage Grandmother

to let AN know that activity is not optional, but that he can choose among these possibilities.

Problem #3: Snacking

- *Parenting dilemma*
  The grandparents want to treat AN to snacks because he is a good kid and does well at school and sometimes feels bad about himself. Grandmother is glad AN is doing well in school and not in any trouble. She likes to have snacks around that AN likes.

- *Strategy: Substitutions and positive reinforcement*
  You give Grandmother a list of low-calorie snacks she can have at home (Table 6.2). You also explore with grandmother and AN other ways she can reinforce AN's good behavior and school achievements. Praise, one-on-one time with Grandmother, and an increase in privileges such as a later bedtime on weekends are some suggestions.

Problem #4: Low Self-esteem

- *Parenting dilemma: Peer teasing*
  Grandmother is worried about AN. She wants him to feel better but doesn't know exactly how to help him. She suspects he is being teased, but he won't talk about what is going on at school.

- *Strategy*
  You ask AN if he is being teased and he says he is. His usual response to the teasing is to ignore it, but you can tell it really bothers him. You reinforce ignoring the teasing and ask specifically about any physical pushing or hitting. He denies any fighting.

  You begin to explore AN's interests and competencies. You encourage Grandmother to pursue the activities you discussed previously to give him an alternate peer group. You encourage AN to try something new and ask him to report back at his next visit.

Second Visit

AN returns to a scheduled visit in 1 month. His weight is down 2 lb (0.9 kg). His blood pressure has decreased to 120/75 mm Hg and he has lost 1" (2.54 cm) from his waist circumference. Grandmother has provided him with lower calorie snacks, which he has accepted. He reports that he has been going to the Boys & Girls Club and playing basketball after school. Grandmother notes that he seems happier and more cooperative at home.

You congratulate AN and Grandmother on the changes they have made and schedule him for another visit in a month.

Third Visit

AN has lost another 2.5 lb (1.1 kg) and 2" (5.08 cm) from his waist and his blood pressure is down to 118/68 mm Hg. He is more talkative and is telling you about his basketball buddies. You order a fasting glucose, insulin, and lipid profile.

When laboratory results come back his insulin is 25 µU/L (mildly elevated), his triglyceride is 150 mg/dL, and his HDL is 35 mg/dL.

You schedule him to come back 1 month from now and plan to repeat his 2-hour GTT at that visit.

References

1. Rogol AD, Roemmich JN, Clark PA. Growth at puberty. *J Adolesc Health.* 2002;31(6 Suppl):192–200
2. Dolan LM, Bean J, D'Alessio D, et al. Frequency of abnormal carbohydrate metabolism and diabetes in a population-based screening of adolescents. *J Pediatr.* 2005;146:751–758
3. Goran MI, Gower BA. Longitudinal study on pubertal insulin resistance. *Diabetes.* 2001;50:2444–2450
4. Remsberg KE, Demerath EW, Schubert CM, Chumlea WC, Sun SS, Siervogel RM. Early menarche and the development of cardiovascular disease risk factors in adolescent girls: the Fels Longitudinal Study. *J Clin Endocrinol Metab.* 2005;90:2718–2724
5. Wang Y. Is obesity associated with early sexual maturation? A comparison of the association in American boys versus girls. *Pediatrics.* 2002;110:903–910
6. Brage S, Wedderkopp N, Ekelund U, et al. Objectively measured physical activity correlates with indices of insulin resistance in Danish children. The European Youth Heart Study (EYHS). *Int J Obes Relat Metab Disord.* 2004;28:1503–1508
7. Thompson AM, Baxter-Jones AD, Mirwald RL, Bailey DA. Comparison of physical activity in male and female children: does maturation matter? *Med Sci Sports Exerc.* 2003;35:1684–1690

8. Trager S. Preventing weight problems before they become too hard to solve. *The State Education Standard.* December 2004;5:13–20. Available at: www.nasbe.org/Standard/17_Dec2004/atkins.pdf. Accessed June 28, 2006

9. Vandewater EA, Shim MS, Caplovitz AG. Linking obesity and activity level with children's television and video game use. *J Adolesc.* 2004;27:71–85

10. Pate RR, Baranowski T, Dowda M, Trost SG. Tracking of physical activity in young children. *Med Sci Sports Exerc.* 1996;28:92–96

11. Kvaavik E, Tell GS, Klepp KI. Predictors and tracking of body mass index from adolescence into adulthood: follow-up of 18 to 20 years in the Oslo Youth Study. *Arch Pediatr Adolesc Med.* 2003;157:1212–1218

12. Kohen-Avramoglu R, Theriault A, Adeli K. Emergence of the metabolic syndrome in childhood: an epidemiological overview and mechanistic link to dyslipidemia. *Clin Biochem.* 2003;36:413–420

13. Hauner H. Insulin resistance and the metabolic syndrome—a challenge of the new millennium. *Eur J Clin Nutr.* 2002;56(Suppl 1):S25–S29

14. Sinaiko AR, Donahue RP, Jacobs DR, Prineas RJ. Relation of weight and rate of increase in weight during childhood and adolescence to body size, blood pressure, fasting insulin, and lipids in young adults. The Minneapolis Children's Blood Pressure Study. *Circulation.* 1999;99:1471–1476

15. Sinha R, Fisch G, Teague B, et al. Prevalence of impaired glucose tolerance among children and adolescents with marked obesity. *N Engl J Med.* 2002; 346:802–810

16. Eisenmann JC, Welk GJ, Wickel EE, Blair SN, Aeorbics Center Longitudinal Study. Stability of variables associated with the metabolic syndrome from adolescence to adulthood: the Aerobics Center Longitudinal Study. *Am J Hum Biol.* 2004;16:690–696

17. D'Angelo SL, Omar HA. Parenting adolescents. *Int J Adoles Med Health.* 2003;15:11–19

Chapter 9

Mid-Adolescent

· ·

9.1 Background

Puberty is thought of as one of the critical periods of adipose tissue differentiation when adipose stromal cells differentiate into triglyceride-filled adipocytes. In pubertal boys, lean body mass tends to increase, decreasing body fat as a percentage of total weight. Pubertal girls tend to have increased fat and fat-free body mass with an increase in body fat as a percentage of body weight. Distribution of body fat also changes during adolescence with an increase in subcutaneous and visceral fat in the abdominal region in boys and additional deposition of fat in breast, gluteal, and thigh regions in girls.[1]

Reversal of this fat accumulation becomes increasingly difficult for many adolescents. The likelihood of adult obesity increases; there is an 80% chance of an obese adolescent becoming an obese adult.[2]

Obesity-related comorbidities increase as obesity persists into adolescence. Features of the metabolic syndrome such as hyperinsulinemia, obesity, hypertension, hyperlipidemia, and dyslipidemia are much more common in adolescents who are overweight.[3] Type 2 diabetes is also increased in obese adolescents; rates exceed those of type 1 diabetes in this population. Sleep apnea and hypertension are also commonly diagnosed and are linked to body mass index (BMI).

Elevated BMI is also related to depression, and obese adolescents who had the highest depression scores had the greatest increase in BMI.[4]

Energy balance continues to be problematic in the mid-adolescent age group. Although recommendations for exercise include 60 minutes of exercise a day,[5] some measures suggest that as few as 30% of teens are meeting this goal.[6] Girls, older adolescents, minority adolescents, and disadvantaged teens are less likely to meet this baseline requirement. Healthy People 2010 sets a goal of 75% for the proportion of adolescents who watch television for fewer than 2 hours per day but as of 1999, only 57% of adolescents met this goal.[5] Obese adolescents have been found to have limited exercise tolerance because of the greater oxygen demand of their excess mass.[7] Exercise recommendations for these adolescents should be tailored to allow for activities that can be sustained without causing fatigue caused by lactate accumulation.[7]

9.2 Prevention: Talking to Parents and Teens (BALANCE)

Prevention touch points for parents and teens include **belief, assessment, lifestyle, activity, nutrition, child/adolescent,** and **environment** (BALANCE).

Belief

- Parents of mid-adolescents often feel that their teens are old enough to take charge of their own nutrition and activity and conversely may complain that their teens are unmotivated to do so. However, people of all ages do better with family support, and nutrition and activity should continue to be discussed openly within the family.
- In enlisting family support, teens and parents often respond to the idea of the parent as coach, and parents need to be encouraged to provide support and positive role modeling of good decision making when it comes to eating and activity.

Assessment

- Going over normal growth and development and sharing height, weight, and BMI measurements are important ways of normalizing the changes the teen is experiencing.
- Providing a short list of some problem behaviors that can interfere with healthy eating and activity can be helpful to introduce the concept of self-assessment (Table 9.1).

Table 9.1. Self-assessment Questions for Teens

I eat in front of the television or computer.	☐ Yes	☐ No
There are times when I skip meals.	☐ Yes	☐ No
I snack at night before bedtime.	☐ Yes	☐ No
I watch more than 2 hours of television or the computer each day.	☐ Yes	☐ No
I find it hard to exercise on a daily basis.	☐ Yes	☐ No

Lifestyle

- It may be helpful at this point to have the teen help with an environmental assessment of nutrition and activity. Going through a kitchen inventory with parents and discussing healthy and unhealthy choices can foster communication and dialogue.
- In the same way, getting together and evaluating what is available inside and outside the home to support activity and what gets in the way of being active can create dialogue and lead to healthier changes.
- Activity alternatives in the community can also be explored together. Parents can partner with their teens as they choose among activities that are within the family's financial and time constraints. This keeps the focus on family partnership in determining healthy eating and activity.

Activity

- At this point in their school and social lives, physical activity often is on the decline for most adolescents, with options for participation in sports giving way to competitive activities in which relatively few teens can take an active role.
- Screen time may correspondingly increase and many teens are at a loss to come up with alternative activities. This is where parents and families can try to offer creative alternatives to electronic media. Sports that the teen may not have tried before such as tennis, golf, karate, or swimming can be offered. Part-time jobs, volunteer work, hobbies, and clubs are good alternatives to screen time.

Nutrition

- Breakfast is a meal that is often omitted during the teen years. In a study of adolescent eating patterns, the 26% of adolescents classified as inconsistent breakfast consumers had significantly higher BMIs and lower iron intake relative to consistent breakfast consumers.[8]
- Lack of time, not being hungry, and an early lunch period are frequently cited reasons to skip breakfast. Troubleshoot possible breakfast options together, such as
  - Portion out cereal in a small plastic bag in the evening to be readily available while getting ready for school.
  - If healthy choices are available, taking advantage of the school breakfast program is an option.

– A breakfast bar with fruit and a glass of milk may be an option as a
way to transition to a more standard breakfast.
– Low-fat yogurt with fruit is also an option.
– Toaster pastries, liquid breakfasts, leftovers, and fast-food breakfasts
should be avoided.

Child/Adolescent

● Most adolescents move through the teen years without major difficulties[9]
and are engaged in the process of negotiating more independent relationships with their parents.
● Parental warmth and involvement have been found to increase adolescents' response to parental influence. When these parental traits are
combined with structure and support, the transition to self-regulation
occurs more smoothly.[10]

Environment

● The nutrition and activity environments of teens expand beyond
home and school to include social gatherings, workplaces, and
community settings.
● Teens need to continue to develop assessment and decision-making
skills that will allow them to make healthy choices as they move outside
the more or less controlled environments of the family and school.
● Providing information on nutritional content of fast foods, discussing
handling of eating at buffets and social events, and helping the teen
look for opportunities for increasing physical activity as part of a
daily routine are all issues that foster critical thinking about eating
and activity.

9.3 Intervention

When an adolescent has a BMI greater than 85% and less than 95% or is
crossing growth percentiles in an upward direction, this is the time for a
more in-depth look at eating and activity, especially related to unregulated
eating, increase in sedentary time, and poor food choices—all of which
can contribute to the risk of becoming an obese adult. In addition to
reemphasizing concepts covered previously, parents and families may need

to give increased attention to their ability to provide and influence nutrition and activity by focusing on **energy balance, structure,** and **modeling healthy behavior.**

Energy Balance

Unregulated eating and activity can quickly undermine energy balance at a time when the peak of the growth spurt may be waning. Overdoing screen time, late-night snacking, and meal skipping all can contribute to weight gain. It is important to get a grasp of the teen's daily diet and activity, which may or may not correspond to the rest of the family's routine. Many adolescents get up to one third of their calories from snacks, which add calories and compromise nutritious eating at meals. Grazing from after school to after dinner is frequently a cause of increased weight gain. Eating from boredom, stress, or depression is also a cause of a rise in weight. Late-night eating usually associated with screen time can also lead to decreased hunger in the morning and further disrupt eating patterns. Unregulated eating can veer off into bingeing and feelings of loss of control over eating, leading to low self-esteem.

Structure

Structured eating and activity continue to be important. At this point parents can support the adolescent by picking out a few areas to focus on to reinstitute healthy eating and activity. Family dinners, an after-school snack prepared in advance, and exercise equipment at home are some ways parents can support their adolescent's efforts. Working with their teen on decision making, creating a schedule for free time, and working on ideas for healthy meals can help create positive communication about food and exercise. Part-time jobs, volunteer work, clubs, and activities are also ways of adding structure to the teen's after-school time and mitigate prolonged screen time with its attendant eating.

Modeling Healthy Behavior

Adolescents may get quite a bit of information about diet and exercise from their peers. Dietary routines that may seem like they make sense, such as skipping meals or using dietary supplements, are common. Helping adolescents sift through information about diets and drugs is one of the important components of enhancing decision making.

9.4 Treatment

When a teen's BMI is greater than 95% and you are dealing with excess adiposity, it is time to initiate a focused treatment strategy. It is important to review the issues discussed in the previous 2 sections because these are building blocks of good nutrition and activity habits. But you will also have to focus on the barriers to change that may have prevented parents, families, and teens from implementing these strategies.

A useful way to begin is to obtain a family history focused on obesity-related comorbidities. This can serve to emphasize the health risks involved and the necessity of taking early action once obesity is identified.

9.5 Family History

Family history (page 143) should be updated at this time with attention to obesity-related comorbidities, the family weight trajectory, eating behaviors, and mental health diagnosis.

9.6 Review of Systems

The review of systems can also serve as a point of departure to discuss obesity-related comorbidities, pointing out particular risk factors as they relate to increasing BMI.

- Skin: Acanthosis nigricans, striae, acne
- Head, eyes, ears, nose, and throat (HEENT): Headache, snoring, sleep disturbance, daytime napping, attention problems, poor school functioning, irritability, visual disturbance
- Lungs: Asthma, shortness of breath during exercise, cough at end of exercise, decreased exercise tolerance
- Cardiac: Hypertension, hyperlipidemia
- Abdomen: Gastroesophageal reflux, stomach pain before or after eating, chronic diarrhea or constipation, morning anorexia, right upper quadrant discomfort or pain
- Musculoskeletal: Limping, hip pain or decreased motion, knee pain, bowing, ankle pain
- Genitourinary: Enuresis, delayed pubertal development
- Psychological: Symptoms of depression, anxiety, low self-esteem, self-injury or suicidal ideation, sleep disturbance

Family History, Mid-Adolescent

Complete or update this family history targeted toward obesity and related comorbidities.

	Mother	Father	Maternal Grandmother	Maternal Grandfather	Paternal Grandmother	Paternal Grandfather	Sibling 1	Sibling 2
Obesity	☐	☐	☐	☐	☐	☐	☐	☐
Cardiovascular disease	☐	☐	☐	☐	☐	☐	☐	☐
High blood pressure	☐	☐	☐	☐	☐	☐	☐	☐
Stroke	☐	☐	☐	☐	☐	☐	☐	☐
High cholesterol	☐	☐	☐	☐	☐	☐	☐	☐
High triglyceride	☐	☐	☐	☐	☐	☐	☐	☐
Type 1 or 2 diabetes	☐	☐	☐	☐	☐	☐	☐	☐
_____	☐	☐	☐	☐	☐	☐	☐	☐
_____	☐	☐	☐	☐	☐	☐	☐	☐
_____	☐	☐	☐	☐	☐	☐	☐	☐
_____	☐	☐	☐	☐	☐	☐	☐	☐
_____	☐	☐	☐	☐	☐	☐	☐	☐
_____	☐	☐	☐	☐	☐	☐	☐	☐

9.7 Physical Examination

- Height
- Weight
- BMI + previous BMI measurements
- Blood pressure
- General: Height deceleration or poor linear growth, centripetal or visceral fat distribution
- Skin: Acanthosis nigricans (neck, axilla, groin), acne, cervical fat pad, striae
- HEENT: Funduscopic examination for papilledema, tonsillar hypertrophy, thyroid enlargement
- Cardiopulmonary: Wheezing, poor ventilation, heart murmur
- Abdominal: Hepatomegaly
- Musculoskeletal: Range of motion, genu varum, limp, hip or knee pain, ankle pain
- Genitourinary: Tanner stage

9.8 Family Constellation and Social History

Information about the family can provide a starting point to discuss how nutrition and activity decisions are made and how changes might take place.

- Who is living at home with the adolescent?
- Who is providing the adolescent with meals and snacks?
- Who is purchasing food for meals and snacks?
- Who is eating with the adolescent at meals?

9.9 Parenting Questions

Parenting styles and skills are important when families are trying to make changes in lifestyle. These questions may help you focus on family factors that may facilitate or hinder change.

	Never	Seldom	Sometimes	Often	Always
1. Parents set clear expectations and limits.	☐	☐	☐	☐	☐
2. Parents set boundaries that are consistent and appropriate for an adolescent's development.	☐	☐	☐	☐	☐
3. Parents provide opportunities for healthy nutrition and activity.	☐	☐	☐	☐	☐

9.10 Parenting and Teen Touch Points

Parenting and teen touch points focus on helping families initiate and maintain change by helping them believe change can occur, identify the change needed, value the outcome of the change, know how to change, and have the energy to change and sustain the change.

- *Believe that change can occur.* Adolescents who have been struggling with their weight are often discouraged about their ability to make change. Starting slowly, being consistent, and having a strategy for dealing with setbacks are all important for ensuring success that will contribute to further change. It is important to help dispel negative attitudes in the teen and family that may have gotten fostered by failed attempts in the past.

- *Identify the change.* An important component of making change is to identify possibilities for change with the teen and parents; for example, eliminating juice and soda, going to the YMCA after school, or cutting down on screen time. Equally important is identifying which change or changes the teen thinks will be doable. Parental support is still crucial. Changes that depend on the adolescent alone have less chance of success than ones that the parents support.

- *Value the outcome.* It is more important than ever to include the adolescent in discussions of the value of change. Reasons for working on weight can vary from "my parents want me to" to "the prom is coming up" to worry about decreased ability to participate in physical activities. Worry about family history and obesity-related comorbidities might not be uppermost in the minds of adolescents. Reducing the effects of obesity-related comorbidities such as diabetes or sleep apnea might also have value if the teen feels that he or she will be directly affected. Validating the teen's concerns as well as those of the parents is helpful. Teens may also be concerned about feelings of eating being out of control and making bad decisions about food. It is important to start wherever the teen is and use this as the fulcrum for making change.

- *Know how to change.* Goal setting is important. Clear goals such as eating breakfast every day or walking home from school are important. It is more important to focus on the behaviors that need to change as goals rather than weight loss only. The concept of consistency is very important because adolescents will often discount exceptions, and the extra snack or hour of screen time will be enough to positively shift energy balance. Remind the teen that an extra 150 kcal a day over a year can result in a 15-lb (6.8-kg) weight gain. Persistence is also important and the concept of permanent change rather than a temporary diet should be addressed.

- *Have energy to change and sustain.* Parents are perhaps most important in helping to provide the emotional energy and support for teens to stick to the changes they are trying to make. Providing healthy foods at home as well as opportunities for activity such as partnering in a walking program are some concrete ways parents can help. Other family members can be very important contributors to supporting the teen.

9.11 Developmental Touch Point

Striving for independence and a separate identity from parents is a normal process of adolescence. Adolescents may resist limit setting but respond to mutual goal setting in the family.

9.12 Nutrition and Activity Questions and Interventions

Nutrition and activity questions (see pages 148–149) can be answered by the parents and provide a focal point for targeted intervention (see pages 150–151) in a brief encounter. Questions answered "Often" or "Always" can be targeted first for change. For example, if the parent answered questions 1, 7, 9, and 13 on pages 148 and 149 with "Often" or "Always," you would ask them to rate the difficulty of change for questions 1, 7, 9, and 13 on pages 150 and 151.

9.13 A Case in Point: BT

BT is a 13-year-old African American girl whose parents schedule an appointment with you so you can talk to BT about her weight and eating. BT's parents are concerned about her weight because of a family history of obesity and diabetes in 3 out of the 4 grandparents and BT's father. They are frustrated with BT because she won't listen to what they say.

At the visit, BT's weight is 230 lb (104.3 kg) and her height is 5'4" (162.6 cm), giving her a BMI of 39.5. You ask BT if she is worried about her health and she says, "No, but my parents are."

On the initial questionnaire, parents have noted that BT always drinks soda between meals (question 1), grazes between meals (question 3), seems depressed (question 5), eats at night (question 9), and seems unmotivated to get active (question 19).

Parents indicate that they "could try" to change from soda or juice to water or diet drinks (intervention 1), could "sometimes" provide BT with healthy snack options (intervention 3), could "easily" have BT evaluated for depression (intervention 5), feel it would be "impossible" to keep BT from eating at night (intervention 9), and feel it would be "impossible" to motivate BT to get active (intervention 19).

On review of systems, BT has acanthosis nigricans and irregular periods and despite being a very good student, seems unmotivated and depressed to her parents. BT herself says that she frequently feels sad and frustrated about her weight and expresses some anger at her parents for not helping her.

On physical examination you note that her blood pressure is 130/82 mm Hg and she has acanthosis nigricans not only of her neck creases, but also in her axilla and groin area. The rest of her physical examination is unremarkable.

When her parents initially scheduled her appointment, you ordered laboratory studies. These show an elevated triglyceride level of 215 mg/dL, high-density lipoprotein (HDL) cholesterol at a low level of 30 mg/dL, and an elevated insulin level of 73 μU/dL, with a normal fasting glucose of 85 mg/dL and a hemoglobin A_{1C} of 5.9%. Total cholesterol and liver enzymes were normal.

You note the combination of elevated blood pressure, increased triglyceride levels, low HDL cholesterol, and high insulin would make the diagnosis of metabolic syndrome. This constellation of signs in addition to the positive family history place her at risk for type 2 diabetes. In addition, the

Nutrition and Activity Questions, Mid-Adolescent

These questions can be answered by the parents and provide a focal point for targeted intervention in a brief encounter. First have the parents answer these questions about the presence or absence of behaviors that promote weight gain, then refer to Nutrition and Activity Interventions, Mid-Adolescent.

	Never	Seldom	Sometimes	Often	Always
1. Drinks juice or sugared beverages between meals.	☐	☐	☐	☐	☐
2. Eats junk food.	☐	☐	☐	☐	☐
3. Grazes between meals.	☐	☐	☐	☐	☐
4. Frequents the snack and soft drink vending machines at school.	☐	☐	☐	☐	☐
5. Seems depressed.	☐	☐	☐	☐	☐
6. Eats at fast-food restaurants.	☐	☐	☐	☐	☐
7. Gets own snacks.	☐	☐	☐	☐	☐
8. Binges.	☐	☐	☐	☐	☐
9. Eats at night.	☐	☐	☐	☐	☐
10. Eats limited variety of food groups.	☐	☐	☐	☐	☐

	Never	Seldom	Sometimes	Often	Always
11. Overeats after school.	☐	☐	☐	☐	☐
12. Eats in front of the television.	☐	☐	☐	☐	☐
13. Skips breakfast.	☐	☐	☐	☐	☐
14. Eats alone.	☐	☐	☐	☐	☐
15. Eats when bored.	☐	☐	☐	☐	☐
16. Watches more than 2 hours of television or the computer each day.	☐	☐	☐	☐	☐
17. Stays indoors after school.	☐	☐	☐	☐	☐
18. Prefers quiet activities.	☐	☐	☐	☐	☐
19. Seems unmotivated to get active.	☐	☐	☐	☐	☐
20. Lacks interest in peer activities.	☐	☐	☐	☐	☐

Nutrition and Activity Interventions, Mid-Adolescent

Questions answered "Often" or "Always" in Nutrition and Activity Questions, Mid-Adolescent, can be targeted first for change. Using these specific questions, ask the parent, "How difficult would it be for you to…?"

	Impossible	Could try	Could do sometimes	Could do most of the time	Easy
1. Change from soda or juice to water or diet drinks between meals.	☐	☐	☐	☐	☐
2. Eliminate junk food.	☐	☐	☐	☐	☐
3. Have only healthy snacks available; discuss snack options when with friends.	☐	☐	☐	☐	☐
4. Discuss making healthier choices.	☐	☐	☐	☐	☐
5. Have pediatrician, counselor, or therapist evaluate.	☐	☐	☐	☐	☐
6. Decrease fast food.	☐	☐	☐	☐	☐
7. Pack healthier school snacks.	☐	☐	☐	☐	☐
8. Explore emotions and food with pediatrician.	☐	☐	☐	☐	☐
9. Keep only healthy snacks in the house; encourage lower calorie snacks.	☐	☐	☐	☐	☐
10. Eat well-balanced meals together as much as possible.	☐	☐	☐	☐	☐

	Impossible	Could try	Could do sometimes	Could do most of the time	Easy
11. Provide healthy snack options for after school; discourage stopping at local stores on the way home from school.	☐	☐	☐	☐	☐
12. Try to turn off the television during meals and snacks.	☐	☐	☐	☐	☐
13. Allow simple on-the-run breakfast choices.	☐	☐	☐	☐	☐
14. Eat meals together.	☐	☐	☐	☐	☐
15. Help your adolescent with a schedule for school and evening time that includes activities outside the house.	☐	☐	☐	☐	☐
16. Try to limit television or computer time to 2 hours a day and provide help in deciding on alternative activities.	☐	☐	☐	☐	☐
17. Encourage extracurricular activities.	☐	☐	☐	☐	☐
18. Try to encourage activities other than screen time such as crafts, chores, and reading.	☐	☐	☐	☐	☐
19. Partner with your teen in a physical activity.	☐	☐	☐	☐	☐
20. Encourage a peer group activity to be part of after-school time.	☐	☐		☐	☐

constellation of acanthosis nigricans, insulin resistance, and irregular periods indicate possible polycystic ovary syndrome (PCOS). You order free and total testosterone, dehydroepiandrosterone levels, and sex hormone binding globulin. Her testosterone is elevated at 80 ng/dL with a normal range of less than 50 mg/dL, her sex hormone binding globulin is decreased, and her dehydroepiandrosterone level is slightly elevated. Luteinizing hormone is low and follicle-stimulating hormone is high, strongly indicating the diagnosis of PCOS. You refer her to the endocrinologist for hormonal treatment and possible treatment with metformin hydrochloride.

Problem #1: Metabolic Syndrome and Polycystic Ovary Syndrome

BT already has both risk factors and comorbidity associated with obesity. You emphasize the health issues to the family (who are already concerned) and BT and offer to work intensely with them to reduce the risk of diabetes and treat the PCOS.

Problem #2: Consumption of Soft Drinks

- *Parenting dilemma: BT won't listen.*
  When this issue is mentioned, BT immediately says to her mother, "You keep buying regular soda at the store for yourself and hide it in your room." Parents say BT is old enough to listen and drink the diet soda they have provided for her.

- *Strategy*
  You go over the family history of diabetes, the parents' concern about BT developing diabetes, and the need for father to follow a diabetic nutrition plan as well. You point out that adolescents do better with their dietary changes if the whole family works with them. Mother notes that she can try diet drinks in an effort to help BT.

Problem #3: Possible Depression

- *Parenting dilemma*
  The parents have been worried about BT and wondered if she was depressed. They say she won't talk about it. Their concern is increased because her mother and grandmother have a history of depression and treatment.

- *Strategy*

  You ask the parents to check and see what counseling options exist in their medical plan. You also perform a brief depression inventory and note that currently BT is feeling sad, but is not depressed or suicidal. Parents agree to counseling and were relieved to have a pathway to address BT's depression.

Problem #4: Grazing Between Meals

- *Parenting dilemma*

  The parents feel BT should be able to control her eating between meals. They are frustrated because she often reaches for snacks while watching television and becomes very irritable and angry when they try to interfere.

- *Strategy*

  You explain the high calorie, sugar, and fat content of most snack foods. You also acknowledge that depression can be a trigger for snacking. You offer the family a list of lower calorie snack options to have available for BT and ask her if she would consider trying these. BT says she would if everyone else would have to eat them too.

  You acknowledge to the family that BT's eating at night and lack of motivation to exercise are very important, but that these issues will be tackled at the next visits as the family moves through making healthy lifestyle changes. You ask the family to try these strategies and return in 3 to 4 weeks.

Second Visit

BT returns having gained only 0.44 lb (0.2 kg) in 1 month, compared with her previous rate of weight gain of 3.3 lb (1.5 kg) per month. Her blood pressure is 126/80 mm Hg.

- *Problem #1: Metabolic syndrome and PCOS.* BT has seen the endocrinologist, been placed on birth control pills, and encouraged in her lifestyle changes with a revisit in 3 months. So far she has had no problems.

- *Problem #2: Consumption of soft drinks.* The family has successfully converted to drinking water or diet drinks between meals. There is no regular soda at home and BT offers that when she is out with her friends, she orders a diet soda instead of a regular one.

- *Problem #3: Possible depression.* Parents have found a counselor for BT and she has had one visit. When asked about how the session went, BT replies, "OK, I guess." She does say she is willing to go again.

- *Problem #4: Grazing between meals.* The parents have provided healthy snacks. BT is eating these snacks at home but is having trouble making good choices when she is out with friends and at family gatherings.

You reinforce the good choices she is able to make, noting her slowed weight gain, and go over strategies to handle exposure to snacks and treats socially.

Problem #5: Lack of Motivation to Be Active

- *Parenting dilemma*
  The parents have become very tired of nagging BT to go out and get involved with no results.

- *Strategy*
  You ask the parents to start by partnering BT in a family activity such as walking, biking, or bowling once a week.

You schedule another visit in 4 weeks and order insulin, glucose, and hemoglobin A_{1C} level tests.

Third Visit

BT's weight on this visit is 227 lb (103.0 kg) and her blood pressure is 122/78 mm Hg. She seems happier and is pleased she has lost weight. Her fasting insulin is 40 µU/mL and her hemoglobin A_{1C} is 5.6%.

- *Problem #1: Metabolic syndrome and PCOS.* Her insulin is starting to come down, as are her hemoglobin A_{1C} and blood pressure. She continues on birth control pills and has an endocrinology revisit appointment in the next month.

- *Problem #2: Consumption of soft drinks.* The consumption of water or diet drinks has become part of the family's routine. Father even says he feels his blood sugars have improved because of it. BT says she is choosing nonsugared beverages in almost all social situations.

- *Problem #3: Possible depression.* BT has had her second counseling visit and feels things are going OK. She reports decreased feelings of sadness and the parents feel her mood has improved.

- *Problem #4: Grazing between meals.* BT seems to be making healthier choices. She noted that one day when she was really upset, she bought candy at the local store, but was able to stay with the healthy snacks the rest of the time. You spend a little time talking about the link between emotions and eating and BT is starting to recognize this connection. You encourage BT to continue making good choices.

- *Problem #5: Lack of motivation to be active.* BT and her parents report that they have had some good times with their family activities and actually look forward to them. You explore with the parents and BT what other possible extracurricular activities are available and encourage them to pick several possibilities and see if BT will try one of them.

You schedule a return visit in 1 month.

References

1. Daniels SR, Arnett DK, Eckel RH, et al. Overweight in children and adolescents: pathophysiology, consequences, prevention, and treatment. *Circulation.* 2005;111:1999–2012

2. Whitaker RC, Wright JA, Pepe MS, Seidel KD, Dietz WH. Predicting obesity in young adulthood from childhood and parental obesity. *N Engl J Med.* 1997;337:869–873

3. Cook S, Weitzman M, Auinger P, Nguyen M, Dietz WH. Prevalence of a metabolic syndrome phenotype in adolescents: findings from the third National Health and Nutrition Examination Survey, 1988-1994. *Arch Pediatr Adolesc Med.* 2003;157:821–827

4. Goodman E, Whitaker RC. A prospective study of the role of depression in the development and persistence of adolescent obesity. *Pediatrics.* 2002;110: 497–504

5. Patrick K, Norman GJ, Calfas KJ, et al. Diet, physical activity, and sedentary behaviors as risk factors for overweight in adolescence. *Arch Pediatr Adolesc Med.* 2004;158:385–390

6. Pate RR, Freedson PS, Sallis JF, et al. Compliance with physical activity guidelines: prevalence in a population of children and youth. *Ann Epidemiol.* 2002; 12:303–308

7. Norman AC, Drinkard B, McDuffie JR, Ghorbani S, Yanoff LB, Yanovski JA. Influence of excess adiposity on exercise fitness and performance in overweight children and adolescents. *Pediatrics.* 2005;115:e690–e696

8. Stockman NK, Schenkel TC, Brown JN, Duncan AM. Comparison of energy and nutrient intakes among meals and snacks of adolescent males. *Prev Med.* 2005;41:203–210

9. Henricson C, Roker D. Support for the parents of adolescents: a review. *J Adolesc.* 2000;23:763–783

10. Steinberg L, Morris AS. Adolescent development. *Annu Rev Psychol.* 2001;52: 83–110

Chapter 10

Late Adolescent and Young Adult

··

10.1 Background

The rising prevalence of obesity and morbid obesity in adolescence means that more adolescents will be experiencing obesity-related comorbid conditions such as type 2 diabetes, nonalcoholic steatohepatitis, dyslipidemia, hypertension, and pulmonary disease than ever before. Almost 80% of adolescents who are obese will go on to become obese adults[1] and in adulthood, obesity also increases risks of cancer of the breast, colon, prostate, endometrium, kidney, and gallbladder[2] and contributes to significant functional disability because of osteoarthritis. All of these will necessitate screening at increasingly earlier ages.

Morbidly obese adults have a 50% to 100% increased risk of premature death compared with normal-weight adults, and even modest weight increases of 10 to 20 lb (4.5–9.1 kg) can increase mortality.[3] A study from Norway of 14- to 19-year-olds who were followed 31.5 years found they had a 30% higher mortality if their body mass index (BMI) was between 85% and 95% and an 80% (for males) to 100% (for females) higher mortality if their BMI was greater than 95% for age in adolescence.[4] Psychologic morbidity is also a significant factor in the life of obese adolescents. In a study of seventh to 12th graders, adolescents who were depressed had a higher rate of obesity at follow-up while baseline obesity did not predict depression, indicating that obesity can be the outcome of psychologic morbidity.[5] The developmental tasks of adolescence need to be taken into account in prevention and treatment of obesity, bearing in mind that family involvement is still crucial to provide support for the teen. Evolution of a healthy self-image is one of the important steps toward adulthood, and self-esteem has been found to be lower in obese adolescents than normal-weight peers.[6] The effects of adolescent obesity on body image may persist into adulthood; women who become obese as adolescents were found to have persistent severe disturbances in body image, in contrast to women who become obese as adults.[7]

Another of the tasks of late adolescence is developing a plan for social and economic stability. Obesity in female adolescents has been linked to lower education levels, lower household incomes, and higher poverty rates in adulthood.[8] Lower college acceptance and less likelihood of marriage were also found among obese women.[2,9]

10.2 Prevention: Conversations With Teens (BALANCE)

Prevention touch points for teens include **belief, assessment, lifestyle, activity, nutrition, child/adolescent,** and **environment** (BALANCE).

Belief

- Obesity prevention continues to be important in this age group because risk for obesity continues into adulthood. Obesity rates continue to rise in adulthood—in a survey of adults older than 20 years in 1999–2000, 65% were overweight or obese while a corresponding 27% of high school students were overweight or obese.[10]
- Teens may need to be reminded that excess weight gain can still occur and continued attention to nutrition and activity is important.
- It may also be helpful to discuss obesity prevention in the overall context of health prevention issues; family history can be a useful entry point into this discussion for the young adult.

Assessment

- Self-monitoring may be a valuable technique to manage weight in this age group.
- Female college freshman who received feedback on their weight change gained little to no weight over a semester compared with a control group that gained an average of 6.6 lb (3.0 kg).[11]

Lifestyle

- Irregular schedules and decreased sleep duration may contribute to weight gain.[12] It is worth going over the importance of scheduling activity, meals, and sleep and the relationship of structure to maintaining healthy behaviors.

- Time management and priority setting are important skills when asking a teen to consider attending to regular meals and exercise.
- Families can provide support by providing a regular dinnertime, healthy available snacks, and opportunities for exercise such as YMCA memberships. The adolescent can be encouraged to set aside time to take advantage of these opportunities.

Activity

- The older teen and young adult may be moving out of competitive activities and looking for options to maintain physical activity in the course of day-to-day activities.
- Optimizing opportunities such as walking to school or work, looking for part-time jobs that involve physical activity, and engaging in social activities that involve physical activity can all be helpful.
- Learning a lifetime sport such as tennis, golf, or biking should be encouraged.

Nutrition

- Frequency of fast-food consumption is associated with greater weight gain and greater increase in insulin resistance.[13] It is important to help adolescents find simple, nutritious alternatives to fast food.
- Unregulated eating often gives rise to increased snacking and fast-food or convenience food consumption and meal skipping.
- Eating patterns may veer off into binge eating, bulimia, grazing, fad diets, or restrictive eating or anorexia. The following questions about binge eating[14] can help to start a conversation about binge eating behavior. Does the adolescent

  1. Eat much more quickly than usual during binge episodes?
  2. Eat until uncomfortably full?
  3. Eat large amounts of food even when not really hungry?
  4. Eat alone because of embarrassment about the amount of food eaten?
  5 Feel disgusted, depressed, or guilty after overeating?

- Patterns of emotional eating may also occur. Attention to a diet history that takes into account dietary behaviors and feelings is important.
- If an eating disorder is suspected, a resource is the American Academy of Pediatrics policy statement, "Identifying and Treating Eating Disorders"[15] (see page 321).

Child/Adolescent

- Attention to mental health is important as teens prepare for the next phase of development. Depression in adolescence is associated with an additional increased risk of obesity in young adulthood.[16]
- High-risk health behaviors may be more common in this age group and include risk for obesity. Late adolescents and young adults (18–24 years) have a higher prevalence of smoking, greater increases in smoking, larger increase in obesity, and higher level of sedentary behavior compared with adults from 25 to 74 years of age.[17]

Environment

- It is helpful to get a picture of the adolescent's day including place and time of eating, structured and unstructured activity, screen time, homework, and job and home responsibilities.
- Working with late adolescents and young adults on strategies to buffer an obesity-promoting environment is important and independent living or entrance to college can be opportunities to have this interaction.

10.3 Intervention

When an adolescent has a BMI greater than 85% and less than 95% or is crossing growth percentiles in an upward direction, it is time for a more in-depth look at eating and activity, especially related to unregulated eating, increase in sedentary time, and poor food choices—all of which can contribute to the risk of becoming an obese adult. In addition to reemphasizing concepts covered previously, teens and families may need to give increased attention to their ability to provide and influence nutrition and activity by focusing on **energy balance, structure,** and **modeling healthy behavior.**

Energy Balance

Change in lifestyle and increased pressures of college, work, and social life may cause shifts in energy balance that are not immediately apparent to the teen. Self-assessment is important; diet and activity records can be a start to focus attention on day-to-day choices. Connections between eating and study habits, workplace environments, and social eating are all important to tease out to allow the teen to begin making conscious choices about nutrition and activity.

Structure

Older adolescents and young adults are becoming increasingly independent of family meal structure, have irregular work hours, and are often juggling the demands of school, work, and social lives. Energy balance may have as much to do with time management as unhealthy eating choices and sedentary behavior. Teens may see increased freedom at college as meaning the absence of structure and may need help seeing that working on scheduling meals, activity, and sleep may help correct a weight gain.

Modeling Healthy Behavior

It is important to ask a teen what is being used as a model for decision making about eating and activity. This can be a thought-provoking question and stimulate discussion about healthy behaviors. In a teen that is already overweight, it is important to continue discussion about health risks and family history, exploring models of health behavior they were exposed to as children as a basis for taking care of their own health.

10.4 Treatment

When a teen's BMI is greater than 95% and you are dealing with excess adiposity, it is time to initiate a focused treatment strategy. It is important to review the issues discussed in the previous 2 sections because these are building blocks of good nutrition and activity habits. But you will also have to focus on the barriers to change that may have prevented parents, families, and teens from implementing these strategies.

A useful way to begin is to obtain a family history focused on obesity-related comorbidities. This can serve to emphasis the health risks involved and the necessity of taking early action once obesity is identified.

10.5 Family History

Family history should be updated at this time with attention to obesity-related comorbidities, the family weight trajectory, eating behaviors, and mental health diagnosis. (See page 163.)

10.6 Review of Systems

The review of systems can also serve as a point of departure to discuss obesity-related comorbidities, pointing out particular risk factors as they relate to increasing BMI.

- Skin: Acanthosis nigricans, striae, acne
- Head, eyes, ears, nose, and throat (HEENT): Headache, snoring, sleep disturbance, daytime napping, attention problems, poor school functioning, irritability, visual disturbance
- Lungs: Asthma, shortness of breath during exercise, cough at end of exercise, decreased exercise tolerance, smoking
- Cardiac: Hypertension, hyperlipidemia
- Abdomen: Gastroesophageal reflux, stomach pain before or after eating, chronic diarrhea or constipation, morning anorexia, right upper quadrant discomfort or pain
- Musculoskeletal: Limping, hip pain or decreased motion, knee pain, bowing, ankle pain
- Genitourinary: Enuresis, delayed pubertal development
- Psychological: Symptoms of depression, anxiety, low self-esteem, self-injury or suicidal ideation, sleep disturbance

10.7 Physical Examination

- Height
- Weight
- BMI + previous BMI measurements
- Blood pressure

- General: Height deceleration or poor linear growth, centripetal or visceral fat distribution
- Skin: Acanthosis nigricans (neck, axilla, groin), acne, cervical fat pad, striae

Family History, Late Adolescent and Young Adult

Complete or update this family history targeted toward obesity and related comorbidities.

	Mother	Father	Maternal Grandmother	Maternal Grandfather	Paternal Grandmother	Paternal Grandfather	Sibling 1	Sibling 2
Obesity	☐	☐	☐	☐	☐	☐	☐	☐
Cardiovascular disease	☐	☐	☐	☐	☐	☐	☐	☐
High blood pressure	☐	☐	☐	☐	☐	☐	☐	☐
Stroke	☐	☐	☐	☐	☐	☐	☐	☐
High cholesterol	☐	☐	☐	☐	☐	☐	☐	☐
High triglyceride	☐	☐	☐	☐	☐	☐	☐	☐
Type 1 or 2 diabetes	☐	☐	☐	☐	☐	☐	☐	☐
_____	☐	☐	☐	☐	☐	☐	☐	☐
_____	☐	☐	☐	☐	☐	☐	☐	☐
_____	☐	☐	☐	☐	☐	☐	☐	☐
_____	☐	☐	☐	☐	☐	☐	☐	☐
_____	☐	☐	☐	☐	☐	☐	☐	☐

- HEENT: Funduscopic examination for papilledema, tonsillar hypertrophy, thyroid enlargement
- Cardiopulmonary: Wheezing, poor ventilation, heart murmur
- Abdominal: Hepatomegaly
- Musculoskeletal: Range of motion, genu varum, limp, hip or knee pain, ankle pain
- Genitourinary: Tanner stage

10.8 Family Constellation and Social History

Information about where the family and adolescent are in terms of decision making and independence can be helpful in working with the adolescent to individualize lifestyle change.

- Who is living at home with the adolescent?
- Who is responsible for purchasing and preparing meals?
- Does the family eat together?
- How much of a priority is improving nutrition and physical activity to the adolescent?

10.9 Questions for the Family

Family dynamics and communication are important when adolescents are trying to make changes in lifestyle. These questions may help you focus on family factors that may facilitate or hamper change.

	Never	Seldom	Sometimes	Often	Always
1. Parents and adolescent agree on nutritional issues.	☐	☐	☐	☐	☐
2. Parents understand the principles of adolescent development.	☐	☐	☐	☐	☐
3. Parents are interacting with the young adult to guide and support responsible decision making.	☐	☐	☐	☐	☐

10.10 Teen Touch Points

Teen touch points focus on helping teens initiate and maintain change by helping them believe change can occur, identify the change needed, value the outcome of the change, know how to change, and have the energy to change and sustain the change.

- *Believe that change can occur.*
  - Building on success is crucial. Finding ways that succeeded in the past and translating skills and behaviors to weight loss can help the young person feel that change is possible.
  - Engaging a support network is also important because teens often feel that they have to do this alone. Parents, extended family, and friends can all be helpful in encouraging the teen.

- *Identify the change.*
  - The concept of incremental change may still be difficult for the teen to grasp in an environment that may give the message of all or nothing. You may need to work with the young person to get the change down to a doable level.
  - Giving background information about nutrition and activity is important, letting the teen decide where to start the change process.

- *Value the outcome.*
  - It is important to help identify what values underpin decision making in this age group.
  - A teen may be more interested and committed initially to stabilizing weight, reducing cholesterol, or feeling more in control of eating than weight loss.
  - It is important to start "where the patient is" when beginning the treatment process.

- *Know how to change.* Goal setting is important, as is developing a strategy for change. Self-knowledge is a key ingredient of establishing a plan. By this age most young adults know how they operate in the world (planners, procrastinators, analytical, emotional decision makers, influenced by friends, independent). Using this self-knowledge can help you and the teen individualize a pathway of activity and nutrition change.

- *Have energy to change and sustain.* Joining a group engaged in activity, volunteering, or a special interest can provide emotional support for the late adolescent and build positive relationships and skills. Adult weight management groups may be appropriate for some older teens as well. The ability to recognize stress and use stress-management techniques is important, and skill building in this area can be taught.

10.11 Developmental Touch Point

At this stage of development adolescents are working on independence and a positive identity allowing for achievement of goals. Sexual identity is established and close personal friendships and relationships are fostered. Vocational decisions are being considered and individual capabilities are being self-assessed.

10.12 Nutrition and Activity Questions and Interventions

Nutrition and activity questions (see pages 168–169) can be answered by the young adult and provide a focal point for targeted intervention (see pages 170–171) in a brief encounter. Questions answered "Often" or "Always" can be targeted first for change. For example, if the young adult answered questions 1, 7, 9, and 13 on pages 168 and 169 with "Often" or "Always," you would ask him or her to rate the difficulty of change for questions 1, 7, 9, and 13 on pages 170 and 171.

10.13 A Case in Point: BL

BL is a 17-year-old white girl who comes with her mother to your office because her mother is concerned about her weight. BL has been overweight since the beginning of first grade; her current weight is 236 lb (107.0 kg) and height is 5'6" (167.6 cm). You calculate her BMI and it is 38.1.

When you ask BL if she is concerned about her weight, she says a fairly emphatic, "No."

BL is a good student, a junior in high school, planning on majoring in English in college. She is not in any extracurricular activities, likes to read, and had in the past been involved in several school plays.

You take a family history and find that Mother's cholesterol was 245 mg/dL before she started taking medication. Father has treated hypertension and the paternal grandfather has had a myocardial infarction and bypass surgery.

BL's review of systems except for her weight is essentially negative. On physical examination you find her blood pressure is elevated at 124/82 mm Hg and she has a minor degree of abdominal striae, but otherwise it is a negative physical examination.

You have asked BL to fill out the questions in section 10.12 and she has answered "Often" or "Always" to

4. Eat a school lunch and snacks at schools.
10. Don't eat any vegetables.
13. Skip breakfast.
18. Have mainly sedentary leisure activities.

When you ask how easy it would be for BL to change any of these behaviors she fills out "Impossible" or "Could try" for all of them, saying she really is not concerned about her weight and doesn't feel she needs to change anything.

Mother feels that BL's weight is keeping her from doing the things she should be doing at her age such as dating and being more involved in extracurricular and social activities. Mother is also worried about what it will be like at college for BL unless she learns to make better food choices.

You acknowledge BL's and Mother's feelings. You point out that obesity-related comorbidities are in BL's family history and that BL's blood pressure is elevated. You express your concerns about BL's current and future health and ask her to get laboratory studies to further evaluate her health status. She agrees, as does her mother, and you give them an appointment to come back in 3 to 4 weeks and review the laboratory work.

Second Visit

BL returns and her weight is unchanged. You have received BL's laboratory studies, which are all normal except for elevated total cholesterol of 276 mg/dL and a low high-density lipoprotein (HDL) of 34 mg/dL.

You begin the visit by reviewing the laboratory data and elevated cholesterol as well as the positive family history for hypercholesterolemia and heart disease. BL is somewhat upset by having a high cholesterol and asks

Nutrition and Activity Questions, Late Adolescent and Young Adult

These questions can be answered by the young adult and provide a focal point for targeted intervention in a brief encounter. First have the young adult answer these questions about the presence or absence of behaviors that promote weight gain, then refer to Nutrition and Activity Interventions, Late Adolescent and Young Adult.

	Never	Seldom	Sometimes	Often	Always
1. Drink juice or sugared beverages between meals.	☐	☐	☐	☐	☐
2. Eat junk food.	☐	☐	☐	☐	☐
3. Eat more than 1 snack between meals a day.	☐	☐	☐	☐	☐
4. Eat a school lunch and snacks at school.	☐	☐	☐	☐	☐
5. Feel bad about myself after I eat.	☐	☐	☐	☐	☐
6. Eat at fast-food restaurants.	☐	☐	☐	☐	☐
7. Get my own meals and snacks.	☐	☐	☐	☐	☐
8. Eat alone at dinner.	☐	☐	☐	☐	☐
9. Crave sweets or snacks even right after eating a meal.	☐	☐	☐	☐	☐
10. Don't eat any vegetables.	☐	☐	☐	☐	☐

	Never	Seldom	Sometimes	Often	Always
11. Overeat after school.	☐	☐	☐	☐	☐
12. Eat in front of the television or computer.	☐	☐	☐	☐	☐
13. Skip breakfast.	☐	☐	☐	☐	☐
14. Have difficulty making healthy food choices when eating out at restaurants or with friends.	☐	☐	☐	☐	☐
15. Eat when bored.	☐	☐	☐	☐	☐
16. Watch more than 2 hours of television or the computer each day.	☐	☐	☐	☐	☐
17. Have no outside time.	☐	☐	☐	☐	☐
18. Have mainly sedentary leisure activities.	☐	☐	☐	☐	☐
19. Am unmotivated to get active.	☐	☐	☐	☐	☐
20. Lack interest in peer or extracurricular activities.	☐	☐	☐	☐	☐

Nutrition and Activity Interventions, Late Adolescent and Young Adult

Questions answered "Often" or "Always" in Nutrition and Activity Questions, Late Adolescent and Young Adult, can be targeted first for change. Using these specific questions, ask the young adult, "How difficult would it be for you to...?"

	Impossible	Could try	Could do sometimes	Could do most of the time	Easy
1. Change from soda or juice to water or diet drinks between meals.	☐	☐	☐	☐	☐
2. Eliminate junk food.	☐	☐	☐	☐	☐
3. Pack a school lunch and snacks.	☐	☐	☐	☐	☐
4. Eat vegetables instead of second helpings.	☐	☐	☐	☐	☐
5. Begin to think about strategies to control my eating.	☐	☐	☐	☐	☐
6. Decrease fast food.	☐	☐	☐	☐	☐
7. Pack healthier school snacks.	☐	☐	☐	☐	☐
8. Try to eat dinner meal with family.	☐	☐	☐	☐	☐
9. Keep only healthy snacks in the house.	☐	☐	☐	☐	☐
10. Eat vegetables at meals.	☐	☐	☐	☐	☐

	Impossible	Could try	Could do sometimes	Could do most of the time	Easy
11. Pack a snack for after school; limit purchase of snack foods.	☐	☐	☐	☐	☐
12. Turn off the television during meals and snacks.	☐	☐	☐	☐	☐
13. Eat on-the-run breakfast choices.	☐	☐	☐	☐	☐
14. Work on planning choices in advance.	☐	☐	☐	☐	☐
15. Think of other activities to engage in when hungry between meals.	☐	☐	☐	☐	☐
16. Reduce television time.	☐	☐	☐	☐	☐
17. Include 30 minutes of outdoor activity in my day.	☐	☐	☐	☐	☐
18. Learn a lifetime activity or increase activities of daily living.	☐	☐	☐	☐	☐
19. Find a family member or friend who can partner in a physical activity.	☐	☐	☐	☐	☐
20. Join a peer group activity.	☐	☐	☐	☐	☐

what she can do about it. Mother reiterates her concern about BL's weight and eating habits. You review the positive family history for hypercholesterolemia and heart disease.

You go back to BL's original questionnaire and point out that school lunches and snacks are generally high in fats and calories, both of which can contribute to elevations in cholesterol, and mention that vegetables are a natural source of fiber that can also help lower cholesterol. You ask if BL could pack a lunch or make a healthier choice at school and she says she thinks she can. You ask BL if she can think of a way she can start to eat more vegetables; she mentions she could eat salad, and you ask Mother to provide salad ingredients instead of snack food for BL's after-school snack. She agrees.

You give BL a diet and activity record to fill out and some background information on recommended food groups and portion sizes and ask BL to schedule a return visit in 1 month.

Third Visit

BL comes back with her diet and activity records. Her weight is 234 lb (106.1 kg), her height is 5'6" (167.6 cm), and her blood pressure is 120/79 mm Hg. Her review of systems and physical examination are unremarkable. She has been packing a lunch most of the time and is not having any problems with this change. She started out eating a salad after school but has been drifting to the snack food her brother eats. Mother is impatient with her and BL says she has been nagging her a lot.

You review BL's choices and reinforce the positive changes she has made. You note her lower weight and blood pressure and encourage her to continue. You reassure Mother that BL is making progress and to try to stay positive. You order a repeat cholesterol test to be done right before her next visit in 4 to 5 weeks.

Fourth Visit

BL returns with her laboratory work. Her cholesterol is 252 mg/dL and HDL is 35 mg/dL. Her weight is 232 lb (105.2 kg) and blood pressure is 120/80 mm Hg. BL's diet records show that she is packing her lunch and has been able to eat salad most days after school. She has also become involved in Spanish club at school. You reinforce BL's positive changes, but Mother notes that she should be doing more, taking more responsibility, and that her weight is not changing enough. You encourage Mother, pointing out that this is the first time since BL was in first grade that she has lost weight.

You ask BL if she is ready to make any more changes and she says she is because she would like to get her cholesterol down. She shares that she is worried about the family history of heart attacks. You review her initial questions and ask if she could begin eating a nonsugared cereal for breakfast. You also go over some ways she could increase her activities of daily living, such as walking around the block before coming in from the bus stop after school, taking on dog-walking chores, and thinking about increasing her walking when she is out with friends. She thinks she will try these ideas and you ask her to schedule an appointment in 4 to 5 weeks.

Fifth Visit

This visit BL comes by herself, having just turned 18. She brings diet records and notes that her mother is still nagging her all the time about her weight and eating habits. BL's weight on this visit is 231 lb (104.8 kg) and her blood pressure is 120/82 mm Hg. Her review of systems and physical examination are normal. You note that she has been eating breakfast and walking off and on. You spend some time talking to BL about how she is handling her mother's nagging. She said it bothers her and she often gets stubborn and eats what she knows she shouldn't. You ask about her own goals for herself and she says she is used to her weight so it doesn't bother her that much, but having her cholesterol normal is important to her. You ask if she can make the changes you have talked about "for her" and not her mother, and schedule her next visit in 6 weeks with repeat laboratory studies.

Sixth Visit

BL comes back with her laboratory values, which show a cholesterol level of 226 mg/dL and HDL cholesterol of 38 mg/dL with a blood pressure of 118/76 mm Hg. Her weight is 225 lb (102.1 kg). She has gotten a summer job at the local mall and is walking with friends during their break. She has been eating breakfast and packing a lunch and notes that she has been making healthy choices when going out with friends. She is pleased with the results of her laboratory work and asks you to write the results down so she can show her mother. She is looking forward to her senior year and you schedule her next visit for 6 to 8 weeks.

References

1. Whitaker RC, Wright JA, Pepe MS, Seidel KD, Dietz WH. Predicting obesity in young adulthood from childhood and parental obesity. *N Engl J Med.* 1997;337:869–873

2. Gortmaker SL, Must A, Perrin JM, Sobol AM, Dietz WH. Social and economic consequences of overweight in adolescence and young adulthood. *N Engl J Med.* 1993;329:1008–1012

3. Warman JL. The application of laparoscopic bariatric surgery for treatment of severe obesity in adolescents using a multidisciplinary adolescent bariatric program. *Crit Care Nurs Q.* 2005;28:276–287

4. Engeland A, Bjorge T, Sogaard AJ, Tverdal A. Body mass index in adolescence in relation to total mortality: 32-year follow-up of 227,000 Norwegian boys and girls. *Am J Epidemiol.* 2003;157:517–523

5. Goodman E, Whitaker RC. A prospective study of the role of depression in the development and persistence of adolescent obesity. *Pediatrics.* 2002; 110:497–504

6. Strauss CC, Smith K, Frame C, Forehand R. Personal and interpersonal characteristics associated with childhood obesity. *J Pediatr Psychol.* 1985; 10:337–343

7. Stunkard A, Mendelson M. Obesity and body image. 1. Characteristics of disturbances in the body image of some obese persons. *Am J Psychiatry.* 1967;123:1296–1300

8. Sargent JD, Blanchflower DG. Obesity and stature in adolescence and earnings in young adulthood. Analysis of a British birth cohort. *Arch Pediatr Adolesc Med.* 1994;148:681–687

9. Dietz WH. Childhood weight affects adult morbidity and mortality. *J Nutr.* 1998;128(2Suppl):411S–414S

10. Centers for Disease Control and Prevention. Overweight among students in grades K-12—Arkansas, 2003-04 and 2004-05 school years. *MMWR Morb Mortal Wkly Rep.* 2006;55:5–8

11. Levitsky DA, Garay J, Nausbaum M, Neighbors L, Dellavalle DM. Monitoring weight daily blocks the freshman weight gain: a model for combating the epidemic of obesity. *In J Obes (Lond).* 2006;30:1003–1010

12. Gangwisch JE, Malaspina D, Boden-Albala B, Heymsfield SB. Inadequate sleep as a risk factor for obesity: analyses of the NHANES I. *Sleep.* 2005;28:1289–1296

13. Pereira MA, Kartashov AI, Ebbeling CB, et al. Fast-food habits, weight gain, and insulin resistance (the CARDIA study): 15-year prospective analysis. *Lancet.* 2005;365:36–42

14. WIN Weight-Control Information Network (NIDDK). Binge eating disorder. Available at: win.niddk.nih.gov/publications/binge.htm. Accessed June 21, 2006

15. American Academy of Pediatrics Committee on Adolescence. Identifying and treating eating disorders. *Pediatrics.* 2003;111:204–211

16. Franko DL, Striegel-Moore RH, Thompson D, Schreiber GB, Daniels SR. Does adolescent depression predict obesity in black and white young adult women? *Psychol Med.* 2005;35:1505–1513

17. Winkleby MA, Cubbin C. Changing patterns in health behaviors and risk factors related to chronic diseases, 1990-2000. *Am J Health Promot.* 2004;19:19–27

Obesity Health Strategies for Practices: Identification, Prevention, Intervention, and Treatment

11.1 Practice Interventions

Every pediatrician will need to address obesity in his or her practice. Pediatric subspecialists are currently engaged in treating the comorbidities of obesity—type 2 diabetes, nonalcoholic steatohepatitis, hypertension and hyperlipidemia, sleep apnea, and polycystic ovarian disease—previously seen only in adults. Hospitalists are caring for seriously ill obese patients and need to prepare to treat obesity-related disease in an inpatient setting. Primary care pediatricians will need to be able to increase their practice capacity to carry out identification, prevention, intervention, and treatment of the obese child and family.

11.2 Identification of Weight Status

Risk Factors

No physician should miss the opportunity to identify the obesity risk status of a child or an adolescent. Risk for obesity can be increased by parental obesity,[1] a history of maternal diabetes,[2] intrauterine growth retardation,[3] and obesity-associated genetic syndromes.[4] Questions about these factors should be routinely incorporated into every child's medical history.

Body Mass Index

Calculating and categorizing a patient's body mass index (BMI) is essential and every child should have BMI and BMI percentile routinely measured and plotted on the BMI curve.[5] Practice patterns should be addressed to incorporate this into the staff's routine. Sharing growth and BMI charts with parents and families is a first step toward bringing up the issue of healthy growth and opening the door to discussion of family patterns of nutrition, activity, and sedentary behavior.

11.3 Prevention

The extent and severity of the obesity epidemic dictates that practice strategies need to be put in place to incorporate obesity prevention into the office routine. Pediatricians and other health care professionals can provide parents and patients with information about the etiology of obesity, developmentally appropriate nutrition and activity balance, and family-based lifestyle change. Adolescents perceive their providers as valuable sources of information about weight.[6] Research on primary care prevention of obesity is still evolving, but some basic recommendations can be made.

Promote Breastfeeding

Breastfeeding should be encouraged and supported for all newborns.[7]

- Pediatricians can advocate for breastfeeding-friendly hospitals.
- Provide lactation support for all mothers, especially mothers who are obese, to encourage initiation and maintenance.
- Encourage mothers and families who formula feed to recognize satiety cues.

Encourage Healthy Eating

Families should be provided with guidelines that explain age-appropriate food group composition, servings, and portions sizes.

- Fruit and vegetable consumption should be increased to meet dietary requirements (5 servings a day).[5]
- Parents and families should be encouraged to model healthy eating.
- Parents should choose what is available to eat at meals and snacks but allow children to choose whether to eat and how much to eat.[5]

Limit Juice and Sugar-Sweetened Beverages

The American Academy of Pediatrics (AAP) recommends that intake of juice be limited, with the following specific suggestions[8]:

- Juice should not be introduced into the diet of infants before 6 months of age.

- Infants should not be given juice from bottles or easily transportable covered cups that allow them to consume juice easily throughout the day. Infants should not be given juice at bedtime.

- Intake of fruit juice should be limited to 4 to 6 oz a day for children 1 to 6 years old. For children 7 to 18 years old, juice intake should be limited to 8 to 12 oz or 2 servings per day.

- Children should be encouraged to eat whole fruits to meet their recommended daily fruit intake.

- The consumption of sugar-sweetened beverages should be reduced.[9]

Reduce Screen Time

Studies in school interventions have shown that reduction in screen time (eg, television, computer) can prevent obesity.[10,11] The AAP recommends[12]

- Limiting children's total time with entertainment media to no more than 1 to 2 hours of quality programming per day

- Removing television sets from children's bedrooms

- Discouraging television viewing for children younger than 2 years and encouraging more interactive activities that will promote proper brain development, such as talking, playing, singing, and reading together

- Encouraging alternative entertainment for children, including reading, athletics, hobbies, and creative play

Encourage Physical Activity

Physical activity is part of healthy development in children and lays the groundwork for lifelong habits that will support activity in adulthood. The AAP recommends encouraging physical activity as part of an obesity-prevention strategy.[13]

- Determine physical activity levels of the child and family members at regular health care visits.

- Encourage children and adolescents to be physically active for at least 60 minutes per day, which may be accumulated by using smaller increments.

- Events should be of moderate intensity and include a wide variety of activities as part of sports, recreation, transportation, chores, work, planned exercise, and school-based physical education classes. These activities should be primarily unstructured and fun if they are to achieve best compliance.
- Identify any barriers the child, youth, or parent might have against increasing physical activity, which might include lack of time, competing interests, perceived lack of motor skills, and fear of injury on the part of the child.
- Parents might be additionally concerned about financial and safety issues. Efforts must be made to work with the family to educate them on the importance of lifelong physical activity and identify potential strategies to overcome some of their barriers.
- Advise parents to support their child or youth in developmentally and age-appropriate sports and recreational activities. The child's favorite types of physical activity should be a priority. These might best occur in the school setting during extracurricular activities, in which parents or grandparents can take part as leaders and coaches.
- Recommend that parents become good role models by increasing their own level of physical activity. Parents should also incorporate physical activities that family members of all ages and abilities can do together.
- Parents should encourage children to play outside as much as possible. Safety should be promoted by the use of appropriate protective equipment (eg, bicycle helmets, life jackets).

These obesity prevention messages should permeate the practice and be delivered at every opportunity.

11.4 Intervention

When a child or teen has a BMI greater than 85% and less then 95% or is crossing growth percentiles in an upward direction, these prevention messages should be intensified. At this point, recommended nutrition and activity lifestyle changes should be coupled with strategies to help parents and families implement them. Several strategies are recommended to help regain control of excess weight gain, including controlling the nutrition and activity environments, setting goals, monitoring behavior, rewarding success, problem solving, and parenting skills.[6]

Controlling the Nutrition and Activity Environments

Micromanaging eating and activity behaviors can be exhausting for families. Family-based environmental change can set new norms for eating and activity that do not need to be renegotiated every time. Examples of managing the environment include

- Eliminating sugar-sweetened beverages from the home
- Increasing the number of meals prepared at home
- Serving food restaurant style—placing appropriate portions on the plate—rather than family style with serving dishes on the table
- Reducing screen time to 2 hours a day for children and family members older than 2 years
- Not eating in front of the television
- Removing the television from the bedroom
- Planning after-school time to include activities and outdoor time

Setting Goals

Help the family set incremental, achievable goals for behavior change in a setting that allows discussion between family members and the pediatrician.

- Goals can be environmental and involve parental behavior.
- Goals can be individual, such as a child committing to spending time outdoors every day or joining one after-school activity.
- Goals can be relational, such as parents and child agreeing to partner with each other on a daily walk or parents increasing praise of the child for following the television schedule.

Monitoring Behavior

Monitoring behavior helps families stay on course with change. Monitoring should occur in a setting where behavior can be discussed in a nonjudgmental way. This will allow setbacks to be identified and needed changes to occur. Examples of monitoring could include keeping track of

- Sugar-sweetened beverages consumed each day
- An activity log
- Screen time
- Outdoor time
- Parents' success in achieving environmental change

Rewarding Success

Managing weight is hard work; parents and families can become focused on what is not being done and forget to reward their successes. Reminding parents to praise and give attention to the positive can help fuel the next steps toward change. For example,

- Rewards should be for short-term gains, ie, something done that day.
- Parents should let the child know what behaviors will be rewarded and how and be consistent.
- Reward with time, attention, and activity.

Problem Solving

Skills families need most are the ones that enable them to evaluate progress, identify problems, come up with solutions, and try out new behaviors. This is similar to the Deming cycle of plan, do, study, act used in quality improvement. Examples of issues that require problem solving are

- After-school hunger
- Emotional eating
- Resistance to change
- Parties
- Eating out
- Eating with friends

Parenting Skills

Initiating and maintaining lifestyle change requires parenting skills. Firm, consistent parenting that supports the child's autonomy and self-sufficiency while setting appropriate boundaries is likely to be the most effective parenting strategy. Parents willing to partner with their child, communicate expectations, and reward progress allow weight management to occur in a positive setting. Examples of helpful parenting skills include

- Setting reasonable boundaries and allowing children to choose within those boundaries
- Setting limits and saying no in a reasonable, consistent way
- Modeling the expected behaviors
- Communicating expectations clearly in a developmentally appropriate manner

Strategies for accomplishing this work in a practice setting need to be developed. Additional visits, group visits, use of nursing personnel, nutritionists, and psychologists can all be considered.

11.5 Treatment

A BMI greater than 95% for age and gender has a high likelihood of identifying obesity in a child with a high correlation with increased adiposity.[14] At this point 3 things must occur: screening for obesity-related comorbidities, treatment of obesity, and treatment of any identified comorbidities.

Screening for Obesity-Related Comorbidities

Appropriate history, review of systems, physical examination, and laboratory testing need to be part of the practice routine when obesity is identified. Remember that presence of one comorbid condition does not rule out additional comorbidities and signs and symptoms of many may be present at the same time (Table 11.1).

In addition to comorbidities, obesity-related emergencies can also occur (see Chapter 1, section 1.2 for additional information).

Treatment of Obesity

The preventive and intervention approaches discussed previously should be intensified in the treatment of the obese child and family. Specific randomized controlled trials for obesity treatment were evaluated by the Cochrane Review.[15]

- Interventions with the main focus on changes in physical activity and sedentary behavior
- Interventions in which the main focus was behavioral therapy compared with usual care or no treatment
- Interventions comparing behavior therapy at varying degrees of family involvement
- Interventions comparing cognitive behavioral therapy with relaxation
- Interventions comparing behavioral therapy with mastery criteria and contingent reinforcement
- Interventions comparing problem solving with usual care or behavioral therapy

Table 11.1. Screening and Treatment for Obesity-Related Comorbidities

Type 2 Diabetes

History	Maternal diabetes during pregnancy, small for gestational age, intrauterine growth retardation, family history of diabetes
Review of systems	Polyuria; polydipsia; nocturia; recurrent vaginal, bladder, or other infections; recent weight loss
Physical examination	Acanthosis nigricans
Laboratory	Elevated fasting glucose, glycosuria, positive glucose tolerance test, hyperinsulinemia
Treatment	Referral to pediatric endocrinologist for treatment with metformin or insulin and lifestyle change

Nonalcoholic Steatohepatitis

History	No specific history; some cases have other family members affected
Review of systems	Possible nausea and right upper quadrant discomfort
Physical examination	Hepatomegaly
Laboratory/imaging	Elevated serum aminotransferases, echogenicity of liver on ultrasound
Treatment	Referral to pediatric gastroenterologist for evaluation and definitive diagnosis, weight loss

Hypertension

History	Family history of hypertension or other obesity-related comorbidity
Review of systems	Usually asymptomatic
Physical examination	Elevated systolic and/or diastolic blood pressure
Laboratory/imaging	Evaluation for other causes of hypertension as indicated
Treatment	Referral to pediatric hypertension specialist, dietary treatment, pharmacologic treatment

Dyslipidemia

History	Family history of lipid disorders, cardiovascular disease
Review of systems	Asymptomatic; other obesity comorbidities, particularly signs of metabolic syndrome
Physical examination	No specific signs; acanthosis nigricans may indicate metabolic syndrome
Laboratory/imaging	Lipid panel
Treatment	Referral to lipid specialist, dietary management

Sleep Apnea

History	Family history of sleep apnea
Review of systems	Snoring, snoring with apnea, daytime tiredness, napping, poor concentration in school, enuresis
Physical examination	Large tonsils or adenoids
Laboratory/imaging	Nighttime polysomnography
Treatment	Referral to pediatric pulmonologist, weight loss

Slipped Capital Femoral Epiphysis

History	Knee or hip pain
Review of systems	Knee or hip pain, limp
Physical examination	Limp, pain in knee or hip
Laboratory/imaging	Hip and knee films
Treatment	Immediate referral to pediatric orthopedist

Blount Disease

History	Bowing
Review of systems	Bowing (tibia vera), knee pain, limp
Physical examination	Bowing, knee pain, limp
Laboratory/imaging	Knee films
Treatment	Referral to pediatric orthopedist

Table 11.1. Screening and Treatment for Obesity-Related Comorbidities, continued

Depression	
History	Family history of depression, history of abuse, psychological trauma, teasing, low self-esteem
Review of systems	Loss of interest, anger, irritability, sadness, suicidal ideation
Physical examination	No signs; may have sad, irritable appearance with lack of self-care
Laboratory/imaging	None
Treatment	Mental health referral for counseling or pharmacologic treatment

Interventions With the Main Focus on Changes in Physical Activity and Sedentary Behavior

Increasing exercise has been a therapeutic strategy in the treatment of obesity; however, few randomized controlled trials have been performed.[15] In a study reviewed by the Cochrane report, obese girls had exercise added to a family-based dietary weight control program.[16] Both groups lost weight, but the exercise group had significantly larger decreases in percent overweight at 6 months; however, this difference did not persist at 12 months. Children in the exercise group had supervised exercise 3 times a week that changed to walking 3 miles with a parent 3 times a week in the maintenance phase.[16] In another reviewed study, exercise was found to increase fat-free mass in a group of adolescents when added to an intervention providing dietary advice.[17]

Exercise has been found to confer a metabolic benefit in obese children, with reductions of adiponectin after a 3-month exercise intervention that also lowered fat mass, insulin resistance, and hyperinsulinemia without significantly altering weight.[18]

Lifestyle activities have been defined as "…interventions [which] allow a person to individualize his/her physical activity programs to include a wide variety of activities that are at least of moderate intensity and to accumulate bouts of these activities in a manner befitting his/her life circumstances."[19] In a randomized controlled study evaluated by the Cochrane review,[15] lifestyle exercise was compared with aerobic exercise and low-intensity calisthenics as an intervention for obesity in 5- to 8-year-old children. All groups were trained in behavioral-therapy–type strategies and all children lost weight during the active treatment period. Lifestyle exercise was found to result in significantly lower percent overweight than in children in the aerobic and calisthenic group.[20]

Decreasing sedentary behavior is also one of the strategies applied to treat obesity in children and has been shown to result in decreased percent overweight.[21] In a study of 8- to 12-year-old obese children, exercise was compared with decreasing sedentary behavior. Parents decreased sedentary behavior by limiting television watching cues (eg, turning television to the wall) and providing physical activity equipment. Children self-monitored their physical activity. At the end of 1 year children in the group that decreased sedentary behavior had greater decreases in percentage overweight and percentage body fat versus the exercise and combined groups. The children whose sedentary activity was decreased also had lower caloric intake and increased likely for high-intensity exercise than those children in the exercise group. All children had increased fitness at the end of the study.

Another study of obese 8- to 12-year-olds compared increased physical activity with decreased sedentary behavior.[22] There were no differences between groups, but both groups showed decreases in percent overweight as a result of the intervention. These studies would suggest that increasing exercise, including lifestyle exercise, and strategies to reduce sedentary time are valuable and necessary additions to obesity treatment plans.

Interventions in Which the Main Focus Was Behavioral Therapy Compared With Usual Care or No Treatment

Obesity treatment plans in children rely on family-based lifestyle change and need to include a behavioral component. Several randomized controlled trials[15] have shown a positive effect when behavioral therapy is added to the intervention. In a study of 5- to 8-year-old obese girls, behavioral treatment (ie, training in self-monitoring, praise, modeling, contracting) was compared with an educational intervention.[20] At 12 months there were significant differences in percent overweight in the behavioral group compared with the educational intervention.

In another study, a behavioral intervention for obese children 6 to 13 years of age was compared to a waiting list control group with no intervention.[23] Both behavioral groups had significantly greater decreases in percent overweight than the control group, but were not different from each other.

An evaluation of the Shapedown program for adolescents showed that a 15-month intervention significantly improved relative weight, weight-related behavior, and depression at 1 year compared with a control group.[24]

In a different study, a comparison was made between obese children in a control group who had medical checkups, dietitian advice, and negotiated changes in dietary behavior and a group who had the addition of family therapy to the conventional treatment. Children in the family therapy group had a smaller increase in BMI and reduced skinfold thickness over 18 months than the conventional group.[25] There was no difference between the conventional therapy group and control group.

Interventions Comparing Behavior Therapy at Varying Degrees of Family Involvement

Parent involvement has been found to be important. When parent behavioral training was added to a multicomponent behavioral weight management program involving obese 8- to 12-year-olds and their parents, there was a greater decrease in percent overweight than in a group without the parent training.[26]

Parents have been found to be more effective as the exclusive agents of changes than when children are responsible for their own weight loss, with greater weight reduction in the parent-only intervention group.[27–29]

When child self-regulation was emphasized in a parent-child multi-component behavioral weight management program, there was a trend toward decreased gain in percent overweight over a 3-year period in the child self-regulation group.[30]

No difference was found in a study of African American girls aged 14 years in a weight management program between treating the child alone, mother and child in the same session, or mother and child in different sessions.[31]

Interventions Comparing Cognitive Behavioral Therapy With Relaxation

The addition of cognitive behavioral therapy did not seem to make a difference in outcome when added to standard behavioral-therapy weight management programs in the studies included in the Cochrane review.[15] In obese children 7 to 13 years of age both groups at 6 months had significant reduction in percent overweight but were not different from each other.[32]

A second study was a 6-week patient rehabilitation program for children and adolescents. Both groups—the standard behavioral group and one with added cognitive behavioral therapy—had significant weight loss at 6 weeks and 1 year but were not different from each other.[33]

Interventions Comparing Behavioral Therapy With Mastery Criteria and Contingent Reinforcement

Addition of mastery of parenting skills to standard behavior change strategies was compared with the standard therapy over 26 weekly and 6 monthly meetings in a group of obese children. Weight loss was better at 1 year in the parenting skills group, but there was no difference between groups at 2 years.[34]

Interventions Comparing Problem Solving With Usual Care or Behavioral Therapy

Family involvement is important in any obesity treatment plan.[5] Specific strategies of including problem-solving skills in the obesity intervention have been reviewed.[15] In a study to investigate the effect of including problem-solving training in a weight-loss group,[35] parents were trained in problem-solving exercises related to weight control in addition to receiving training in self-monitoring, stimulus control strategies, family support, cognitive restructuring, peer relations, and maintenance strategies as well as diet and exercise information that was also received by the control group. A third group received only instructional materials. Six months after the 8-week intervention the problem-solving and behavioral groups had significantly decreased their percent overweight compared with the instruction-only group. Children in the problem-solving group had significantly greater decreases in percent overweight than children in the behavioral group.[35] Results of another study showed no difference between groups in a family-based behavioral program and either child or child-parent teaching of problem solving.[36]

As a result of this review, the Cochrane reviewers stated that practitioners need to consider issues that affect sustainability and environmental change while addressing behavior change in a complex set of circumstances in which families currently find themselves. Family involvement and support of families is crucial.[15]

References

1. Whitaker RC, Wright JA, Pepe MS, Seidel KD, Dietz WH. Predicting obesity in young adulthood from childhood and parental obesity. *N Engl J Med.* 1997;337:869–873

2. Pettitt DJ, Aleck KA, Baird HR, Carraher MJ, Bennett PH, Knowler WC. Congenital susceptibility to NIDDM. Role of intrauterine environment. *Diabetes.* 1988;37:622–628

3. Gluckman PD, Hanson MA. The consequences of being born small—an adaptive perspective. *Horm Res.* 2006;65(Suppl 3):5–14

4. Hassink S. Problems in childhood obesity. In: Bray GA, ed. *Office Management of Childhood Obesity.* Philadelphia, PA: Saunders; 2004:73–90

5. Dietz WH, Robinson TN. Clinical practice. Overweight children and adolescents. *N Engl J Med.* 2005;352:2100–2109

6. Marks A, Malizio J, Hoch J, Brody R, Fisher M. Assessment of health needs and willingness to utilize health care resources of adolescents in a suburban population. *J Pediatr.* 1983;102:456–460

7. Arenz S, Ruckerl R, Koletzko B, von Kries R. Breast-feeding and childhood obesity—a systematic review. *Int J Obes Relat Metab Disord.* 2004;28:1247–1256

8. American Academy of Pediatrics Committee on Nutrition. The use and misuse of fruit juice in pediatrics. *Pediatrics.* 2001;107:1210–1213

9. Ludwig DS, Peterson KE, Gortmaker SL. Relation between consumption of sugar-sweetened drinks and childhood obesity: a prospective, observational analysis. *Lancet.* 2001;357:505–508

10. Robinson TN. Reducing children's television viewing to prevent obesity: a randomized controlled trial. *JAMA.* 1999;282:1561–1567

11. Gortmaker SL, Peterson K, Wiecha J, et al. Reducing obesity via a school-based interdisciplinary intervention among youth: Planet Health. *Arch Pediatr Adolesc Med.* 1999;153:409–418

12. American Academy of Pediatrics Committee on Public Education. Children, adolescents, and television. *Pediatrics.* 2001;107:423–426

13. American Academy of Pediatrics Council on Sports Medicine and Fitness and Council on School Health. Active healthy living: prevention of childhood obesity through increased physical activity. *Pediatrics.* 2006;117:1834–1842

14. Freedman DS, Wang J, Maynard LM, et al. Relation of BMI to fat and fat-free mass among children and adolescents. *Int J Obes (Lond).* 2005;29:1–8

15. Summerbell CD, Ashton V, Campbell KJ, Edmunds L, Kelly S, Waters E. Interventions for treating obesity in children. *Cochrane Database Syst Rev.* 2003;3:CD001872

16. Epstein LH, Wing RR, Penner BC, Kress MJ. Effect of diet and controlled exercise on weight loss in obese children. *J Pediatr.* 1985;107:358–361

17. Schwingshandl J, Sudi K, Eibl B, Wallner S, Borkenstein M. Effect of an individualised training programme during weight reduction on body composition: a randomised trial. *Arch Dis Child.* 1999;81:426–428

18. Balagopal P, George D, Yarandi H, Funanage V, Bayne E. Reversal of obesity-related hypoadiponectinemia by lifestyle intervention: a controlled, randomized study in obese adolescents. *J Clin Endocrinol Metab.* 2005;90:6192–6197

19. Dunn AL, Andersen RE, Jakicic JM. Lifestyle physical activity interventions. Hstory, short- and long-term effects, and recommendations. *Am J Prev Med.* 1998;15:398–412

20. Epstein LH, Wing RR, Woodall K, Penner BC, Kress MJ, Koeske R. Effects of family-based behavioral treatment on obese 5- to 8-year-old children. *Behav Ther.* 1985;16:205–212

21. Epstein LH, Valoski AM, Vara LS, et al. Effects of decreasing sedentary behavior and increasing activity on weight change in obese children. *Health Psychol.* 1995;14:109–115

22. Epstein LH, Paluch RA, Gordy CC, Dorn J. Decreasing sedentary behaviors in treating pediatric obesity. *Arch Pediatr Adolesc Med.* 2000;154:220–226

23. Senediak C, Spence SH. Rapid versus gradual scheduling of therapeutic contact in a family based behavioural weight control programme for children. *Behav Psychother.* 1985;13:265–287

24. Mellin LM, Slinkard LA, Irwin CE. Adolescent obesity intervention: validation of the SHAPEDOWN program. *J Am Diet Assoc.* 1987;87:333–338

25. Flodmark CE, Ohlsson T, Ryden O, Sveger T. Prevention of progression to severe obesity in a group of obese schoolchildren treated with family therapy. *Pediatrics.* 1993;91:880–884

26. Israel AC, Stolmaker L, Andrian CA. The effects of training parents in general child management skills on a behavioral weight loss program for children. *Behav Ther.* 1985;16:169–180

27. Golan M, Fainaru M, Weizman A. Role of behaviour modification in the treatment of childhood obesity with the parents as the exclusive agents of change. *Int J Obes Relat Metab Disord.* 1998;22:1217–1224

28. Golan M, Weizman A, Apter A, Fainaru M. Parents as the exclusive agents of change in the treatment of childhood obesity. *Am J Clin Nutr.* 1998; 67:1130–1135

29. Golan M, Weizman A, Fainaru M. Impact of treatment for childhood obesity on parental risk factors for cardiovascular disease. *Prev Med.* 1999;29:519–526

30. Israel AC, Guile CA, Baker JE, Silverman WK. An evaluation of enhanced self-regulation training in the treatment of childhood obesity. *J Pediatr Psychol.* 1994;19:737–749

31. Wadden TA, Stunkard AJ, Rich L, Rubin CJ, Sweidel G, McKinney S. Obesity in black adolescent girls: a controlled clinical trial of treatment by diet, behavior modification, and parental support. *Pediatrics.* 1990;85:345–352

32. Duffy G, Spence SH. The effectiveness of cognitive self-management as an adjunct to a behavioural intervention for childhood obesity: a research note. *J Child Psychol Psychiatry.* 1993;34:1043–1050

33. Warschburger P, Fromme C, Petermann F, Wojtalla N, Oepen J. Conceptualization and evaluation of a cognitive-behavioural training programme for children and adolescents with obesity. *Int J Obes Relat Disord.* 2001;25(Suppl 1):S93–S95

34. Epstein LH, McKenzie SJ, Valoski A, Klein KR, Wing RR. Effects of mastery criteria and contingent reinforcement for family-based child weight control. *Addict Behav.* 1994;19:135–145

35. Graves T, Meyers AW, Clark L. An evaluation of parental problem-solving training in the behavioral treatment of childhood obesity. *J Consult Clin Psychol.* 1988;56:246–250

36. Epstein LH, Paluch RA, Gordy CC, Saelens BE, Ernst MM. Problem solving in the treatment of childhood obesity. *J Consult Clin Psychol.* 2000;68:717–721

Chapter 12

School and Community Efforts

12.1 The Overweight or Obese Child and the School Setting

Schools provide a daily nutrition and activity environment for more than 95% of US children.[1] A variety of obesity prevention and treatment strategies have been tried in schools, including improving nutrition education, increasing physical activity, television reduction efforts, and decreasing availability of high-calorie drinks and snacks. Somewhat similar to the family setting, issues of access, knowledge, attitudes, beliefs, and behavior play a role in shaping these environments for children. To engage in obesity prevention and treatment, it is important for the pediatrician to understand the role that school is playing in the daily lives of children and their families.

12.2 The Individual Patient

Each obese child will have a unique interaction with the school environment. It is important to understand the particular school-based nutrition and activity factors that affect energy balance in each individual situation.

Access to Food

School breakfast and lunch programs are important to many children. It is critical for families and pediatricians to know what is served, in what portions, and what discretion children have over choices and amounts of foods. School menus can be very helpful, but it is always important to ask the child or adolescent what is actually eaten and what food is left from the school meal. Trading food and buying extra snacks are not unusual behaviors and should be asked about. Some schools use plastic credit cards for food purchases that the parents fund on a monthly basis; asking about how fast this money is being spent can also give an idea of extra food consumption. Meal skipping can occur and disrupt eating patterns. Some children simply don't like what is offered and will wait until they get home to eat or will feel self-conscious about eating in front of others; still others will feel rushed by long lines and little time, grab a snack, and skip a regular meal. It is important to understand these meal patterns so you can help families find solutions. Packing a lunch can be helpful in providing needed nutritional changes. Families may need suggestions for selecting healthy options in a packed lunch. Pediatricians should also be advocates for providing the healthiest possible breakfast and lunch options.

Snacking can occur as a planned part of the school day. Many schools provide morning snacks for younger children. Snacks and sweetened beverages can also be provided as special treats and rewards such as birthday parties or class achievements. Snacking is a routine part of afterschool programs and can often be purchased from school stores or vending machines. Families can pack a snack to substitute for the one at school, lobby with schools to remove vending machines or provide healthier alternatives, or limit money the child has available to purchase these items.

Access to Physical Activity

Physical education classes may range from every day to not at all. It is important to ask about frequency of physical education as well as time spent in actual activity and skill development. These classes, in addition to regular curriculum, should provide an opportunity for honing ageappropriate skills and developing interest in noncompetitive activities that could provide lifelong activity. Children like activity to be fun, geared to their skill level, and inclusive. Pediatricians should make every effort to keep obese children involved in physical education. Adaptive gym and alternatives such as participating in walking club or walking during class can be used as ways to encourage obese children to stay active.

Extracurricular sports can play a large role in providing daily physical activity for children. However, for an obese child, these competitive sports may quickly move out of reach. Pediatricians should encourage schools to maintain intramural sports and provide as many lifestyle activities after school as possible. Sometimes reengaging the obese child or adolescent needs to start with any planned after-school activity, club, or group to break the cycle of television, computer, and sedentary time. Families may need to be encouraged to find options available at school for extracurricular activities that go beyond competitive sports.

Educational Opportunities

Opportunities for increasing students' knowledge of good nutrition, importance of activity, media savvy, and importance of television reduction have been studied in schools. Changing knowledge and beliefs of children may be one of the more powerful tools that school programs can provide to combat obesity. Curriculum changes, extracurricular classes, and support groups have all been mechanisms used to accomplish these goals. Pediatricians can play a role as invited classroom speakers, in training faculty, and meeting with parents to get the message out about obesity prevention and treatment. Pediatricians can also be available as resources for school boards and encourage needed policy changes such as reducing soda and juice availability. Many schools are beginning to report body mass index (BMI) percentiles; pediatricians have a clear role in helping school nurses and the families who receive this information interpret and act on it.

12.3 Advocacy

Pediatricians are often in a position to advocate for change in schools and provide support and expertise to school personnel. There are challenges facing schools in providing healthy meals and snacks. Competitive foods, defined as any foods of minimal nutritional value sold in competition with school meals in snack bars, school stores, and vending machines, tempt students. Offering these foods also sends a mixed message to students and may devalue lessons given in class about good nutrition. Food service personnel may often have limited training, space, and time as well as inadequate facilities in which to prepare food.[2] Some specific school programs will be reviewed to provide background for the kinds of changes and implementation strategies that have been used. In a review of studies of obesity prevention programs in school, the Cochrane review published an analysis of obesity prevention trials lasting at least 12 weeks.[3] These studies were all randomized, controlled trials performed in the school setting.

12.4 Early Childhood Settings[3]

Special Supplemental Nutrition Program for Women, Infants, and Children

The Special Supplemental Nutrition Program for Women, Infants, and Children (WIC) programs would seem a logical site for obesity prevention. Most studies in this population to date have been feasibility studies. In one study, Bright Futures guidelines were incorporated into the content of every 2-month educational group and twice-yearly session with a nutritionist. Six key messages were used: 1) increase physical activity, 2) monitor mealtime behavior, 3) limit household television viewing, 4) drink water instead of sweetened beverages, 5) consume 5 fruits or vegetables daily, and 6) increase family activities to promote fitness. Parents were encouraged to serve as role models. Compared with a control group, participants reported increased frequency of active play with the child and of offering the child water instead of sweetened beverages.[4]

Preschool[3]

In the preschool group (aged 2.6–5.5 years), a study in a child care setting involved 7 one-hour sessions on reducing television viewing by encouraging reading with informational packets sent home to parents. Children were watching 11.9 hours (intervention group) and 14.0 hours (control group) per week of television and videos before the intervention. Although body mass index did not change, children reduced their television viewing by 3.1 hours per week, while the control group increased their viewing by 1.6 hours per week.[5]

Home Visits

A trial of a group of boys with an average age of 22±8 months studied home visiting focused on parenting skills to develop appropriate diet and activity behavior added to a parenting skills intervention in a Native American population compared with a parenting skills intervention alone. At the end of 12 weeks, energy intake was increasing for controls and decreasing for the intervention group, although there were no differences in BMI. Mothers in the intervention group were also engaging in less-restrictive feeding.[6]

12.5 School Settings[3]

Sweetened Beverage Reduction

In a study, 644 UK schoolchildren aged 7 to 11 years received 3 one-hour sessions (1 per term) focused on reducing carbonated beverage consumption. Self-reported soft drink consumption decreased approximately 58 mL per day, but there was no significant difference in BMI Z score between groups.[7]

Increased Physical Activity[3]

For a trial of 292 kindergarten children in Thailand (mean age, 4.5 years), 35 minutes of aerobic exercise (15-minute walk before school and 20-minute aerobic dance following afternoon nap) was added 3 times a week for 29.6 weeks to the usual physical education. Thirteen months after the intervention there was a suggestion of a greater decrease in BMI of the control versus the intervention group, but no statistically significant difference between groups in BMI or triceps skinfold was found.[8]

In another trial, this time in the United States, called project SPARK, 549 children (mean age, 9.25 years) were provided with high levels of physical activity in three 30-minute sessions a week. There was a trend toward lower triceps and calve skinfolds in the control group, but there were no significant differences between groups at 2 years.[9]

Improved Nutrition and Increased Physical Activity[3]

The APPLES study[10] included 634 children aged 7 to 11 years in 10 schools. This was a 1-year study targeting parents, teachers, and food service staff. Schools individualized plans to include modifying meals, physical education and recess, and classroom education. The intervention team included a dietitian, pediatrician, health promotion specialist, psychologist, obesity physician, and nutritional epidemiologist. There was no difference in BMI at 1 year, but intervention children had higher vegetable consumption than the control group.

A school study from England[11] tracked the independent effects of nutrition intervention alone, physical activity alone, a combined intervention, and a control group for children 5 to 7 years of age. The intervention took place at lunchtime clubs and was delivered by the intervention team, which included parents. Reinforcing health messages, food tasting, and noncompetitive activities were targeted. After 20 weeks there was no change in overweight or obesity. Physical activity did increase on the playground and fruit and vegetable consumption increased, but there was no decrease in snack food.

A 24-week obesity prevention program in the United States[12] included 201 girls aged 9 to 12 years with BMI greater than 75%. This intervention included social support and nutrition education that occurred 4 times a week for 16 weeks. Once a week community instructors led groups in dance, self-defense, and swimming. Nutrition advice was to avoid dieting, increase fruit and vegetable intake, and decrease sugar intake. The girls meet weekly for 2 months following the intervention for lunch and discussion. At the end of the study there was no difference in BMI between the control and intervention groups, but the intervention group did progress toward physical activity on the stages of change model.

Six hundred six children aged 9 to 10 years[13] were randomized to a play, play and physical education, physical education only, and control group. The intervention promoted more walking; teachers taught play activities and encouraged self-directed activities with the goal of 30 minutes of activity outside school a day. At 12 weeks there was no difference in BMI among groups, but the intervention group had an increase in physical activity, especially among girls.

Television Viewing Reduction[3]

In a study to reduce television viewing, children aged 8 to 10 years[14] were exposed to 18 lessons of 30 to 50 minutes incorporated into the curriculum. Self-monitoring, self-reporting of television and video use, and adoption of a 7-hour-a-week budget were encouraged. After 6 months, the intervention group showed a significant decrease in television viewing and meals eaten in front of the television as well as in all measures of body fatness, BMI, waist circumference, and waist-hip ratio.

Improved Nutrition, Increased Physical Activity, and Decreased Television Viewing[3]

Planet Health[15] is a school obesity prevention intervention that included 1,295 children aged 11 to 12 years. The intervention was designed to be delivered by teachers in multiple subject areas—language arts, math, science, social studies, and physical education—and included information on promotion of physical activity, modification of dietary intake, and a strong emphasis on reducing television viewing. After 18 months the percentage of obese girls in intervention schools was reduced compared with controls. There was no significant difference in outcome for the boys. There was also greater remission of obesity in intervention girls than the control. Television viewing hours were reduced among boys and girls, and girls increased their fruit and vegetable consumption. Television reduction predicted obesity change in the girls but not boys. Analysis of cost benefit was performed and worked out to a cost of $4,305 per quality of life year saved, with a net savings of $7,313 to society.[16]

Teachers found Planet Health to be feasible and acceptable. Difficulties in implementation mentioned were lack of time for planning, lack of curriculum reinforcement in school meal programs, vending machines in schools, and lack of reinforcement in the child's home.[17]

A study of 410 German children aged 5 to 7 years incorporated nutrition education and activity breaks into the school curriculum. Emphasis was on increased fruit and vegetable consumption, reduced high-fat food consumption, 1 hour of activity a day, and decreased television viewing to less than 1 hour a day. At 1 year there was no change in BMI, but triceps skinfold measurements deceased in the intervention group. There was no difference in percentage overweight in either group.[18]

12.6 Comprehensive School Health Program Changes

A review of schools following Centers for Disease Control and Prevention (CDC) guidelines for healthy eating programs, which include recommendations for school policies, curriculum change, instructions to students, integration of school food services and nutrition education, staff training, family and community involvement, and program evaluation,[19] was conducted to determine effectiveness of these recommendations. Students from schools following these guidelines had lower rates of overweight and obesity, higher consumption of fruits and vegetables, less caloric intake from fat, higher dietary quality, more participation in physical activities, and less participation in sedentary activities compared with students that were only provided healthier menu alternatives or no nutritional plan.[20]

In summary, the Cochrane reviewers[3] felt that sustainability and environmental change combined with behavior change and family support are factors that were important in determining a positive outcome for these interventions. In a recent review of obesity interventions, the CDC stated, "When planning future interventions aimed at weight-control outcomes, considering interventions that produced modest but positive changes in weight-related measures might be useful. These interventions are 1) including nutrition and physical activity components in combination, 2) allotting additional time to physical activity during the school day, 3) including noncompetitive sports (eg, dance), and 4) reducing sedentary activities, especially television viewing."[21]

Programs that have been successful in a research setting need to be translated into the wider school environment. Factors felt to be important in terms of initiating and maintaining a school-based obesity program are the following[22]:

- The program has a relative advantage—innovation is better that the status quo.
- Compatibility—innovation is consistent with current values of the school.
- Low complexity—the innovation is not difficult to understand and use.
- Observability—the results are noticeable to others.
- "Trialability"—the innovation can be tried out on a partial or temporary basis.

References

1. Resnicow K. School-based obesity prevention. Population versus high-risk interventions. *Ann NY Acad Sci.* 1993;699:154–166
2. Gross SM, Cinelli B. Coordinated school health program and dietetics professionals: partners in promoting healthful eating. *J Am Diet Assoc.* 2004;104:793–798
3. Summerbell CD, Waters E, Edmunds LD, Kelly S, Brown T, Campbell KJ. Interventions for preventing obesity in children. *Cochrane Database Syst Rev.* 2005;3:CD001871
4. McGarvy E, Keller A, Forrester M, Williams E, Seward D, Suttle DE. Feasibility and benefits of a parent-focused preschool child obesity intervention. *Am J Public Health.* 2004;94:1490–1495

5. Dennison BA, Russo TJ, Burdick PA, Jenkins PL. An intervention to reduce television viewing by preschool children. *Arch Pediatr Adolesc Med.* 2004; 158:170–176

6. Harvey-Berino J, Rourke J. Obesity prevention in preschool Native-American children: a pilot study using home visiting. *Obes Res.* 2003;11:606–611

7. James J, Thomas P, Cavan D, Kerr D. Preventing childhood obesity by reducing consumption of carbonated drinks: cluster randomized controlled trial. *BMJ.* 2004;328:1237

8. Mo-suwan L, Pongprapai S, Junjana C, Peutpaiboon A. Effects of a controlled trial of a school-based exercise program on the obesity indexes of preschool children. *Am J Clin Nutr.* 1998;68:1006–1111

9. Sallis JF, McKenzie TL, Alcaraz JE, Kolody B, Hovell MF, Nader PR. Project SPARK. Effects of physical education on adiposity in children. *Ann N Y Acad Sci.* 1993;699:127–136

10. Sahota P, Rudolf MC, Dixey R, Hill AJ, Barth JH, Cade J. Randomised controlled trial of primary school based intervention to reduce risk factors for obesity. *BMJ.* 2001;323:1029–1032

11. Warren JM, Henry CJ, Lightowler HJ, Bradshaw SM, Perwaiz S. Evaluation of a pilot school programme aimed at the prevention of obesity in children. *Health Promot Int.* 2003;18:287–296

12. Neumark-Sztainer D, Story M, Hannan PJ, Rex J. New Moves: a school-based obesity prevention program for adolescent girls. *Prev Med.* 2003;37:41–51

13. Pangrazi RP, Beighle A, Vehige T, Vack C. Impact of Promoting Lifestyle Activity for Youth (PLAY) on children's physical activity. *J Sch Health.* 2003;73:317–321

14. Robinson TN. Reducing children's television viewing to prevent obesity: a randomized controlled trial. *JAMA.* 1999;282:1561–1567

15. Gortmaker SL, Peterson K, Wiecha J, et al. Reducing obesity via a school-based interdisciplinary intervention among youth: Planet Health. *Arch Pediatr Adolesc Med.* 1999;153:409–418

16. Wang LY, Yang Q, Lowry R, Wechsler H. Economic analysis of a school-based obesity prevention program. *Obes Res.* 2003;11:1313–1324

17. Wiecha JL, El Ayadi AM, Fuemmeler BF, et al. Diffusion of an integrated health education program in an urban school system: Planet Health. *J Pediatr Psychol.* 2004;29:467–474

18. Muller MJ, Asbeck I, Mast M, Lagnase L, Grund A. Prevention of obesity—more than an intention. Concept and first results of the Kiel Obesity Prevention Study (KOPS). *Int J Obes Relat Metab Disord.* 2001;25(Suppl 1):S66–S74

19. Centers for Disease Control and Prevention. Guidelines for school health programs to promote lifelong healthy eating. *MMWR Recomm Rep.* 1996; 45(RR-9):1–41

20. Veugelers PJ, Fitzgerald AL. Effectiveness of school programs in preventing childhood obesity: a multilevel comparison. *Am J Public Health.* 2005; 95:432–435

21. Katz DL, O'Connell M, Yeh MC, et al. Public health strategies for preventing and controlling overweight and obesity in school and worksite settings: a report on recommendations of the Task Force on Community Preventive Services. *MMWR Recomm Rep.* 2005;54(RR-10):1–12

22. Rogers EM. Diffusion of preventive innovations. *Addict Behav.* 2002; 27:989–999

Appendices

Appendix A.1

BALANCE for a Healthy Life: Patient Handouts for Your Practice

....

Index

Avoiding Food Traps

Food traps are situations and places that make it difficult to eat right. We all find them. The following tips may help you avoid some of the most common traps.

Food trap #1: Vacations, holidays, and other family gatherings

Vacations

When on a trip, don't take a vacation from healthy eating and exercise.

What you can do

- [ ] **Plan your meals.** Will all your meals be from restaurants? If so, can you split entrees and desserts to keep portions from getting too large? Can you avoid fast food? Can you bring along your own healthy snacks?
- [ ] **Stay active.** Schedule time for physical activities such as taking a walk or swimming in the hotel pool.

Holidays

It's easy to overeat during holidays. But you don't need to fear or avoid them.

What you can do

- [ ] **Approach the holidays with extra care.** Don't lose sight of what you and your child are eating. Plan to have healthy foods and snacks on hand.
- [ ] **Celebrate for the day,** not an entire month! Be sure to return to healthy eating the next day.

Other family gatherings

In some cultures, when extended families get together, it can turn into an food feast, from morning to night.

What you can do

- [ ] **Eat smaller portions.** Avoid overeating whenever you get together with family. Try taking small portions instead.
- [ ] **Get family support.** Grandparents, aunts, and uncles can have an enormous effect on your child's health. Let them know that you'd like their help in keeping your child on the road to good health.

Food trap #2: Snack time

The biggest time for snacking is after school. Kids come home wound up, stressed out, or simply bored, so they reach for food.

What you can do

- ☐ **Offer healthy snacks** like raw vegetables, fruit, light microwave popcorn, vegetable soup, sugar-free gelatin, or fruit snacks.

- ☐ **You pick the snack.** When children are allowed to pick their own snacks, they often make unhealthy choices. Talk to your child about why healthy snacks are important. Come up with a list of snacks that you can both agree on and have them on hand.

- ☐ **Keep your child entertained.** Help your child come up with other things to do instead of eating such as playing outside, dancing, painting a picture, flying a kite, or taking a walk with you.

- ☐ **Make sure your child eats 3 well-balanced meals a day.** This will help cut down on the number of times she needs a snack.

Food trap #3: Running out of time

Finding time every day to be physically active can be very difficult. However, if you plan ahead, there are ways to fit it in.

What you can do

- ☐ **Make a plan.** Sit down with your child and plan in advance for those days when it seems impossible to find even 15 minutes for physical activity.

- ☐ **Have a plan B** ready that your child can do after dark such as exercising to a workout video.

- ☐ **Make easy dinners.** If you run out of time to make dinner, don't run to the nearest fast-food restaurant. Remember, dinners don't have to be elaborate. They can be as simple as a sandwich, bowl of soup, piece of fruit, and glass of milk.

Remember

Your job is to provide good nutrition to your child and family and encourage regular physical activity. Stay positive and focus on how well your child is doing in all areas of life. It can help keep nutrition and activity change moving along.

BELIEF, ASSESSMENT, LIFESTYLE, ACTIVITY, NUTRITION, CHILD, ENVIRONMENT

Adapted from American Academy of Pediatrics. *A Parent's Guide to Childhood Obesity: A Road Map to Health.* Hassink SG, ed. Elk Grove Village, IL: American Academy of Pediatrics; 2006

Everyone Get Fit

A generation ago, most kids came home from school, had a snack, and then went outside until they were called in for dinner. Most children, it seemed, were active without being told to do so. Today we are seeing an epidemic of obesity, and the lack of interest in physical activity is a big reason why. Use the following to help your child be more physically active.

Encouraging physical activity

All children need to do some physical activity every day. If your child is overweight, you may need to help your child get moving. Your goal should be to turn exercise into a lifelong habit.

What you can do

- **Encourage your child** to set a goal of doing some kind of exercise each day, even if it's walking for only a few minutes at a time.
- **Make sure your child has things to play with** that are right for his age, from balls to plastic bats, to make exercise fun.
- **Let your child choose** what to play with at any given time.

A family affair

Spend family time doing physical activities that all of you like. When you do things together, your child will see how important exercise is to you. You'll become her most important role model.

What you can do

- **Play catch** in the yard or spend time hitting a tennis ball at the neighborhood courts.
- **Take a family hike** or bike ride.
- **Go to the park** and throw the football back and forth.
- **Play tag** in the front yard.
- **Go to the community pool** for a family swim.
- **Go to the mall and walk** from one end to the other (without spend any time at the food court).
- **Do household chores together** such as cleaning, raking leaves, or waxing the car.

Peer group activities

Most children can get involved in organized sports such as Little League, soccer, martial arts, or basketball, hockey, or football leagues. Team sports are fun and the perfect fit for many children. However, some obese children may feel self-conscious about playing team sports and are much more comfortable getting their exercise in other ways.

What you can do

☐ **Let your child choose** something that he enjoys, and encourage him to make it a regular part of life.

☐ **Limit TV watching** or time spent on the computer or playing video games to no more than 1 to 2 hours a day (for children older than 2 years).

☐ **Try to find activities that fit the family's budget** and schedule and give your child several choices.

☐ **Help your child choose** activities that stress participation, not competition.

☐ **Don't forget the lifetime sports** that can last for decades, including golf, tennis, skating, and skiing.

Remember

Regular activity not only burns calories, but also strengthens the cardiovascular system, builds strong bones and muscles, and increases flexibility. It can also relieve stress, teach teamwork and sportsmanship, boost self-esteem, and improve a person's overall sense of well-being.

BELIEF, ASSESSMENT, LIFESTYLE, ACTIVITY, NUTRITION, CHILD, ENVIRONMENT

Adapted from American Academy of Pediatrics. *A Parent's Guide to Childhood Obesity: A Road Map to Health.* Hassink SG, ed. Elk Grove Village, IL: American Academy of Pediatrics; 2006

The information contained in this publication should not be used as a substitute for the medical care and advice of your pediatrician. There may be variations in treatment that your pediatrician may recommend based on individual facts and circumstances.

Family Meals

Eating together as a family is a great way to

- Help your child learn healthy eating habits.
- Model healthy eating for your child.
- Spend valuable time together as a family.

Read on to find out how regular family meals can make a difference in your child's life.

The power of family

Helping your child lose weight should be a family project. You can't expect your obese child to change her eating habits on her own while others in the family continue to reach for candy and ice cream.

What you can do

☐ **Get your entire family on board** and support the weight-loss efforts of your obese child.

☐ **Be sure everyone in the family models** healthy eating behaviors.

☐ **Avoid making your overweight child feel singled out** and isolated. It will make her resentful and increase the chances of failure.

☐ **Explain that the entire family,** whether they have a weight problem or not, is going to work at getting healthier.

☐ **Turn mealtime into family time** whenever possible.

Structured eating

When you have a child trying to lose weight, you need to pay particular attention to mealtimes. They should be firmly structured, not only for your obese child, but for the entire family.

What you can do

☐ **Have set times for meals.** If your child knows that dinner is going to be served at 6:00 pm, he'll be less likely to start searching for a snack at 5:30 pm. If dinner is served at a different time every night, he might grab a snack rather than risk having to wait 2 or 3 hours to eat.

☐ **Offer your family 3 well-balanced meals each day.** Avoid meal skipping. If your child skips a meal, he'll become over-hungry and set himself up for overeating.

....

☐ **Offer your child 1 to 2 healthy snacks** per day. Discourage grazing (when your child has access to and grabs food all day long).

☐ **Prepare meals that are balanced** and have portion sizes that are right for your child's age.

☐ **Provide** at least one fruit or vegetable with every meal.

☐ **Let your child help** choose what will be on the menu. Encourage and praise him for making healthy food choices.

Mealtime as family time

In too many homes, families rarely sit down for a meal together. Having regular meals together as a family is an important way for families to grow closer. Family meals give everyone the chance to talk about their day. They are also an opportunity for you to keep an eye on what your child is eating.

What you can do

☐ **Try to have as many meals together** as a family as possible.

☐ **Set a no-TV rule** during family meals. The TV is a disruption that you should avoid while you're eating.

☐ **Keep meals pleasant** and focus on the positives. Celebrate your child's successes and praise her for her efforts.

Remember

Children learn more about good food choices and healthy nutrition when family members join one another for meals. Research also shows that kids eat more vegetables and fruits and less fried foods and sugary drinks when they eat with the entire family.

Belief, Assessment, Lifestyle, Activity, Nutrition, Child, Environment

Adapted from American Academy of Pediatrics. *A Parent's Guide to Childhood Obesity: A Road Map to Health.* Hassink SG, ed. Elk Grove Village, IL: American Academy of Pediatrics; 2006

The First 2 Years: Focus on Good Nutrition

If you're worried that your young child is overweight or becoming obese, you might be thinking about feeding her only low-fat foods. Here's the bottom line—do *not* restrict your child's dietary fat and calories in the first 2 years of life. Read on to find out why.

Fat is important

The first 2 years of life are critical for normal development of the brain and body. Dietary fat not only helps in that development, it also provides energy and helps the body absorb certain vitamins.

What you can do

- **For the first year of life,** babies should only drink breast milk or formula, not cow's milk.

- **After age 1 year,** offer your child whole milk to ensure he is getting enough fat in his diet.

- **After age 2 years,** you can switch from whole milk to skim or fat-free milk. You can make this easier on your family by gradually changing from whole milk to 2%, then to 1%, and then to skim milk. You might even try mixing them together to make the changes even easier for your family.

Using formula correctly

Formula is designed to provide about 20 calories per ounce and includes the proper amount of fat to ensure healthy growth.

What you can do

- **When preparing formula,** be sure to follow the instructions carefully.

- **Be sure to add the correct amount of water.** If you add too much water, you can interfere with your baby's normal physical growth and brain development.

How much fat is enough?

During the first 2 years, about half of your child's calories should come from fat. After age 2, you can modify your child's diet gradually until dietary fat makes up about one third of the total calories.

What you can do

☐ **Establish healthy eating habits early** by giving your child well-balanced meals and snacks.

☐ **Focus on good nutrition,** not reducing calories.

☐ **Discourage grazing** (this is when your child has access to and grabs food all day long).

☐ **Offer your child meals** that have a balance of fats, protein, carbohydrates, vitamins, and minerals and include foods from the major food groups each day.

☐ **Limit sweets.**

Remember

Healthy eating for the first 2 years of your child's life should focus on good nutrition, not calories. Do not limit the amount of dietary fat on your toddler's plate. Instead, help her form healthy eating habits by giving her well-balanced meals and snacks.

BELIEF, ASSESSMENT, LIFESTYLE, ACTIVITY, NUTRITION, CHILD, ENVIRONMENT

Adapted from American Academy of Pediatrics. *A Parent's Guide to Childhood Obesity: A Road Map to Health.* Hassink SG, ed. Elk Grove Village, IL: American Academy of Pediatrics; 2006

Food and TV: Not a Healthy Mix

TV is an important part of our lives—it entertains us and has much to teach. But too much TV can make eating right very difficult. Limiting TV time can help your child stay on the path to healthy living. Here's how.

TV and babies

Studies have shown that excessive TV watching is associated with obesity and overweight in children. The best way to avoid this is to limit how much TV your baby watches.

What you can do

☐ **Do not place your baby in front of the TV.** TV isn't appropriate for children younger than 2 years because it takes time away from real interactions with you and other family members.

☐ **Avoid using the TV as a babysitter.** Instead, look for ways to interact with your child face-to-face.

Where the American Academy of Pediatrics stands

In the first 2 years of life, your child's brain and body are growing and developing very quickly. During this time, it is important for your child to have *real* interactions with people and not sit idly in front of the TV.

For that reason, the American Academy of Pediatrics currently recommends that TV should not be watched by children 2 years and younger. For older children, TV watching (of educational, nonviolent programming) should be limited to no more than 1 to 2 hours a day.

TV and the family meal

There is plenty of unconscious eating that can take place in front of the TV. It's easy for kids to simply eat their way from one program to the next. Distracted by the TV, they'll often eat long beyond when they're full. The result? Weight gain.

What you can do

☐ **Set a no-TV rule** during meals.

☐ **Serve all your meals** at the dining room or kitchen table with other family members as often as possible. Mealtime is an important time for family conversations and sharing the day's experiences without the TV getting in the way.

TV and obesity

Here's another important reason to limit your child's TV watching: the steady stream of ads for high-sugar, high-fat foods aimed directly at children. Studies have shown that children who watch a lot of TV have a greater likelihood of becoming obese. The commercials targeted at children are one of the reasons why.

What you can do

- ☐ **Do not allow** children younger than 2 years to watch TV.

- ☐ **Limit** TV watching (as well as video and computer game playing) to 1 to 2 hours a day for older children.

- ☐ **Talk about the ads** your child sees on TV and explain how they encourage unhealthy eating.

- ☐ **Stay strong** when your child begs for the latest food or candy he sees on TV. Explain why you think it's not healthy for him.

Remember

Even if your child doesn't eat in front of the TV, you still need to restrict her TV watching. A daily limit of TV viewing and playing computer or video games should not exceed 1 to 2 hours.

BELIEF, ASSESSMENT, LIFESTYLE, ACTIVITY, NUTRITION, CHILD, ENVIRONMENT

Adapted from American Academy of Pediatrics. *A Parent's Guide to Childhood Obesity: A Road Map to Health.* Hassink SG, ed. Elk Grove Village, IL: American Academy of Pediatrics; 2006

The information contained in this publication should not be used as a substitute for the medical care and advice of your pediatrician. There may be variations in treatment that your pediatrician may recommend based on individual facts and circumstances.

Fruits and Vegetables: How to Get More Every Day

We all know that eating fruits and vegetables is important. But how do you get kids to eat more of these foods? The following tips might help.

What to include

Adding fruits and vegetables to your child's meals is not as difficult as you may think.

What you can do

☐ **Use fruits and vegetables as snacks.**

☐ **Serve salads more often.** Teach your child what an appropriate amount of salad dressing is and how she can order it on the side at restaurants.

☐ **Try out child-friendly vegetarian recipes** for spaghetti, lasagna, chili, or other foods using vegetables instead of meat.

☐ **Include** one green leafy or yellow vegetable for vitamin A such as spinach, broccoli, winter squash, greens, or carrots.

☐ **Include** one vitamin-C–rich fruit, vegetable, or juice such as citrus juices, orange, grapefruit, strawberries, melon, tomato, and broccoli.

☐ **Include a fruit or vegetable as part of every meal or snack.** For example, you could put fruit on cereal, add a piece of fruit or small salad to your child's lunch, use vegetables and dip for an after-school snack, or add a vegetable or two you want to try to the family's dinner.

☐ **Be a role model**—eat more fruits and vegetables yourself.

Fruit and vegetable choking hazards

Children don't fully develop the grinding motion involved in chewing until they're about 4 years old. Until that time, stick with fruits and vegetables that are small and easy to chew and avoid those that might be swallowed whole and get stuck in your toddler's windpipe such as

- Raw carrots
- Raw celery
- Whole grapes
- Raw cherries with pits

How much is enough?

Be sure your child is getting the recommended amount of fruits and vegetables each day.

What you can do

- ☐ **Visit MyPyramid** at www.mypyramid.gov to find out how much of each food group your child should be getting.

- ☐ **When shopping** for food, start in the area of the store where they keep fresh fruits and vegetables. Stock up. That way you know you always have some on hand to serve your child.

- ☐ **Avoid buying high-calorie foods** such as chips, cookies, and candy bars. Your child may not ask for these treats if they are not in sight.

- ☐ **Limit or eliminate how much fruit juice** you give your child and make sure it is 100% juice, not juice "drinks."

- ☐ **Eat as a family** whenever possible. Research shows that kids eat more vegetables and fruits and less fried foods and sugary drinks when they eat with the entire family.

Remember

By choosing health-promoting foods, you can establish good nutritional habits in your child that will last for the rest of his life.

BELIEF, ASSESSMENT, LIFESTYLE, ACTIVITY, NUTRITION, CHILD, ENVIRONMENT

Adapted from American Academy of Pediatrics. *A Parent's Guide to Childhood Obesity: A Road Map to Health.* Hassink SG, ed. Elk Grove Village, IL: American Academy of Pediatrics; 2006

The information contained in this publication should not be used as a substitute for the medical care and advice of your pediatrician. There may be variations in treatment that your pediatrician may recommend based on individual facts and circumstances.

Getting Started

Are you worried about your child's weight? Have you felt helpless as your child gained 2, 5, or 10 extra pounds a year—one year after the next? Maybe you've tried putting your child on a diet, only to be met with frustration and failure. The good news is you can help your child. If you and your child are ready to start on the path to good health, the following tips might help.

Where to start

An important place to start is with your pediatrician. The doctor has the tools and the expertise to help you on this journey.

What you can do

☐ **Talk with your pediatrician** about where your child falls on the growth charts. Growth charts show how your child compares with her peers. Does she fall within the normal range of height and weight for her age?

☐ **Find out your child's body mass index (BMI).** BMI is a calculation of your child's body weight relative to her height. It's an important way to determine if your child is overweight. **Use this formula** or visit www.cdc.gov to measure your child's BMI.

- Multiply her weight (in pounds) by 703.
  Example: 110 pounds x 703 = 77,330 (A)

- Multiply her height (in inches) by itself.
  Example: 48 inches x 48 = 2,304 (B)

- Divide A by B. This will give you her BMI score.
  Example: 77,330 ÷ 2,304 = 33.56

☐ **Talk with your pediatrician** to find out if your child's BMI indicates she is at risk of being overweight or already is overweight.

☐ **Get a sense of your child's current weight, nutrition, and activity level** and where you'd like her to be headed. Talk to your pediatrician about how best to meet those goals.

....

You are not alone

Parents often feel guilty and blame themselves for their children's extra weight. But obesity is a problem that's bigger than one child, parent, or family. It affects boys and girls of all ages, races, ethnic groups, and socioeconomic classes.

What you can do

☐ **Don't feel you have to deal with this by yourself.** Your pediatrician cares about your child's health and can help you and your child on this journey.

☐ **Get your entire family on board** and support the weight-loss efforts of your obese child. Be sure everyone in the family models healthy eating behaviors.

☐ **Talk with others** in your child's life about supporting his efforts. This includes relatives, friends, school, and child care. Your child is more likely to succeed if he knows everyone is supporting him.

Remember

You and your child can succeed. It may not be easy, but you have already taken the first step. Getting the information and skills you need to help your child adopt good nutrition and activity habits will ease the journey to good health.

BELIEF, ASSESSMENT, LIFESTYLE, ACTIVITY, NUTRITION, CHILD, ENVIRONMENT

Adapted from American Academy of Pediatrics. *A Parent's Guide to Childhood Obesity: A Road Map to Health.* Hassink SG, ed. Elk Grove Village, IL: American Academy of Pediatrics; 2006

Hungry or Just Bored?

Children (as well as adults) often use food for reasons other than to satisfy hunger. Obese children often eat in response to their emotions and feelings. If your child seems hungry all the time, use the following tips to get a better idea of what is really going on.

What triggers hunger?

If your child is eating 3 well-balanced meals a day but still claims to be hungry, there may be other reasons beyond hunger that make her want to eat.

What you can do

Ask yourself the following questions:

☐ **Does your child sometimes reach for food** when she's experiencing any of the following?

- Boredom
- Depression
- Stress
- Frustration
- Insecurity
- Loneliness
- Fatigue
- Resentment
- Anger
- Happiness

☐ **Does your child eat at times other than regular mealtimes** and snacks? Is she munching at every opportunity?

☐ **Do you reward your child with food** (does an A on a test sometimes lead to a trip to the ice cream shop)? This can inadvertently contribute to your child's obesity.

☐ **When your child is doing things right, do you tell her?** Words of approval can boost a child's self-esteem. They can also help keep her motivated to continue making the right decisions for her health and weight.

☐ **How are you speaking to your child?** Is it mostly negative? Is it often critical? It's hard for anyone, including children, to make changes in that kind of environment.

Healthy alternatives

If you suspect your child is eating out of boredom, you may need to steer him toward other activities to get his mind off his stomach.

What you can do

☐ **Make sure your child is eating 3 well-balanced meals a day.** This will keep him from feeling hungry between meals.

☐ **Help your child choose** other things to do instead of eating, such as
- Walking the dog
- Running through the sprinklers
- Playing a game of badminton
- Kicking a soccer ball
- Painting a picture
- Going in-line skating
- Dancing
- Planting a flower in the garden
- Flying a kite
- Joining you for a walk through the mall (without stopping at the ice cream shop)

☐ **Offer healthy snacks** like raw vegetables, fruit, light microwave popcorn, vegetable soup, sugar-free gelatin, and fruit snacks. Snacks like chips and candy bars have empty calories that will not make your child feel full.

☐ **You pick the snack.** When children are allowed to pick their own snacks, they often make unhealthy choices. Talk to your child about why healthy snacks are important. Come up with a list of snacks that you can both agree on and have them on hand.

Remember

Your own relationship with food and weight, dating back to your childhood, can influence the way you parent your own overweight child. One of your biggest challenges is to determine whether your child is eating for the right reasons.

BELIEF, ASSESSMENT, LIFESTYLE, ACTIVITY, NUTRITION, CHILD, ENVIRONMENT

Adapted from American Academy of Pediatrics. *A Parent's Guide to Childhood Obesity: A Road Map to Health.* Hassink SG, ed. Elk Grove Village, IL: American Academy of Pediatrics; 2006

Managing Setbacks and Detours on the Way to Healthy Eating and Activity

No matter how strongly your child tries to gain control over her food and activity choices, she'll likely have some backsliding from time to time. When you meet a few roadblocks on the journey to better health, the following tips might help.

Stay positive

Mistakes will happen. Maybe your child will overeat for a few days in a row. Maybe he'll sneak some junk food when you are not looking. But focusing on the mistake is not usually helpful.

What you can do

☐ **Try not to view mistakes as total failure.** Instead, think of them as minor stumbling blocks, which is exactly what they are.

☐ **Don't let disappointment be a reason to give up.** Remind him of all the successes he has had so far.

☐ **Think about what went wrong** and how you can help your child avoid it happening again.

☐ **Avoid scolding your child** or other family members for these inevitable detours. Remember that none of us are perfect. Stay optimistic and return your attention to healthier living.

Team effort

No one likes to feel alone. Your child will feel much better knowing that there are others who are there to help when the going gets rough.

What you can do

☐ **Reassure your child** that you are there for her and want to help her in any way you can.

☐ **Let your child help figure out what went wrong** and work together on how to prevent it from happening again.

☐ **Let your child in on meal planning,** food shopping and preparation, and family activity planning. This will help her learn to make good decisions from your example.

....

Identify the problem

Give some thought to what might be the problem. You'd be surprised at how often parents and children know that something isn't going right, but never take the time to evaluate what's really happening.

What you can do

- ☐ **Write down what your child is eating** and what his activity level is. This can help you identify specific problem areas and why they might be taking place.

- ☐ **Try to figure out** if the setbacks happen at certain times. For example, does grandma bring sweets every time she visits? Did you run out of time to make dinner and stop at a fast-food restaurant?

- ☐ **As a family, return to your commitment** to eating healthy.

- ☐ **Keep monitoring your child's progress** in the weeks and months ahead. Make sure he doesn't fall back into old habits.

Remember

Learning how to make good decisions about nutrition and activity is important. Help your child understand that it's a process that takes time. The journey will not always be easy. There may be plenty of obstacles along the way that could temporarily derail your child from the path toward better health.

BELIEF, ASSESSMENT, LIFESTYLE, ACTIVITY, NUTRITION, CHILD, ENVIRONMENT

Adapted from American Academy of Pediatrics. *A Parent's Guide to Childhood Obesity: A Road Map to Health.* Hassink SG, ed. Elk Grove Village, IL: American Academy of Pediatrics; 2006

The information contained in this publication should not be used as a substitute for the medical care and advice of your pediatrician. There may be variations in treatment that your pediatrician may recommend based on individual facts and circumstances.

Setting Goals

If you've ever tried to lose weight, you know how hard it is. Being overweight is no less challenging for children. But your child can succeed. If you and your child are ready to start on the road to better health, the following tips may be helpful.

Start small

Weight loss is a journey. And like every other road on which we travel, there may be bumps and detours along the way.

What you can do

☐ **Don't expect instant results.** That's just not realistic and will only set you and your child up for disappointment.

☐ **Help your child make small changes** at first. These small steps can lead to bigger steps that are more likely to be kept up over time.

☐ **Start with the basics.** Help your child choose healthier foods and cut down on high-fat or sugary snacks.

☐ **Have your child do some kind of physical activity every day,** even if it's only for a few minutes to start.

Family goals

There are many ways in which you and other family members can help your child's success in losing weight.

What you can do

☐ **Become a role model.** That means getting out the door and being active yourself, perhaps along with your child.

☐ **Be supportive,** not critical in how you help your child make good decisions about eating and being active. Be sure other family members follow this as well.

☐ **Keep only those foods in the house** that fit into your child's nutritional plan. Even if other family members do not need to lose weight, they can still benefit from healthier eating.

☐ **Eat meals together** as a family whenever possible away from the TV and help your child choose appropriate portion sizes.

· ·

Remember

The changes that will help your child manage her weight today could also keep a serious illness from developing later. Modeling good eating habits and setting daily physical activity goals will serve her well for the rest of her life.

BELIEF, ASSESSMENT, LIFESTYLE, ACTIVITY, NUTRITION, CHILD, ENVIRONMENT

Adapted from American Academy of Pediatrics. *A Parent's Guide to Childhood Obesity: A Road Map to Health.* Hassink SG, ed. Elk Grove Village, IL: American Academy of Pediatrics; 2006

The information contained in this publication should not be used as a substitute for the medical care and advice of your pediatrician. There may be variations in treatment that your pediatrician may recommend based on individual facts and circumstances.

Sneaking Food

Plenty of children sneak food, often believing (or hoping) that they'll never get caught. In most families, sneaking food doesn't go undetected for long. If your child sneaks food, the following tips may help.

Why kids sneak food

It's important to understand why a child might feel the need to sneak food. Sometimes children find emotions simply too hard to handle and they find food soothing and comforting. Other times, children might be feeling anxious, stressed, bored, or sad.

What you can do

- ☐ **Explain that you know** your child is sneaking food. Encourage her to talk to you about why. Let her do most of the talking, and really listen to what she has to say.

- ☐ **Reassure your child** that you love her and that you will do anything you can to help her work on the problem.

Ask, don't sneak

Rather than simply telling your child, "Don't sneak!" encourage him to ask for food when he wants it. Set up a reward system to encourage him to stop sneaking.

What you should do

- ☐ **For a young child,** reward him with a sticker or star each time he asks you for something to eat. Other ideas are to read him an extra bedtime story or give him points he can put toward a low-cost toy or school supplies.

- ☐ **For an older child,** let him build up points for a ticket to the movies, a day at the skating rink or zoo, or renting a DVD or video game.

- ☐ **Suggest other things to do** instead of eating such as bike riding, going for a walk, playing with friends, or exercising with a workout video.

Remember

It is very important to help your child adopt healthy eating and activity habits that can last a lifetime. By taking steps like serving your child appropriate foods and encouraging her to be physically active every day, any weight concerns that exist now will become less of a problem as she gets older.

BELIEF, ASSESSMENT, LIFESTYLE, ACTIVITY, NUTRITION, CHILD, ENVIRONMENT

Adapted from American Academy of Pediatrics. *A Parent's Guide to Childhood Obesity: A Road Map to Health.* Hassink SG, ed. Elk Grove Village, IL: American Academy of Pediatrics; 2006

The information contained in this publication should not be used as a substitute for the medical care and advice of your pediatrician. There may be variations in treatment that your pediatrician may recommend based on individual facts and circumstances.

What About Juice?

Fruit is one of the 5 food groups and an important part of every child's diet. Offering fruit juice is an easy way for kids to get the recommended amount of fruit in their diets. But too much juice can have its problems. If your child drinks juice, the following tips may be helpful to you.

How much is OK?

Because juice tastes good, it's easy to give your child too much. Too much juice in a child's diet is linked to obesity. It can also cause diarrhea, poor nutrition, and tooth decay.

What you can do

☐ **Do not give juice to infants** younger than 6 months.

☐ **Give only 4 to 6 ounces** of fruit juice per day to children between the ages of 1 to 6 years.

☐ **Give only 8 to 12 ounces** of fruit juice per day to children between the ages of 7 to 18 years.

☐ **Give juice only to infants who can drink from a cup,** never in a bottle.

☐ **Do not allow your child to carry** a cup or box of juice around throughout the day.

How can you tell it's juice?

It's not always easy to tell fruit juice from fruit "drinks." However, the information should be on the label if you know what to look for.

What you can do

☐ **Look for the word "juice"** on the label. It can't be called juice if it's not 100% fruit juice.

☐ **Avoid products that are called "drinks," "beverages," or "cocktails."** They do not contain 100% real fruit juice. If you do buy these products for your child, look for ones with the highest percentage of juice. This information is on the label.

☐ **Read the ingredients** on the label. Juice drinks often add sweeteners and artificial flavors.

Alternatives to juice

Like adults, children need variety in their diets. Instead of relying on juice as your child's only drink, consider other drinks as well.

What you can do

☐ **Offer your child water.** Water is a healthy drink for children of all ages. To make drinking water more interesting to your child, try adding a slice of lemon or lime.

☐ **Offer your child low-fat milk** rather than juice.

☐ **Try a piece of fruit instead of juice.** While a 6-ounce glass of fruit juice equals one fruit serving, a piece of whole fruit such as an apple is healthier. Fruit provides more fiber than fruit juice.

Remember

The nutritional choices you make for your child today will help determine her health not only now, but in the future. If you make an effort to feed her primarily healthy meals, drinks, and snacks, you have a much better chance of helping her attain a healthy weight.

BELIEF, ASSESSMENT, LIFESTYLE, ACTIVITY, NUTRITION, CHILD, ENVIRONMENT

Adapted from American Academy of Pediatrics. *A Parent's Guide to Childhood Obesity: A Road Map to Health.* Hassink SG, ed. Elk Grove Village, IL: American Academy of Pediatrics; 2006

Growth Charts

· ·

Index

Boys

Birth to 36 months: Length-for-age and Weight-for-age percentiles

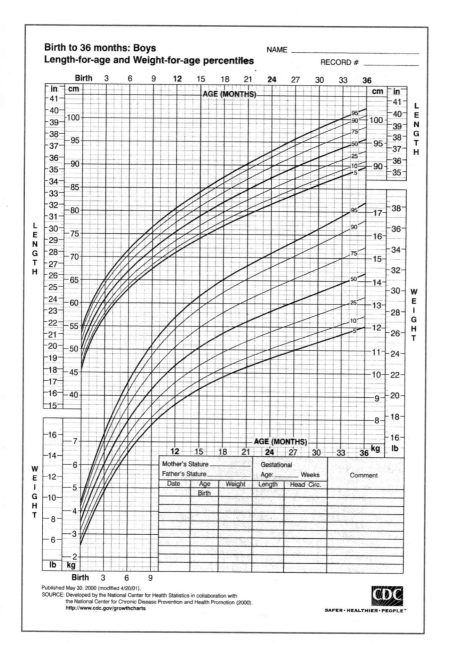

Boys

Birth to 36 months: Head circumference–for-age and
Weight-for-length percentiles

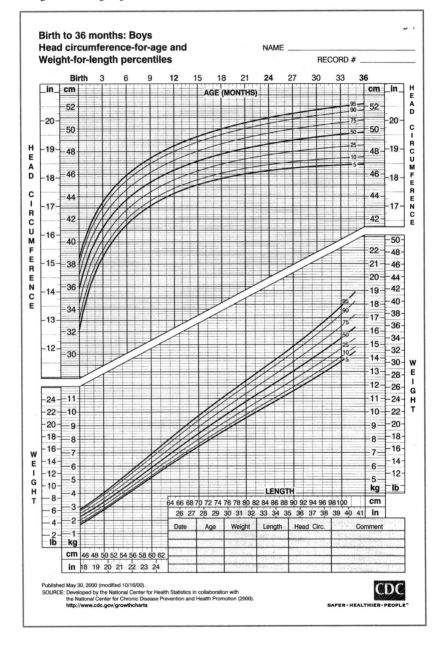

Boys

2 to 20 years: Stature-for-age and Weight-for-age percentiles

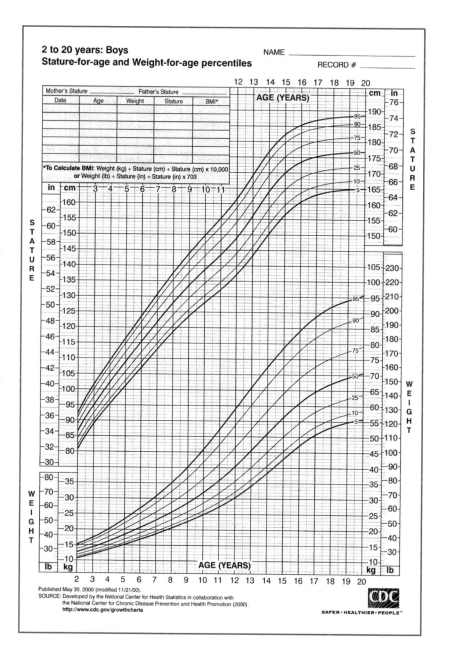

Boys

2 to 20 years: Body mass index–for-age percentiles

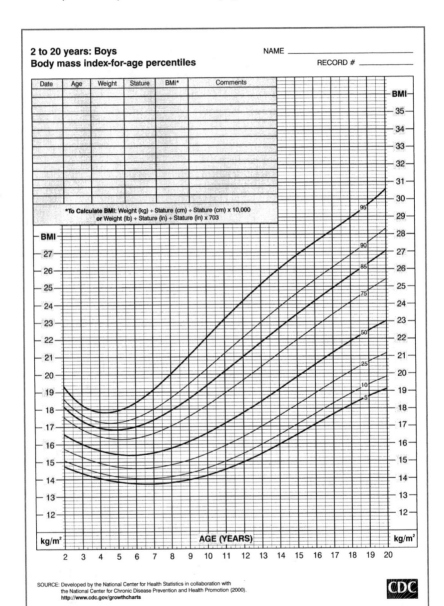

Boys

Weight-for-stature percentiles

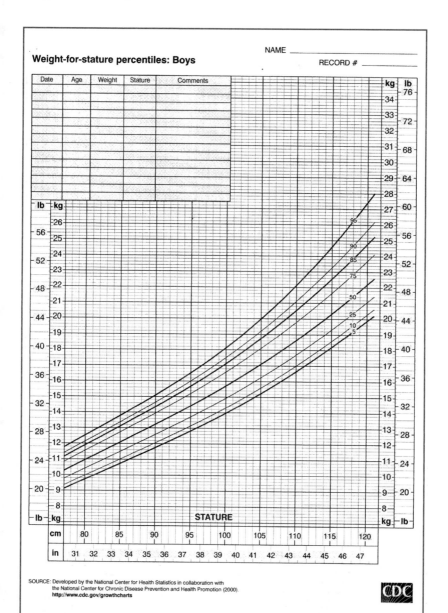

Weight-for-stature percentiles: Boys

NAME _____

RECORD # _____

Date	Age	Weight	Stature	Comments

STATURE

cm	80	85	90	95	100	105	110	115	120
in	31 32 33 34 35 36 37 38 39 40 41 42 43 44 45 46 47

SOURCE: Developed by the National Center for Health Statistics in collaboration with
the National Center for Chronic Disease Prevention and Health Promotion (2000).
http://www.cdc.gov/growthcharts

CDC

Girls

Birth to 36 months: Length-for-age and Weight-for-age percentiles

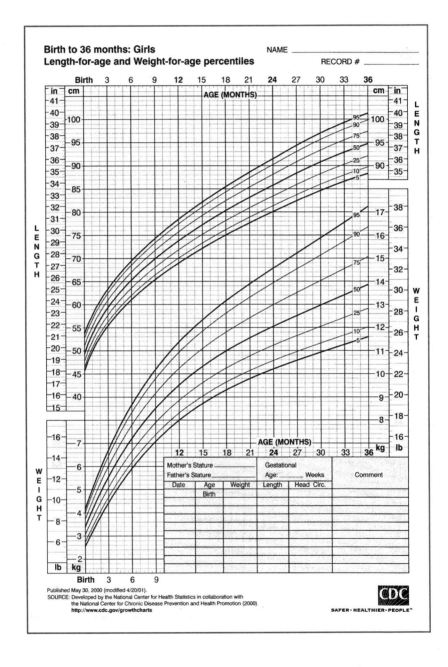

Birth to 36 months: Girls
Length-for-age and Weight-for-age percentiles

NAME _____

RECORD # _____

Published May 30, 2000 (modified 4/20/01).
SOURCE: Developed by the National Center for Health Statistics in collaboration with
the National Center for Chronic Disease Prevention and Health Promotion (2000).
http://www.cdc.gov/growthcharts

CDC
SAFER · HEALTHIER · PEOPLE™

Girls

Birth to 36 months: Head circumference–for-age and
Weight-for-length percentiles

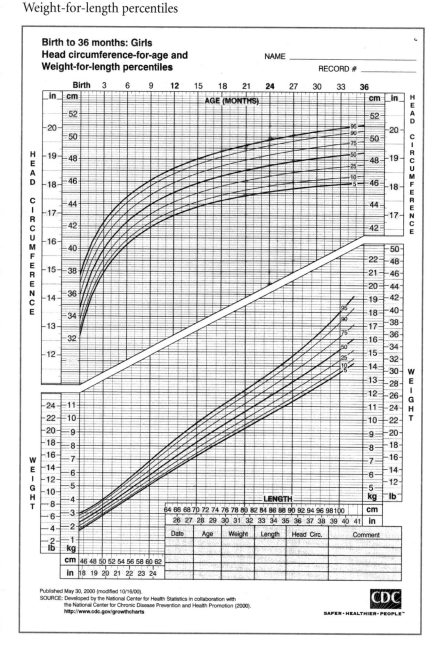

Birth to 36 months: Girls
Head circumference-for-age and
Weight-for-length percentiles

NAME _____

RECORD # _____

Published May 30, 2000 (modified 10/16/00).
SOURCE: Developed by the National Center for Health Statistics in collaboration with
the National Center for Chronic Disease Prevention and Health Promotion (2000).
http://www.cdc.gov/growthcharts

CDC
SAFER · HEALTHIER · PEOPLE™

Girls

2 to 20 years: Stature-for-age and Weight-for-age percentiles

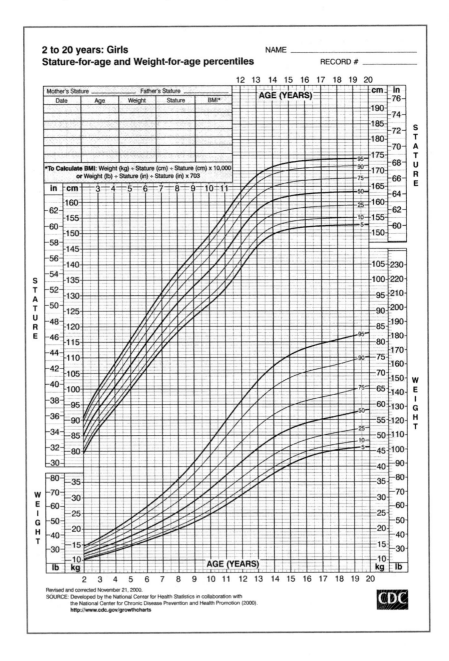

Girls

2 to 20 years: Body mass index–for-age percentiles

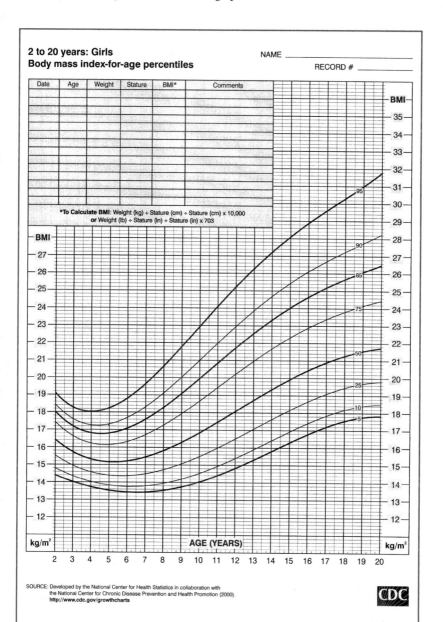

2 to 20 years: Girls
Body mass index-for-age percentiles

NAME _____

RECORD # _____

Date	Age	Weight	Stature	BMI*	Comments

*To Calculate BMI: Weight (kg) ÷ Stature (cm) ÷ Stature (cm) x 10,000
or Weight (lb) ÷ Stature (in) ÷ Stature (in) x 703

AGE (YEARS)

SOURCE: Developed by the National Center for Health Statistics in collaboration with
the National Center for Chronic Disease Prevention and Health Promotion (2000).
http://www.cdc.gov/growthcharts

CDC

Girls

Weight-for-stature percentiles

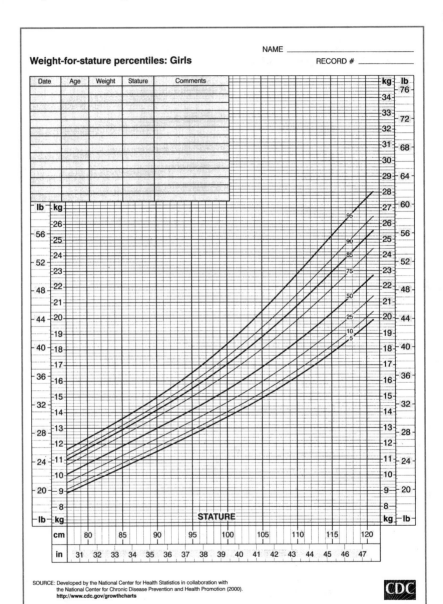

Guide to Food Portions and Servings for Children

Feeding Guide for Children*

Food	2 to 3 Portion Size	2 to 3 Servings	4 to 6 Portion Size	4 to 6 Servings	7 to 12 Portion Size	7 to 12 Servings	Comments
Milk and dairy	½ c (4 oz)	4–5 16–20 oz total	½–¾ c (4–6 oz)	3–4 24–32 oz total	½–1 c (4–8 oz)	3–4 24–32 oz total	The following may be substituted for ½ c fluid milk: ½–¾ oz cheese, ½ cup yogurt, 2½ tbsp nonfat dry milk
Meat, fish, poultry, or equivalent	1–2 oz	2 2–4 oz total	1–2 oz	2 2–4 oz total	2 oz	3–4 6–8 oz total	The following may be substituted for 1 oz meat, fish, or poultry: 1 egg, 2 tbsp peanut butter, 4–5 tbsp cooked legumes
Vegetables and fruit *Vegetables*							
Cooked	2–3 tbsp	4–5	3–4 tbsp	4–5	¼–½ c	3–4	Include one green leafy or yellow vegetable for vitamin A, such as carrots, spinach, broccoli, winter squash, or greens
Raw†	Few pieces		Few Pieces		Several pieces		
Fruit							
Raw	½–1 small		½–1 small		1 medium		Include one vitamin C-rich fruit, vegetable, or juice, such as citrus juices, orange, grapefruit, strawberries, melon, tomato, or broccoli
Canned	2–4 tbsp		4–6 tbsp		¼–½ c		
Juice	3–4 oz		4 oz		4 oz		
Grain products							
Whole grain or enriched bread	½–1 slice	3–4	1 slice	3–4	1 slice	4–5	The following may be substituted for 1 slice of bread: ½ c spaghetti, macaroni, noodles, or rice; 5 saltines; ½ English muffin or bagel; 1 tortilla; corn grits or posole
Cooked cereal	¼–½ c		½ c		½–1 c		
Dry cereal	½–1 c		1 c		1 c		

*Adapted from Lowenberg ME. Development of food patterns in young children. In: Pipes PL, Trahms CM, eds. *Nutrition Infancy and Childhood*. 5th ed. St Louis, MO: Mosby-Year Book; 1993:168–169. With permission of Elsevier.

†Do not give to young children until they can chew well.

Appendix A.4

Patient Worksheets and Self-assessment Forms

....

Index

Adapted from American Academy of Pediatrics. *A Parent's Guide to Childhood Obesity: A Road Map to Health.* Hassink SG, ed. Elk Grove Village, IL: American Academy of Pediatrics; 2006

WORKSHEET TO TAKE TO YOUR PEDIATRICIAN

ENVIRONMENTAL FACTORS

The following assessment will help you understand the environmental influences associated with your child's weight problem.

What Problems Exist Today (Home, School)?
Are there problems in your child's school/child care environment? _____

Are snacks healthy and portions controlled? _____

Is there time for outdoor play/recess? _____

Is there regular physical education at school? _____

Is there more than 1 to 2 hours of screen time (TV, computer)? _____

The Community Environment
Are there safe playgrounds and places to play outside in
the neighborhood? _____

Are there after-school programs nearby that provide activity alternatives? _____

Are there opportunities to play sports/games at community centers? _____

Is it safe for your child to walk to school, activities, and friends' houses? _____

The Home Environment
Does the family have regularly scheduled TV/computer time? _____

Do family members regularly engage in physical activity together? _____

Is there an indoor and outdoor play space for the children? _____

Are there indoor activities your child can do at home instead of
watching TV or using the computer? _____

Family Behavior
With family members in mind (including you, your spouse, and your child's
siblings and grandparents), which of them

Overeats regularly _____

Binges on food _____

Rushes through meals _____

Insists on keeping high-calorie snacks in the house _____

Eats while watching TV _____

Eats frequently at fast-food restaurants _____

Overeats to calm anxiety _____

Gets little or no physical activity each day _____

Your Child's Behavior
Does your overweight child demonstrate the following behaviors that can contribute to an obesity problem? (Answer yes or no.)

Overeats regularly _____

Binges on food _____

Rushes through meals _____

Chooses high-calorie snacks _____

Selects high-sugar drinks _____

Eats while watching TV _____

Eats frequently at fast-food restaurants _____

Overeats to calm anxiety _____

Gets little or no physical activity each day _____

Sneaks or hides food _____

Seems hungry all the time _____

Gets upset when you try to limit portions or snacks _____

Watches more than 1 hour of TV/computer per day _____

Gets own food or snacks _____

Eats alone _____

Drinks a lot of sweetened beverages _____

WORKSHEET TO TAKE TO YOUR PEDIATRICIAN
YOUR CHILD'S GENETICS AND FAMILY HISTORY

How Does Family History Currently Influence Your Child's Health?
Let's look more closely at your own family. In the tables that follow, place a check mark beside the conditions and diseases of each family member. The more check marks you make, the greater your child's risk is of not only becoming overweight, but also of developing the serious diseases associated with it.

	Mother	Father	Sibling #1	Sibling #2	Sibling #3
Obese/overweight	☐	☐	☐	☐	☐
High blood pressure	☐	☐	☐	☐	☐
High cholesterol	☐	☐	☐	☐	☐
High triglycerides	☐	☐	☐	☐	☐
Diabetes	☐	☐	☐	☐	☐
Heart disease	☐	☐	☐	☐	☐
Asthma	☐	☐	☐	☐	☐
Joint pain	☐	☐	☐	☐	☐
Sleep apnea	☐	☐	☐	☐	☐
Liver disease	☐	☐	☐	☐	☐
Other _____	☐	☐	☐	☐	☐

Next, fill out a similar chart for your child's grandparents. Which of the following conditions apply to your youngster's grandfathers and grandmothers?

	Maternal Grandmother	Maternal Grandfather	Paternal Grandmother	Paternal Grandfather
Obese/overweight	☐	☐	☐	☐
High blood pressure	☐	☐	☐	☐
High cholesterol	☐	☐	☐	☐
High triglycerides	☐	☐	☐	☐
Diabetes	☐	☐	☐	☐
Heart disease	☐	☐	☐	☐
Asthma	☐	☐	☐	☐
Sleep apnea	☐	☐	☐	☐
Liver disease	☐	☐	☐	☐
Joint pain	☐	☐	☐	☐
Other _____	☐	☐	☐	☐

WORKSHEET TO TAKE TO YOUR PEDIATRICIAN

HOW IS YOUR CHILD EATING NOW?

To help produce lasting improvements in a child's weight, many parents find it helpful to keep a food diary to monitor exactly what the child is eating. Toward that end, use this worksheet for the next 4 days to record what your child eats, from the time he or she awakens to when he or she goes to sleep.

Foods Eaten Today (enter date): _____

Under each meal and snack write down *what* and *how much* your child ate.

Breakfast _____

Mid-morning Snack _____

Lunch _____

Afternoon Snack _____

Juice or Soda _____

Dinner _____

Late-night Snack _____

Foods Eaten Today (enter date): _____

Under each meal and snack write down *what* and *how much* your child ate.

Breakfast _____

Mid-morning Snack _____

Lunch _____

Afternoon Snack _____

Juice or Soda _____

Dinner _____

Late-night Snack _____

Foods Eaten Today (enter date): _____

Under each meal and snack write down *what* and *how much* your child ate.

Breakfast _____

Mid-morning Snack _____

Lunch _____

Afternoon Snack _____

Juice or Soda _____

Dinner _____

Late-night Snack _____

Foods Eaten Today (enter date): _____

Under each meal and snack write down *what* and *how much* your child ate.

Breakfast _____

Mid-morning Snack _____

Lunch _____

Afternoon Snack _____

Juice or Soda _____

Dinner _____

Late-night Snack _____

· ·

WORKSHEET TO TAKE TO YOUR PEDIATRICIAN
HOW WILL YOU AND YOUR CHILD GET THERE?

Let's be more specific about the goals for your youngster.

As you get started, what short-term goals do you and your child have?

Specifically, how does your family plan to eat healthier, meal by meal?

Specifically, how does your family plan to become more active, day by day?

What other short-term and intermediate goals do you and your child have?

Do you think that making behavioral changes associated with these goals will be easy or difficult?

Who is going to go with you on this weight-loss journey? Who can help you and your child achieve your goals? (Check all that apply.)

- ☐ Other family members
- ☐ Spouse
- ☐ Siblings
- ☐ Grandparents
- ☐ Friends
- ☐ School
- ☐ Parent groups
- ☐ Child care staff
- ☒ Your pediatrician
- ☐ Others

What information do you need to help you achieve these goals? (Check those that apply.)

- ☐ More knowledge of proper nutrition
- ☐ Help with activity alternatives
- ☐ Skills to help your child and family make healthy changes
- ☐ Information about age-appropriate diet and activity
- ☐ Information about the health consequences of obesity

WORKSHEET TO TAKE TO YOUR PEDIATRICIAN
WHERE DO YOU AND YOUR CHILD WANT TO GO?

With this worksheet, you'll begin to look toward your child's future.

What are your child's health goals relative to his or her weight (these should be health goals, rather than being related primarily to weight)?

Is there a health problem associated with your child's weight that you'd like to improve or correct?

- ☐ Lower cholesterol level
- ☐ Lower blood pressure
- ☐ Improve blood sugar glucose level
- ☐ Be able to run or be physically active and keep up with friends without becoming winded so quickly

Are there eating behaviors you would like to help your child improve? (Check those that apply.)

- ☐ Overeating at meals
- ☐ Too many snacks
- ☐ Unhealthy food choices
- ☐ Eating at night
- ☐ Eating in front of TV
- ☐ Too many fast-food meals
- ☐ Very limited diet choices
- ☐ Unhealthy food choices

Are there activity behaviors you would like to help your child improve? (Check all that apply.)

- ☐ Limiting TV/computer use
- ☐ Being more motivated to be active
- ☐ Participating in more peer-group activities
- ☐ Others: _____

What are the long-term goals that you and your child have relative to your child's weight? (Check all that apply.)

- ☐ Improve your child's overall health.
- ☐ Decrease the chances that your child will be an overweight/obese adult.
- ☐ Increase your child's self-esteem.
- ☐ Reduce family conflict around food and activity.
- ☐ Decrease teasing.

●●●

WORKSHEET TO TAKE TO YOUR PEDIATRICIAN
ASSESSING YOUR HOME ENVIRONMENT

Let's continue the journey toward helping your child manage his or her weight by pausing at this checkpoint to make another assessment. This time, you'll evaluate the following components of this part of the road trip toward controlling his obesity:

- Your home environment
- Your parenting role within this environment
- Areas in which improvements may be needed

What Is Currently Happening at Home?
In answering the following questions, you'll get a clearer sense of what is taking place in your home environment that may play a role in your youngster's health.

Does your family mostly eat well-balanced meals? During a typical week, how many well-balanced meals are prepared in the home?

Breakfast _____   Lunch _____   Dinner _____

On average, how many times a week does the family eat fast-food meals that are brought into the home or eaten at restaurants? _____

Who does the grocery shopping in your family? _____

Do other family members (for example, parents, children) contribute to the decisions on what will be purchased in the supermarket? If so, who? Is most of the food brought into the home healthy? _____

Who is giving your child snacks at home (or elsewhere)?
- ☐ Parent(s)   ☐ Other family members
- ☐ Other children   ☐ Child care staff

Does your overweight child and/or family use food
- ☐ As a reward?   ☐ For comfort?   ☐ To relieve boredom?

Is your child physically active every day? _____

How much time does your child spend in physical activities each day? _____

How many hours do family members spend watching TV or on the computer every day? _____

How many TVs/computers do you have in the house? _____

Do family members have TVs/computers in their bedrooms? _____

Does your child have a TV/computer in his or her bedroom? _____

Who sets limits on your child's TV/computer use? _____

How many hours does your child watch TV or play computer or video games during a typical day? _____

What Is Going Well in Your Household?
Based on your previous answers, what areas are you pleased with in your home life that contribute to your child's health? Specifically, check off what is going well in your household.

- ☐ Well-balanced meals
- ☐ Healthy snacking
- ☐ Limiting fast-food meals
- ☐ Regularly participating in physical activity
- ☐ Limiting TV watching and video or computer games

Use this space to elaborate on any of the above:

_____

_____

What Problems Exist in Your Household?
What problem areas are present in your home environment that may need changing or improving (place a check mark by those that apply)?

- ☐ Poor food/meal selection
- ☐ Poor snack food choices
- ☐ Too many fast-food meals
- ☐ Not enough physical activity or time outdoors
- ☐ Too much computer, TV, or video game time

Others: _____

What Change(s) Do You Need to Make and How Will You Make Them?
As the next step in your journey toward better health, identify the specific obstacles that are contributing to your household problems. Which of the following apply to you and your family?

- ☐ Family preferences (for example, unhealthy favorite foods)
- ☐ Not enough available time (to prepare meals, for physical activity)
- ☐ Not enough money
- ☐ Not enough time spent outdoors
- ☐ No safe places to play
- ☐ Your child won't go to activities or play outside
- ☐ Other

Next, select a single, specific change that you'd like to work on with your child and the rest of the family (for example, improving the snacks available in your house and chosen by your family).

_____

_____

To make this change possible, identify who can support you in this process. In addition to your and your child, who else can go on this journey with you, and can help your child reach this goal?

☐ Your spouse
☐ Your other children
☐ Grandparents
☐ Others

Now, use the following space to create a plan to make possible the change you've chosen.

_____

_____

In the past, how has your child reacted and how did you respond to your child when you tried to make changes (for example, did you give in to your child's complaints or demands)?

_____

_____

What could you do differently this time? How can you change your own actions to produce more positive results?

_____

_____

From a parenting point of view, is there anything else standing in the way of making healthier changes in your home environment?

_____

_____

_____

_____

WORKSHEET TO TAKE TO YOUR PEDIATRICIAN
YOUR CHILD AND HIS OR HER WEIGHT

For this assessment, answer the following questions about your youngster:

How does your child feel about his or her weight? (Explain.)

Does your child worry about how much he or she weighs?

What kinds of things concern your child?

Does your child worry about taking gym class at school?

Does your child worry about keeping up with other children on the playground?

Is your child concerned about being teased?

Is your child worried about how he or she looks in clothes?

Is your child concerned about his or her health?

Other concerns:

How do you feel about your child's weight?

Are you concerned about your child being teased by peers? _____

Are you anxious about the short- and long-term consequences of your child's weight gain and eating behaviors?

Other worries:

WORKSHEET TO TAKE TO YOUR PEDIATRICIAN
WHERE DOES YOUR CHILD STAND?

What's Currently Happening With Physical Activity?
Let's take a few moments to determine how your child is currently faring in terms of physical activity. The answers to the following questions will help you identify how much time your child spends in structured and unstructured activities and areas in which your child may need to improve.

How many days a week does your child participate in physical education (PE) classes at school? _____

On those days, approximately how many minutes does your child spend moving or doing activity (as opposed to standing around) in those PE classes? _____

How many days a week does your child play outdoors? _____

About how many minutes (or hours) does your child spend playing outdoors on a typical weekday? _____ On a typical Saturday or Sunday? _____

What structured physical activities does your child participate in (for example, a youth sports team or organized activities at an after-school program)?

_____

_____

In a typical week, how many minutes (or hours) does your child spend in these structured activities? _____

On average, how many hours a day does your child watch TV or play video or computer games? _____

Does your child often snack while in front of the TV or computer screen? _____

What outdoor physical activities does your child enjoy doing?

_____

_____

What other outdoor physical activities would you like to introduce to your child?

_____

_____

What is Going Well?

Use the answers to the previous questions to determine those areas in which your child is already doing well incorporating physical activity in his or her life. In the following space, write down the ways in which your child is active:

_____

_____

_____

What Changes Need to Be Made?

Next, take a few minutes to determine areas in which your child needs to improve. For example,

Does your child need to spend more time playing outdoors? _____

Would your child benefit from participating in youth sports or other organized activities? Would your child get more benefit and be more successful with activities in a small group or with his family?

_____

Does your child need to spend less time in front of the TV or computer or playing video games? _____

Choose a way in which your child can become more active, and write down a strategy for incorporating that activity into his or her life. For example, you may feel your child is watching too much TV after school and explore after-school activities at the local YMCA or Boys & Girls Club. Or you may find that your child is more comfortable increasing activity with a family member by taking a walk or shooting some hoops with a sibling.

_____

_____

What additional improvements would you like to help your child make in his or her efforts to become more active?

_____

_____

_____

· ·

WORKSHEET TO TAKE TO YOUR PEDIATRICIAN
CONQUERING SETBACKS

Has your overweight child experienced a lapse in his or her progress toward better health? If a setback does take place, use this worksheet to help both of you understand and overcome the obstacles that may have tripped your child up. Remember, when trying to work through a setback, it's important to partner with your pediatrician.

What's Currently Happening?
What setback has occurred in your child's life that has interfered with his or her weight-loss efforts?

_____

_____

Did it happen just once, or repeatedly? _____ Is it still going on? _____

Why do you think this backsliding has occurred? Is there an event, a person, or a behavior that has contributed to the problem?

_____

_____

What Changes Need to Be Made and How Will You Make Them?
In the following space, write down a specific area in which a setback has occurred and where you and your child would like to make a change.

_____

_____

Are there obstacles that you and your youngster need to deal with effectively to ensure success in preventing this setback from recurring in the future?

_____

_____

What specific steps can you and your youngster take to make this change and minimize the risk of future setbacks?

_____

_____

Who can support you and your child in making these changes?

_____

WORKSHEET TO TAKE TO YOUR PEDIATRICIAN
EVALUATING SNACKING BEHAVIORS

In this worksheet, we'll look at your child's snacking and ways in which problems can be effectively managed as the family navigates its way toward a healthier life.

What's Currently Happening With Snacking?
Are there certain times of day when your child snacks? _____

Does your child appear to snack because he or she is genuinely hungry? _____

Does your child make mostly healthy choices when he or she reaches for snacks?
_____

If so, what kinds of healthy snacks does your child choose?
_____

What Problems Exist With Snacking?
Does your child sometimes select snacks that provide poor nutrition? _____

If so, what kinds of snacks does your child tend to choose?
_____

Does your child's urge to snack, and do the snacking choices your child makes, seem to be affected by his or her mood or external events to which your child is reacting (for example, stressful situations, particular times of the day)?
_____

What Changes Need to Be Made and How Will You Make Them?
What obstacles are interfering with your child snacking on healthy foods and appropriate portion sizes?
_____

Select a problem area related to snacking with which your child is having difficulty (for example, snacking excessively when watching TV or doing homework). You and your child should create a specific plan for attacking this problem. Write down this approach here.
_____

_____

Who can support you in making this change?
_____

Responding to Common Parental Concerns

Adapted from *A Parent's Guide to Childhood Obesity: A Road Map to Health*, the following are questions or statements commonly posed by parents during clinical visits. So often, the questions or statements are in the format of, "Yes...but." For example, "*Yes*, my child should exercise more, *but* there's just no time," or "*Yes*, I'd like to get the cookies out of our house, *but* what should I tell the other kids who still want cookies here?"

Reviewing these questions or statements and their responses may assist health care professionals in addressing parental concerns.

"Yes, I'd like to give my kids more fruits and vegetables, but fresh produce is too expensive!"
Fresh fruits and vegetables may be more affordable than you think. Particularly if you buy them when they're in season, they'll be much more reasonably priced than at other times of the year. Also, compare the costs of produce to other foods that you may already be buying for your child. For example, processed foods—from cookies to potato chips—are not only more expensive, but they certainly aren't as nutritious as fresh fruits and vegetables.

A number of studies have confirmed that fresh produce is more affordable than you might think. In 2004, the US Department of Agriculture analyzed and released data from household food purchases made in 1999, including multiple types of fruits and vegetables. The researchers concluded that the average American can purchase 4 servings of vegetables and 3 servings of fruits for just 64 cents a day. If this figure were adjusted to today's costs, the price might be an average of less than a dollar a day. No matter how you analyze the numbers, that's a great deal.

By the way, the same study found that two thirds of all fresh fruits and more than half of all fresh vegetables are less costly than processed versions of the same produce.

"Yes, I'd prefer to feed a variety of vegetables to my overweight child, but he absolutely hates vegetables. The only 'vegetables' he'll eat are french fries. That's it!"
As a parent, your job is to provide your child with well-balanced meals, including a variety of vegetables. Once the food is on the plate in front of him, he may choose whether to eat it. Sure, it can be frustrating when kids

push the plate away and refuse to even try something new, but be persistent. The good news is that over time, most children will develop a taste for enough healthy foods—even some vegetables—to be eating a balanced diet.

Some children may be more agreeable to consuming vegetables if you ask them to help you in the kitchen while you're preparing meals. They may be more receptive if you add vegetables to a pasta dish or put them in soups or meat loaf. Some youngsters prefer raw vegetables over cooked, and they'll often snack on cherry tomatoes or cut-up vegetables with yogurt dip. When eating in restaurants, accompany children on trips through the salad bar; expose them to vegetables they may never have tried at home.

Meanwhile, continue to serve as a role model. If your child sees you eating vegetables, he's more likely to try them. Have him get used to the idea that vegetables are part of every lunch and dinner. Remember your child will need to have at least 1 serving of fruits and vegetables with every meal and snack to meet the recommended 5 servings a day.

"Yes, I know my overweight child shouldn't have dessert with dinner every night or sweetened juices whenever he wants them, but I feel terrible if he complains about feeling deprived."
Don't lose sight of why you're making these dietary changes. As a parent, your child's health must be a top priority, and that may require making some adjustments in what he eats and the amount of physical activity he gets.

Of course, you don't want your youngster to feel deprived, and there's no need for you to completely eliminate his favorite desserts from his life. However, save those treats, like rich ice cream or chocolate chip cookies, for special occasions and serve appropriate portion sizes when you do. At the same time, introduce him to healthier desserts such as a dish of strawberries or a piece of angel food cake. When beverages are concerned, rely more often on low-fat milk or water rather than sugar-laden soft drinks or juices. Before long, he'll stop demanding the high-calorie, high-fat treats that he once craved.

"Yes, I'm willing to get unhealthy foods out of the house, but other adults in the home haven't come onboard yet. They tell me that they've been drinking sugary soft drinks all their lives, and they're not willing to give them up."

If other adults in the home insist on keeping high-fat snacks or high-calorie drinks in the cupboard or refrigerator, those kinds of temptations aren't fair to your child. To support your youngster's efforts to lose weight, it's essential for the entire family to get involved. The family needs to sit down and discuss the implications of continuing to live a lifestyle of poor eating choices. If the others still can't be convinced of the potential consequences of doing their own things, perhaps your pediatrician can talk to them. With your youngster's health at stake, your pediatrician may be able to motivate the others to give some ground. If they need to have sugary soft drinks, ask them to indulge at work and leave those kinds of snacks out of the house.

"Yes, my own mother seems to understand how important it is for my child to lose weight, but she still thinks it's a grandmother's prerogative to give my child candy whenever we visit. How can I convince her to get rid of that candy dish?"

The answer to this question is not much different than the previous one about others in the home having an attachment to soft drinks. You need to talk to your child's grandmother about the health risks your youngster faces unless he eats more nutritiously, one meal and one snack after another. As accustomed as grandma may be to baking cookies when the grandchildren visit, you can probably appeal to her strong desire to give your child the best possible chance of living a healthy life. Let grandma know about the nutritious food choices she can have available for the next family visit (see the patient handout, "Avoiding Food Traps").

"Yes, I realize that when the family goes out to dinner, we should stay away from fast-food restaurants most of the time, but whenever we drive by one of those places, my child pleads with me to stop."

It's fine to eat at fast-food restaurants once in a while. Because of their high-fat fare, though, don't make it a habit. Try and encourage lower fat options at fast-food restaurants.

When you visit these types of restaurants, order carefully for the family, finding choices to keep your child happy without sabotaging his healthier eating efforts. Whenever possible, for example, select a grilled chicken sandwich without any dressing for your youngster. If he insists on a hamburger, choose the smaller size, not the supersized double burger that looks like it could feed the entire family. Order a salad with low-fat dressing that he can eat as part of his meal.

Rather than overrelying on fast-food restaurants, choose to eat at sit-down family restaurants more frequently and look for healthy options on the menu. Split a dinner between the two of you. You will save money and eat healthier!

"Yes, snacking before bedtime may not be a good idea for my child while he's trying to lose weight, but when I was growing up, my mother always gave us cookies and milk before we went to bed. It's just something that I feel comfortable doing, and it would be hard to do things differently." Habits may be difficult to break, but for the well-being of your child, you need to make some adjustments. Nothing's inherently wrong with a bedtime snack, but you may need to adjust the kinds of snacks you're offering your youngster.

In general, try to limit the number of snacks to 2 per day. For those late-night munchies, make choices that contribute to overall healthy eating. You might turn to

- Air-popped popcorn rather than high-fat cheeses on crackers
- Frozen yogurt instead of ice cream
- Baked tortilla chips rather than potato chips
- Graham crackers (and milk) instead of chocolate chip cookies
- A piece of fruit rather than sugary cereal

"Yes, I understand that healthy eating is the best way for my child to lose weight, but I sometimes think that he could benefit from a little kick start, and the latest fad diets promise fast results. What's wrong with following one of these diets for a few weeks to get him off to a good start?" Most people have lost weight at some point in their lives—but then gained it all back. They know that fad diets don't work, at least over the long term, but the alluring promises on magazine covers and book jackets are often too tempting to resist.

Unfortunately, fad diets can be dangerous. They often emphasize a single food or food group, and they can be particularly risky for growing children for whom balanced nutrition is extremely important.

You need to put your child's health and well-being first. Don't be persuaded by promises of overnight weight loss. Instead, stick with a plan for good nutrition and physical activity. Your child's weight loss will be gradual and safe and have the best chance for permanent success.

"Yes, I feel that I can control what my child eats at home, but when he's at child care, I have no control over what the child care provider gives him. He's served whatever the other kids eat."
Express your concerns to the child care staff. Even if the facility serves identical meals to all the children, make some suggestions for fine-tuning the menu in the direction of healthier foods. The staff may turn out to be much more flexible than you expected and might be willing to bend to your requests, perhaps serving your youngster a turkey sandwich and small salad for lunch instead of a hamburger and french fries.

If you're sensing some reluctance on their part, offer to pack your child's lunch and/or snacks to make sure that he's eating foods supportive of the family's commitment to more nutritious eating.

"Yes, I'd love to sign my overweight child up for a fitness program at the Y, but we just can't afford it."
Kids can enjoy the benefits of physical activity without busting the family budget. Play is the major way kids can increase their activity. You don't need costly exercise equipment like treadmills, nor do you have to enroll them in classes with expensive sign-up fees. Outdoor play in a safe area can be a major help to increasing physical activity.

There are plenty of activities that won't cause financial stress (see the patient handout, "Everyone Get Fit"). Walking, for example, is one of the best forms of exercise, and it doesn't require any special equipment, other than a good pair of walking shoes. If the entire family gets involved, your overweight child is more likely to be motivated to walk regularly. In fact, the best forms of physical activity are family activities. Keep them fun, and your child won't feel that he's missing out on the formal program at the Y.

"Yes, my child knows that he needs to become more physically active, but he has so much homework, plus piano lessons after school, and there's just no time for exercise."
So many of today's kids lead very busy lives. It seems as though their planned activities start immediately after school and continue until well after nightfall. If you think about it, there's probably some time in your child's afternoon and evening, even just 15 or 20 minutes, when he could fit in some physical activity.

Remember, activity needs to become a priority in your child's life. That means that exercise wins out over video games or surfing the Web almost every time. After school, can he play catch with the neighborhood kids in the park down the block, or work out to an exercise video that you put into the VCR?

Frankly, there aren't too many kids who don't have a few minutes to spare each day for squeezing in some physical activity. Physical activity promotes motor and mental development and is essential for developing coordination.

"Yes, my overweight child should be getting more physical activity, but in our neighborhood, I just don't think it's safe for him to be playing outdoors."
Don't let safety concerns keep your child sedentary. There are plenty of ways for him to stay active other than playing in your front yard or on the neighborhood playground. He can participate in a swimming program at the Boys & Girls Club or join a karate class. He can stay active indoors at home by dancing to his favorite music, spinning a hula hoop, jumping rope, or doing chores like straightening up his room.

"Yes, eating right and being active makes sense, but my teenager has so much weight to lose that we've been talking about weight-loss surgery. Is that something we should consider?"
Although the overwhelming majority of gastric-bypass surgeries are being performed in adults, a relatively small number of teenagers have undergone the procedure. However, this is major surgery, and the decision to have the operation should not be made hastily.

Weight-loss surgery is only advisable for extremely overweight adolescents for whom more conservative weight-loss measures haven't worked, particularly if they also have developed serious obesity-related medical conditions such as high blood pressure, diabetes, and sleep apnea.

Your pediatrician can provide an initial assessment of whether your teenager might be a candidate for surgery. If the pediatrician refers you for a consultation to a weight-loss surgeon who performs these procedures, you and your adolescent will meet with the surgeon as well as a number of other specialists, including clinical psychologists and nutritionists. You and your teenager will have the opportunity to discuss the potential benefits of the operation, plus get your questions answered about the complications sometimes associated with the operation like infections, bleeding, and blood clots.

Obesity and Related Comorbidities Coding Fact Sheet for Primary Care Pediatricians

While coding for the care of children with obesity and related comorbidities is relatively straightforward, ensuring that appropriate reimbursement is received for such services is a more complicated matter. Many insurance carriers will deny claims submitted with "obesity" codes (eg, **278.00**), essentially carving out obesity-related care from the scope of benefits. Therefore, coding for obesity services is fundamentally a two-tiered system in which the first tier requires health care professionals to submit claims using appropriate codes and the second tier involves the practice-level issues of denial management and contract negotiation.

This coding fact sheet provides a guide to coding for obesity-related health care services. Strategies and a template letter for pediatric practices to handle carrier denials and contractual issues are given in "Denial Management and Contract Negotiation for Obesity Services" (Appendix A.7) and "Obesity Services: Sample Carrier Letter" (Appendix A.8).

Procedure Codes

Current Procedural Terminology (CPT®) *Codes*

Body Fat Composition Testing
There is no separate *Current Procedural Terminology (CPT®)* code for body fat composition testing. This service would be included in the examination component of the evaluation and management (E/M) code reported.

Calorimetry
94690   Oxygen uptake, expired gas analysis; rest, indirect (separate procedure)
            or
94799   Unlisted pulmonary service or procedure
            [Note: Special report required.]

Glucose Monitoring

95250 Ambulatory continuous glucose monitoring of interstitial tissue fluid via a subcutaneous sensor for up to 72 hours; sensor placement, hookup, calibration of monitor, patient training, removal of sensor, and printout of recording

95251 Ambulatory continuous glucose monitoring of interstitial tissue fluid via a subcutaneous sensor for up to 72 hours; physician interpretation and report

Routine Venipuncture

36415 Collection of venous blood by venipuncture

36416 Collection of capillary blood specimen (eg, finger, heel, ear stick)

Venipuncture Necessitating Physician's Skill

36406 Venipuncture, younger than 3 years, necessitating physician's skill, not to be used for routine venipuncture; other vein

36410 Venipuncture, 3 years or older, necessitating physician's skill (separate procedure), for diagnostic or therapeutic purposes (not to be used for routine venipuncture)

Digestive System Surgery Codes

43644 Laparoscopy, surgical, gastric restrictive procedure; with gastric bypass and Roux-en-Y gastroenterostomy (Roux limb 150 cm or less)

43645 Laparoscopy, surgical, gastric restrictive procedure; with gastric bypass and small intestine reconstruction to limit absorption

43842 Gastric restrictive procedure, without gastric bypass, for morbid obesity; vertical-banded gastroplasty

43843 Gastric restrictive procedure, without gastric bypass, for morbid obesity; other than vertical-banded gastroplasty

43845 Gastric restrictive procedure with partial gastrectomy, pylorus-preserving duodenoileostomy and ileoileostomy (50 to 100 cm common channel) to limit absorption (biliopancreatic diversion with duodenal switch)

43846 Gastric restrictive procedure, with gastric bypass for morbid obesity; with short limb (150 cm or less) Roux-en-Y gastroenterostomy

43847 Gastric restrictive procedure, with gastric bypass for morbid obesity; with small intestine reconstruction to limit absorption

43848 Revision, open, of gastric restrictive procedure for morbid obesity; other than adjustable gastric band (separate procedure)

Health and Behavior Assessment/Intervention Codes

These codes cannot be reported by a physician, nor can they be reported on the same day as preventive medicine counseling codes (**99401–99412**).

96150 Health and behavior assessment (eg, health-focused clinical interview, behavioral observations, psychophysiologic monitoring, health-oriented questionnaires), each 15 minutes face-to-face with the patient; initial assessment

96151 Health and behavior assessment (eg, health-focused clinical interview, behavioral observations, psychophysiologic monitoring, health-oriented questionnaires), each 15 minutes face-to-face with the patient; reassessment

The focus of the assessment is not on mental health, but on the biopsychosocial factors important to physical health problems and treatments.

96152 Health and behavior intervention, each 15 minutes, face-to-face; individual

96153 Health and behavior intervention, each 15 minutes, face-to-face; group (2 or more patients)

96154 Health and behavior intervention, each 15 minutes, face-to-face; family (with patient present)

96155 Health and behavior intervention, each 15 minutes, face-to-face; family (without patient present)

The focus of the intervention is to improve the patient's health and well-being using cognitive, behavioral, social, and/or psychophysiologic procedures designed to ameliorate the specific obesity-related problems.

Medical Nutrition Therapy Codes

These codes cannot be reported by a physician.

97802 Medical nutrition therapy; initial assessment and intervention, individual, face-to-face with patient, each 15 minutes

97803   Medical nutrition therapy; reassessment and intervention, individual, face-to-face with the patient, each 15 minutes

97804   Medical nutrition therapy; group (2 or more individuals), each 30 minutes

Healthcare Common Procedural Coding System (HCPCS) Level II Procedure and Supply Codes

Current Procedural Terminology codes are also known as Healthcare Common Procedure Coding System (HCPCS) Level I codes. HCPCS also contains Level II codes. Level II codes (commonly referred to as HCPCS ["hick-picks"] codes) are national codes that are included as part of the Health Insurance Portability and Accountability Act of 1996 (HIPAA) standard procedural transaction coding set along with *CPT* codes.

Healthcare Common Procedure Coding System Level II codes were developed to fill gaps in the *CPT* nomenclature. While they are reported in the same way as *CPT* codes, they consist of 1 alphabetic character (A–V) followed by 4 digits. In the past, insurance carriers did not uniformly recognize HCPCS Level II codes. However, with the advent of HIPAA, carrier software systems must now be able to recognize all HCPCS Level I *(CPT)* and Level II codes.

HCPCS Education and Counseling Codes

S9445   Patient education, not otherwise classified, nonphysician provider, individual, per session

S9446   Patient education, not otherwise classified, nonphysician provider, group, per session

S9449   Weight management classes, nonphysician provider, per session

S9451   Exercise class, nonphysician provider, per session

S9452   Nutrition class, nonphysician provider, per session

S9454   Stress management class, nonphysician provider, per session

S9455   Diabetic management program, group session

S9460   Diabetic management program, nurse visit

S9465   Diabetic management program, dietitian visit

S9470   Nutritional counseling, dietitian visit

Diagnosis Codes

International Classification of Diseases, Ninth Revision, Clinical Modification (ICD-9-CM) *Codes*

Circulatory System

401.9	Essential hypertension; unspecified
429.3	Cardiomegaly

Congenital Anomalies

758.0	Down syndrome
759.81	Prader-Willi syndrome
759.83	Fragile X syndrome
759.89	Other specified anomalies (Laurence-Moon-Biedl syndrome)

Digestive System

530.81	Esophageal reflux
564.00	Constipation, unspecified
571.8	Other chronic nonalcoholic liver disease

Endocrine, Nutritional, Metabolic

244.8	Other specified acquired hypothyroidism
244.9	Unspecified hypothyroidism
250.00	Diabetes mellitus without mention of complication, type II or unspecified type, not stated as uncontrolled
250.02	Diabetes mellitus without mention of complication, type II or unspecified type, uncontrolled
253.8	Other disorders of the pituitary and other syndromes of diencephalohypophysial origin
255.8	Other specified disorders of adrenal glands
256.4	Polycystic ovaries
259.1	Precocious sexual development and puberty, not elsewhere specified
259.9	Unspecified endocrine disorder
272.0	Pure hypercholesterolemia
272.1	Pure hyperglyceridemia
272.2	Mixed hyperlipidemia
272.4	Other and unspecified hyperlipidemia

. . . .

272.9   Unspecified disorder of lipoid metabolism
277.7   Dysmetabolic syndrome X/metabolic syndrome
278.00 Obesity, unspecified
278.01 Morbid obesity
278.02 Overweight
278.1   Localized adiposity
278.8   Other hyperalimentation

Genitourinary System

611.1   Hypertrophy of the breast

Mental Disorders

300.00 Anxiety state, unspecified
300.02 Generalized anxiety disorder
300.4   Dysthymic disorder
307.50 Eating disorder, unspecified
307.51 Bulimia nervosa
307.59 Other and unspecified disorders of eating
308.3   Other acute reactions to stress
308.9   Unspecified acute reaction to stress
311   Depressive disorder, not elsewhere classified
313.1   Misery and unhappiness disorder
313.81 Oppositional defiant disorder

Musculoskeletal System and Connective Tissue

732.4   Juvenile osteochondrosis of lower extremity, excluding foot

Nervous System and Sense Organs

327.23 Obstructive sleep apnea (adult) (pediatric)
348.2   Benign intracranial hypertension

Skin and Subcutaneous Tissue

701.2   Acquired acanthosis nigricans

Symptoms, Signs, and Ill-Defined Conditions

780.51 Insomnia with sleep apnea, unspecified
780.53 Hypersomnia with sleep apnea, unspecified
780.54 Hypersomnia, unspecified

780.57	Unspecified sleep apnea
780.59	Sleep disturbance; other
780.71	Chronic fatigue syndrome
780.79	Other malaise and fatigue
783.1	Abnormal weight gain
783.3	Feeding difficulties and mismanagement
783.40	Lack of normal physiological development, unspecified
783.43	Short stature
783.5	Polydipsia
783.6	Polyphagia
783.9	Other symptoms concerning nutrition, metabolism, and development
786.05	Shortness of breath
789.1	Hepatomegaly
790.22	Impaired glucose tolerance test (oral)
790.29	Other abnormal glucose; prediabetes not otherwise specified
790.4	Nonspecific elevation of levels of transaminase or lactic acid dehydrogenase (LDH)
790.6	Other abnormal blood chemistry (hyperglycemia)

Other

NOTE: The *ICD-9-CM* codes that follow are used to deal with occasions in which circumstances other than a disease or injury are recorded as diagnoses or problems. Some carriers may request supporting documentation for the reporting of V codes.

V18.0	Family history of diabetes mellitus
V18.1	Family history of endocrine and metabolic diseases
V49.89	Other specified conditions influencing health status
V58.67	Long-term (current) use of insulin
V58.69	Long-term (current) use of other medications
V61.0	Family disruption
V61.20	Counseling for parent-child problem, unspecified
V61.29	Parent-child problems; other
V61.49	Health problems with family; other
V61.8	Health problems within family; other specified family circumstances

V61.9   Health problems within family; unspecified family circumstances
V62.81   Interpersonal problems, not elsewhere classified
V62.89   Other psychological or physical stress not elsewhere
classified; other
V62.9   Unspecified psychosocial circumstance
V65.19   Other person consulting on behalf of another person
V65.3   Dietary surveillance and counseling
V65.41   Exercise counseling
V65.49   Other specified counseling
V69.0   Lack of physical exercise
V69.1   Inappropriate diet and eating habits
V69.8   Other problems relating to lifestyle; self-damaging behavior
V69.9   Problem related to lifestyle, unspecified

NOTE: The following codes become effective October 1, 2006.
V85.51   Body mass index, pediatric, less than 5th percentile for age
V85.52   Body mass index, pediatric, 5th percentile to less than
85th percentile for age
V85.53   Body mass index, pediatric, 85th percentile to less than
95th percentile for age
V85.54   Body mass index, pediatric, greater than or equal to
95th percentile for age

American Academy of Pediatrics Activities

Some chapters have created pediatric councils that meet with carrier medical directors to discuss pediatric issues. American Academy of Pediatrics (AAP) members may contact their chapters to report issues related to coverage for obesity with carriers. Members may also report carrier issues using the AAP Hassle Factor Form, available on the Member Center of the AAP Web site (www.aap.org/moc) under the "More Resources" link.

The AAP Private Payer Advocacy Advisory Committee and Task Force on Obesity are addressing coverage and reimbursement issues for primary care and developmental and behavioral pediatricians including carve-outs, health plan provider networks, and coverage and compensation for evaluation and treatment, and will be developing strategies and resources to help pediatric practices advocate for enhanced coverage and compensation for obesity. Refer to the AAP "Prevention of Pediatric Overweight and Obesity" policy statement (aappolicy.aappublications.org/cgi/content/full/pediatrics; 112/2/424) for recommendations for health care professionals on the clinical assessment, prevention, and treatment of obesity.

For more information on coding, contact the AAP Division of Health Care Finance and Quality Improvement at dhcfqi@aap.org.

Denial Management and Contract Negotiation for Obesity Services

The current private carrier coverage environment for obesity services is mixed. Private carriers may have health plans that do not cover obesity-related services under the medical plan; they may be carved out of the benefits package completely or part of disease management programs.

The key is to determine the level of coverage by the health plan for obesity evaluation and treatment. If the health plan denies an appropriately coded service for obesity,

- Determine the nature of the denial to determine the appropriate follow-up.

- Review the carrier's denial letter or explanation of benefits (EOB) for the reason for the denial. Most commonly provided reasons are *bundling* of services, it is a *carve-out* from the medical plan benefits, or it is a *noncovered* service.
  - **Bundling.** Obesity evaluation and treatment services may be bundled with the evaluation and management (E/M) services by the carrier. The *Current Procedural Terminology (CPT®)* codes listed in Appendix A.6 represent separately identifiable services and should be reported as such. While there is no legal mandate requiring private carriers to adhere to *CPT* guidelines, it is considered a good faith gesture for them to do so, given that the guidelines are the current standard within organized medicine. All inappropriate bundling of services should be appealed by the pediatric practice to the carrier.
  - **Carve-out.** Some carriers may carve out obesity-related services from the provider network to a smaller specialty network or disease management program. The pediatrician may consider contacting the carrier to determine the extent of the carve-out and to what degree coverage and payment are available for obesity-related services. As a contractual issue between the health plan and pediatric practice, the pediatrician may discuss with the carrier becoming part of the network or disease management program.
  - **Noncovered service.** Carriers may have different levels of health plan benefits, and the family may be covered by a health plan with limited benefits coverage that does not provide any benefits coverage for obesity-related services. In these situations, the family would be financially responsible for services provided to evaluate and treat obesity.

. . . .

Strategies to Enhance Coverage

In addressing issues with carriers, strategies include *filing appeals* and *negotiating contractual provisions*. A sample letter to send to carriers addressing bundling and carve-outs is included in Appendix A.8.

- Filing appeals. Pediatric practices can follow these general guidelines when appealing claim denials or partially paid claims (excerpted from AAP Division of Health Care Finance and Practice. Appealing claim denials can improve the bottom line. *AAP News.* June 2004;24:257):

  1. Review all carrier EOBs. Compare the billed amount and *CPT* codes with the EOBs to determine the level of discounts, denials, inappropriate carrier recoding, or partial payments.
  2. Make sure the claim was prepared properly, all information is correct, and documentation supports the *CPT* codes. Once assured the denial was not caused by an error on the practice's part, proceed with the appeal.
  3. Send appeals in writing and to the right person—look up the contact person in the contract or call the carrier and explain the situation and what is coming so it can be on the lookout. If you are not satisfied with the response, contact the plan's medical director.
  4. Send the appeal by certified mail to verify receipt by the health plan.
  5. List the member's name, carrier identification number, and claim number on all documentation.
  6. State your case in objective and factual terms. Identify the result you want and provide medical justification and *CPT* coding guidelines to support your case (keep in mind, most claim processors do not have a medical or coding background, so be clear and specific). Sample appeal letters that can be used as templates are available on the Member Center of the American Academy of Pediatrics (AAP) Web site (www.aap.org/moc) on the Private Payer Advocacy page.
  7. Suggest how denials can be avoided in the future, particularly if they are a recurring problem.
  8. Monitor for a response. If the carrier does not respond within the time frame specified in your initial appeal, follow up with a second letter.
  9. Create a spreadsheet to track appeals to each carrier so at contract renewal time, you can determine whether to continue to work with that carrier and identify items to modify in the contract.

10. Each health plan should have a written statement explaining the procedures required for first- and second-level appeals. If services are not excluded in the contract and the practice has correctly coded and properly documented them, continue to appeal. Should further action be required, contact the state department of insurance or, depending on the state in which you practice, the state department of banking and insurance or health. Most states have prompt pay laws. If a managed care organization violates the prompt pay law, the physician may be eligible for interest payments on the amount owed, depending on state law.

11. If a claim is denied and the health plan informs that it is a non-covered service or the plan member's responsibility, bill the plan member and include a copy of the EOB and denial with the bill.

12. Contact your AAP chapter to keep it aware of your issues. Some chapters have pediatric councils that meet regularly with health plan medical directors and Medicaid representatives to address coverage issues. Use the AAP Hassle Factor Form to report problems with carriers. (Some chapters have made the Hassle Factor Form available on their Web sites; it also can be accessed on the Member Center under the "More Resources" link.)

- Negotiating contractual provisions. In contacts with health plans to discuss contractual issues, the keys are to

  1. Address this issue with the person who has the authority to make decisions about payment. The carrier provider representative may not have the decision-making authority in this type of matter.

  2. Focus the argument on how this is cost-effective to the family and health plan as well as how it relates to quality care (provide documentation supporting your position).

  3. Frame your position on how it affects the quality of care, cost-effectiveness, and patient satisfaction. Carriers are very conscious of quality issues, how a proposed change will affect overall expenses and efficiency, and market share. The carrier's current policy may not cover obesity-related services and the carrier needs to be made aware of the effect on the patient, family, pediatrician, and carrier.

  4. Consider notifying the family and employer because they may bring pressure on the carrier and employer to expand health plan coverage.

American Academy of Pediatrics Activities

Some chapters have created pediatric councils that meet with carrier medical directors to discuss pediatric issues. American Academy of Pediatrics members may contact their chapters to report issues related to coverage for obesity with carriers. Members may also report carrier issues using the AAP Hassle Factor Form, available on the Member Center of the AAP Web site (www.aap.org/moc) under the "More Resources" link.

The AAP Private Payer Advocacy Advisory Committee and Task Force on Obesity are addressing coverage and reimbursement issues for primary care and developmental and behavioral pediatricians including carve-outs, health plan provider networks, and coverage and compensation for evaluation and treatment, and will be developing strategies and resources to help pediatric practices advocate for enhanced coverage and compensation for obesity. Refer to the AAP "Prevention of Pediatric Overweight and Obesity" policy statement (aappolicy.aappublications.org/cgi/content/full/pediatrics; 112/2/424) for recommendations for health care professionals on the clinical assessment, prevention, and treatment of obesity.

For more information on coding, contact the AAP Division of Health Care Finance and Quality Improvement at dhcfqi@aap.org.

Obesity Services:
Sample Carrier Letter

To: Claims Processing Department or Health Plan Medical Director

RE: Bundling services related to obesity evaluation and treatment

Claim # _____

The above referenced claim inappropriately bundled separately reported services. I would like to clarify that *Current Procedural Terminology (CPT®)* guidelines indicate that services that are identified with specific codes should be reported separately from any other code(s) and therefore, they should not be bundled into any other code(s). Unfortunately, many carriers are unaware that they are violating *CPT* guidelines when they inappropriately bundle 2 services together when each of the involved services has a separate *CPT* code. This concept is found throughout *CPT* guidelines. Some examples include

- "If an abnormality/ies is encountered or a preexisting problem is addressed in the process of performing this preventive medicine service, and if the problem/abnormality is significant enough to require additional work to perform the key components of a problem-oriented E/M service, then the appropriate Office or Other Outpatient code **99201–99215** should also be reported. Modifier **25** should be appended to the Office or Other Outpatient code to indicate that a significant, separately identifiable E/M service was provided by the same physician on the same day as the preventive medicine service." (American Medical Association. *CPT 2006 Professional Edition.* Chicago, IL: American Medical Association; 2005:31)

- "Immunizations and ancillary studies involving laboratory, radiology, other procedures, or screening tests identified with a specific *CPT* code are reported separately." (American Medical Association. *CPT 2006 Professional Edition.* Chicago, IL: American Medical Association; 2005:31)

The *CPT* guidelines are applicable to any other screening tests or procedures that are identified with a specific *CPT* code such as calorimetry, glucose monitoring, and venipuncture. Therefore, physicians are correct in reporting such services separately from any accompanying evaluation and management service. Those separately reportable services that are not recognized by a carrier should be designated as noncovered benefits and billable to the patient.

Enclosed is a copy of the original claim that was submitted with a request that you process reimbursement as indicated on the claim. I look forward to receiving your response. If you have any questions, please feel free to contact me at _____.

Sincerely,

Physician Tracking Form for Pediatric Obesity

Physician Tracking Form for Pediatric Obesity

	For Office Use Only
Patient Name	
	Date of Visit

Patient Assessment

Family History

Obesity

Diabetes

Hypertension

Renal disease

Cardiac disease

Dyslipidemia

Thyroid

Liver disease

Review of Systems

HEENT

Headache

Vision change

Respiratory

Asthma

Snoring

Apnea

Daytime tiredness

Napping

Dyspnea

Cardiovascular

Hypertension

Dyslipidemia

Exercise intolerance

Physician Tracking Form for Pediatric Obesity, continued

	Date of Visit			
Gastrointestinal				
Stomach pain after eating	_____	_____	_____	_____
Nausea/vomiting after eating	_____	_____	_____	_____
Reflux	_____	_____	_____	_____
Liver disease	_____	_____	_____	_____
Genitourinary				
Premature adrenarche	_____	_____	_____	_____
Gynecomastia	_____	_____	_____	_____
Enuresis	_____	_____	_____	_____
Urinary frequency	_____	_____	_____	_____
Musculoskeletal				
Limp	_____	_____	_____	_____
Hip pain	_____	_____	_____	_____
Knee pain	_____	_____	_____	_____
Physical Examination				
Plot weight (%)	_____	_____	_____	_____
Plot height (%)	_____	_____	_____	_____
Plot body mass index (%)	_____	_____	_____	_____
Blood pressure (%)	_____	_____	_____	_____
Waist/hip measurement	_____	_____	_____	_____
Funduscopic eye examination	_____	_____	_____	_____
Skin				
– Acanthosis nigricans	_____	_____	_____	_____
– Facial hair	_____	_____	_____	_____
– Acne	_____	_____	_____	_____
Upper and lower airway				
– Wheezing	_____	_____	_____	_____
– Tonsillar hypertrophy	_____	_____	_____	_____

	Date of Visit			
Cardiac				
– Murmur	_____	_____	_____	_____
Abdomen				
– Striae	_____	_____	_____	_____
– Hepatomegaly	_____	_____	_____	_____
Pubertal stage				
– Pubic hair stage	_____	_____	_____	_____
– Breast stage	_____	_____	_____	_____
– Gynecomastia	_____	_____	_____	_____
Orthopedic				
– Limp	_____	_____	_____	_____
– Hip pain	_____	_____	_____	_____
– Knee pain	_____	_____	_____	_____
Psychosocial Assessment/ Behavioral Issues				
Family stress	_____	_____	_____	_____
Hunger management	_____	_____	_____	_____
Food sneaking	_____	_____	_____	_____
Limit setting	_____	_____	_____	_____
Nutritional Assessment				
Soda/juice intake	_____	_____	_____	_____
Structured meals	_____	_____	_____	_____
Vegetable intake	_____	_____	_____	_____
Snacking	_____	_____	_____	_____
Activity/Inactivity Assessment				
Amount of television/computer	_____	_____	_____	_____
Amount of daily physical activity	_____	_____	_____	_____
Organized physical activity	_____	_____	_____	_____

Physician Tracking Form for Pediatric Obesity, continued

	Date of Visit			
School				
School lunch	_____	_____	_____	_____
Recess	_____	_____	_____	_____
Physical education	_____	_____	_____	_____
Snacks	_____	_____	_____	_____
Laboratory Evaluation				
HbA$_{1C}$ (optional)	_____	_____	_____	_____
Fasting glucose/insulin	_____	_____	_____	_____
Postprandial glucose (if indicated)	_____	_____	_____	_____
Oral glucose tolerance test (if indicated)	_____	_____	_____	_____
Urine for microalbumin (if indicated)	_____	_____	_____	_____
Lipids: cholesterol, HDL, LDL, triglyceride	_____	_____	_____	_____
Liver function profile AST/ALT/GTP	_____	_____	_____	_____
Thyroid: Free T$_4$ and TSH	_____	_____	_____	_____
am cortisol	_____	_____	_____	_____
Management Plan and Patient Education				
Problem-oriented nutritional/ activity/inactivity assessment				
– Diet record: meals, beverages, snacks	_____	_____	_____	_____
– Activity record: physical education, extracurricular activity, family activity	_____	_____	_____	_____
– Inactivity record: hours of TV, computer, games, movies	_____	_____	_____	_____
– Problem-oriented review of behavioral response to change, parenting style, and family system	_____	_____	_____	_____
– Review of complications of obesity and specific treatment ie, hyperlipidemia, hypertension	_____	_____	_____	_____

	Date of Visit			
– Review of comorbidities of obesity and specific treatment ie, asthma, sleep apnea, Blount disease	_____	_____	_____	_____
Specialty Referrals				
Nutritionist (for diet education/ diet plan?)	_____	_____	_____	_____
As indicated for patients with advanced needs or complications				
– Pulmonologist (for sleep apnea/asthma)	_____	_____	_____	_____
– Endocrinologist (for diabetes, PCOS, hypothyroidism)	_____	_____	_____	_____
– Gastroenterologist (for elevated liver function studies)	_____	_____	_____	_____
– Orthopedic surgeon (Blount disease, slipped capital femoral epiphysis, hip or knee pain, limp)	_____	_____	_____	_____
– Psychiatrist (depression, ADHD, anxiety disorder, bipolar)	_____	_____	_____	_____
Treatment Goals				
Weight stability	_____	_____	_____	_____
Weight loss	_____	_____	_____	_____
Normalize metabolic parameters	_____	_____	_____	_____
Improve comorbidities	_____	_____	_____	_____
Family able to initiate lifestyle changes suggested	_____	_____	_____	_____
Conflict around food and lifestyle change decreasing	_____	_____	_____	_____
Family able to problem-solve independently	_____	_____	_____	_____

Form developed by Sandra G. Hassink, MD, and George A. Datto, MD.

Appendix A.10

American Academy of Pediatrics Policy Statements

American Academy
of Pediatrics

DEDICATED TO THE HEALTH OF ALL CHILDREN™

POLICY STATEMENT

Active Healthy Living: Prevention of Childhood Obesity Through Increased Physical Activity

Council on Sports Medicine and Fitness and Council on School Health

Organizational Principles to Guide and Define the Child Health Care System and/or Improve the Health of All Children

ABSTRACT

The current epidemic of inactivity and the associated epidemic of obesity are being driven by multiple factors (societal, technologic, industrial, commercial, financial) and must be addressed likewise on several fronts. Foremost among these are the expansion of school physical education, dissuading children from pursuing sedentary activities, providing suitable role models for physical activity, and making activity-promoting changes in the environment. This statement outlines ways that pediatric health care providers and public health officials can encourage, monitor, and advocate for increased physical activity for children and teenagers.

INTRODUCTION

IN 1997, THE World Health Organization declared obesity a global epidemic with major health implications.[1] According to the 1999–2000 National Health and Nutrition Examination Survey (www.cdc.gov/nchs/nhanes.htm), the prevalence of overweight or obesity in children and youth in the United States is over 15%, a value that has tripled since the 1960s.[2] The health implications of this epidemic are profound. Insulin resistance, type 2 diabetes mellitus, hypertension, obstructive sleep apnea, nonalcoholic steatohepatitis, poor self-esteem, and a lower health-related quality of life are among the comorbidities seen more commonly in affected children and youth than in their unaffected counterparts.[3–7] In addition, up to 80% of obese youth continue this trend into adulthood.[8,9] Adult obesity is associated with higher rates of hypertension, dyslipidemia, and insulin resistance, which are risk factors for coronary artery disease, the leading cause of death in North America.[10]

Assessment of Overweight

Ideally, methods of measuring body fat should be accurate, inexpensive, and easy to use; have small measurement error; and be well documented with published reference values. Direct measures of body composition, such as underwater weighing, magnetic resonance imaging, computed axial tomography, and dual-energy radiograph absorptiometry, provide an estimate of total body fat mass. These techniques, however, are used mainly in tertiary care centers for research purposes. Anthropometric measures of relative fatness may be inexpensive and easy to use but rely on the skill of the measurer, and their relative accuracy must be validated against a "gold-standard" measure of adiposity. Such indirect methods of

www.pediatrics.org/cgi/doi/10.1542/peds.2006-0472

doi:10.1542/peds.2006-0472

All policy statements from the American Academy of Pediatrics automatically expire 5 years after publication unless reaffirmed, revised, or retired at or before that time.

Key Words
healthy living, physical activity, obesity, overweight, advocacy, children, youth

Abbreviations
PE—physical education
AAP—American Academy of Pediatrics

PEDIATRICS (ISSN Numbers: Print, 0031-4005; Online, 1098-4275). Copyright © 2006 by the American Academy of Pediatrics

estimating body composition include measuring weight and weight for height, body mass index (BMI), waist circumference, skinfold thickness, and ponderal index.[11] Of these, perhaps the most convenient is BMI, which can be calculated according to the following formulas (www.cdc.gov/growthcharts):

BMI = weight (kg)/(height) (m²) or

BMI = weight (kg)/height (cm)/height (cm) × 10 000

BMI = weight (lb)/height (in)/height (in) × 703

BMI varies with age and gender. It typically increases during the first months of life, decreases after the first year, and increases again around 6 years of age.[11] A specific BMI value, therefore, should be evaluated against age- and gender-specific reference values. In the United States, such reference charts based on early 1970s survey data of children 2 to 20 years of age are readily available for clinical use.[12] Children and youth with a BMI greater than the 95th percentile are classified as overweight or obese, and those between the 85th and 95th percentiles are designated at risk of overweight.[13] Although BMI tends to underestimate overweight in tall individuals and overestimate overweight in short individuals and those with high lean body mass (ie, athletes), it generally correlates well with more precise measures of adiposity in individuals with BMI in the 95th percentile or greater.[14]

Factors Contributing to Obesity

Some children have medical conditions associated with obesity and/or require pharmacologic treatments resulting in significant weight gain. Others (1%–2% of obese children) have underlying genetic conditions such as Down, Prader-Willi, or Bardet-Biedle syndrome, which can be associated with obesity. Rarely, single-gene disorders, including congenital leptin deficiency and defects in the melanocortin 4 receptor, cause morbid childhood obesity.

Observations on twin, sibling, and family studies suggest that children are more likely to be overweight if relatives are similarly affected and that heritability may play a role in as many as 25% to 85% of cases. However, to suggest that only genetic factors have caused the recent global epidemic of childhood obesity would not be realistic. It is more likely that most of the world's population carries a combination of genes that may have evolved to cope with food scarcity. In obesogenic environments in which calorie-dense foods are readily available and low-energy expenditure is commonplace, this genetic predisposition would be maladaptive and could lead to an obese population.[11]

Nutritional factors contributing to the increase in obesity rates include, in no particular order, (1) insufficient infant breastfeeding, (2) a reduction in cereal fiber, fruit,

and vegetable intake by children and youth, and (3) the excessive consumption of oversized fast foods and soda, which are encouraged by fast-food advertising during children's television programming and a greater availability of fast foods and sugar-containing beverages in school vending machines.[15,16] Although nutritional issues have a significant role to play, this statement focuses on factors associated with decreased energy expenditure, namely excessive sedentary behaviors and lack of adequate physical activity.

Children and youth are more sedentary than ever with the widespread availability of television, videos, computers, and video games. Data from the 1988–1994 National Health and Nutrition Examination Survey indicated that 26% of American children (up to 33% of Mexican American and 43% of non-Hispanic black children) watched at least 4 hours of television per day, and these children were less likely to participate in vigorous physical activity. They also had greater BMIs and skinfold measurements than those who watched <2 hours of television per day.[17]

Not only are the rates of sedentary activities rising, but participation in physical activity is not optimal. In a 2002 Youth Media Campaign Longitudinal Survey, 4500 children 9 to 13 years of age and their parents were polled about physical activity levels outside of school hours. The report indicated that 61.5% of 9- to 13-year-olds did not participate in any organized physical activities and 22.6% did not partake in nonorganized physical activity during nonschool hours.[18]

Youth at Risk of Decreased Physical Activity

Particular individuals at increased risk of having low levels of physical activity have been identified and include children who are from ethnic minorities (especially girls) in the preadolescent/adolescent age groups, children living in poverty, children with disabilities, children residing in apartments or public housing, and children living in neighborhoods where outdoor physical activity is restricted by climate, safety concerns, or lack of facilities.[19,20] According to the Centers for Disease Control and Prevention (www.cdc.gov/nccdphp/sgr/ados.htm), inactivity is twice as common among females (14%) as males (7%) and among black females (21%) as white females (12%). In a meta-analysis that evaluated physical activity and cardiorespiratory fitness, 6- to 7-year-olds were more active in moderate to vigorous physical activity (46 minutes/day) compared with 10- to 16-year-olds (16–45 minutes/day). Boys were approximately 20% more active than girls, and mean activity levels decreased with age by 2.7% per year in boys compared with 7.4% per year in girls.[21] Many reasons are stated for the general lack of physical activity among children and youth. These reasons include inactive role models (eg, parents and other caregivers), competing demands/time pressures, unsafe environments, lack of recreation facilities or insufficient funds to begin recreation programs, and inadequate access to quality daily physical education (PE).

Physical Activity in Schools

Children and youth spend most of their waking hours at school, so the availability of regular physical activity in that setting is critical. Although the *Healthy People 2010* report recommends increasing the amount of daily PE for all students in a larger proportion of US schools, such changes do not seem to be forthcoming.[19] In 2000, a school health policies and program study[22] looked at a nationally representative sample of private and public schools and found that only 8% of American elementary schools, 6.4% of middle schools, and 5.8% of high schools with existing PE requirements provided daily PE classes for all grades for the entire year. In addition, although approximately 80% of states have policies calling for students to participate in PE in all schools, 40% of elementary schools, 52% of middle schools, and 60% of high schools allow exemption from PE classes, particularly for students with permanent physical disabilities and those having religious reasons.[22] The National Association of State Boards of Education recommends 150 minutes per week of PE for elementary students and 225 minutes per week for middle and high school students.[23] Unfortunately, these requirements are not being implemented. In a study of 814 third-grade students from 10 different US data-collection sites, the mean duration of PE was 33 minutes twice a week, with only 25 minutes per week at a moderate to vigorous intensity level.[24] In addition, 1991–2003 Youth Risk Behavior Surveillance data showed that although the percentage of high school students enrolled in PE class remained constant (48.9%–55.7%), the percentage of students with daily PE attendance decreased from 41.6% in 1991 to 25.4% in 1995 and remained stable thereafter (25.4%–28.4%).[25]

Management of the Obese Child

The successful treatment of obesity in the pediatric age group has been somewhat obscure to date. Studies have shown that younger children seem to respond better to treatment than adolescents and adults.[11,26] Reasons given for this include greater motivation, more influence of the family on behavioral change, and the ability to take advantage of longitudinal growth, which allows children to "grow into their weight." Treatment programs that include nutritional intervention in combination with exercise have higher success rates than diet modification alone. Indeed, a research program that included dietary modification, exercise, and family-based behavioral modification demonstrated enhanced weight loss and better maintenance of lost weight over 5 years.[27] Successful activity-related interventions include a reduction in sedentary behavior and an increase in energy expenditure. Improvements in BMI have been shown to occur

when television viewing is restricted.[28] In this regard, the American Academy of Pediatrics (AAP) recommends no more than 2 hours of quality television programming per day for children older than 2 years.[29] Lifestyle-related physical activity, as opposed to calisthenics or programmed aerobic exercise, seems to be more important for sustained weight loss.[30] Such treatment programs should be individually tailored to each child, and their success should be measured not just in terms of weight loss but also in terms of the effects of the programs on associated morbidities.

Health Benefits of Physical Activity

Regular physical activity is important in weight reduction and improving insulin sensitivity in youth with type 2 diabetes.[31] Aerobic exercise has been shown in a prospective randomized, controlled study of 64 children (9–11 years old) with hypertension to reduce systolic and diastolic blood pressure over 8 months.[32] Resistance training (eg, weight lifting) after aerobic exercise seems to prevent the return of blood pressure to preintervention levels in hypertensive adolescents.[33] Weight loss through moderate aerobic exercise has been shown to reduce the hyperinsulinemia, hepatomegaly, and liver enzyme elevation seen in patients with steatohepatitis.[6,34] Regular physical activity is also beneficial psychologically for all youth regardless of weight. It is associated with an increase in self-esteem and self-concept and a decrease in anxiety and depression.[35]

Prevention of Overweight in Children and Youth

Given the challenges of reversing existing obesity in the pediatric population, preventive tactics are likely to be the key to success. Unfortunately, controlled prevention trials have been somewhat disappointing to date. In a systematic Cochrane Database review,[36] 3 of 4 long-term studies combining dietary education with physical activity showed no difference in overweight, and 1 long-term physical activity intervention study showed a slight reduction in overweight. However, the randomized control design may not be ideal for the study of most health-promotion interventions. This is because these are typically population-based programs, which tend to be complex, are delivered over long periods of time, and present some difficulties in controlling all variables.[11] Solution-oriented research, which evaluates promising interventions, often in a quasi-experimental manner, may be more appropriate in the long run.[37] It is unlikely, however, that any single strategy will be sufficient to reverse current trends in pediatric obesity. Success is more likely to be achieved by the implementation of sustainable, economically viable, culturally acceptable active-living policies that can be integrated into multiple sectors of society.

Increasing Physical Activity Levels in Children and Youth
Physical activity needs to be promoted at home, in the community, and at school, but school is perhaps the most encompassing way for all children to benefit. As of June 2005, there is a new opportunity for pediatricians to get involved with school districts. Section 204 of the Child Nutrition and WIC [Supplemental Nutrition Program for Women, Infants, and Children] Reauthorization Act of 2004 (Public Law 108–265) requires that every school receiving funding through the National School Lunch and/or Breakfast Program develop a local wellness policy that promotes the health of students, with a particular emphasis on addressing the problem of childhood obesity. By the 2006–2007 school year, each school or school district is required to set goals for healthy nutrition, physical activity, and other strategies to promote student wellness. Parents, students, school personnel, and members of the community are required to be involved in the policy development. Pediatricians can take advantage of this requirement to get involved. In light of the school wellness policy, many schools are looking to modify their present PE programs to improve their physical activity standards.

In past years, PE classes used calisthenics and sport-specific skill acquisition to promote fitness. This approach did not meet the needs of all students, such as those with obesity or physical disabilities. PE curricula and instruction should emphasize the knowledge, attitudes, and motor and behavioral skills required to adopt and maintain lifelong habits of physical activity.[38] Cross-sectional school-based studies have shown modest correlation between physical activity and lower BMI, although long-term follow-up data are lacking. In an observational study of 9751 kindergarten students, an increase in PE instruction time was associated with a significant reduction in BMI among overweight girls.[39] Project SPARK (Sports, Play, and Active Recreation for Kids Curriculum) looked at increasing physical activity through modified PE and classroom-based teaching on health and skill fitness. Physical activity levels increased during PE classes, and fitness levels in girls improved as a result.[40] It is interesting to note that, despite a significant increase in PE class time, there was no interference with academic attainment, and some achievement test results improved. A recent review of the literature suggests that school-based physical activity programs may modestly enhance academic performance in the short-term, but additional research is required to establish any long-term improvements. There does not seem to be sufficient evidence to suggest that daily physical activity detracts from academic success.[41]

An increase in school PE participation alone is not likely to be sufficient to reverse the childhood obesity epidemic. A 2-year study of elementary students showed that those who had enhanced physical activity education as well as modified PE classes to increase lifestyle aerobic activity increased their physical activity inside the classroom, but lower levels were noted outside the classroom in their leisure time, and no improvements on fitness testing or body fat percentage were seen.[42] The PLAY (Promoting Lifestyle Activity for Youth) program, which encourages the accumulation of 30 to 60 minutes of moderate to vigorous physical activity daily beyond school time and during regular school hours outside of PE classes, has been shown to increase the physical activity levels of children, especially girls.[43] Children can increase their physical activity levels in many other ways during school and nonschool hours, including active transportation, unorganized outdoor free play, personal fitness and recreational activities, and organized sports. Parents of children in organized sports should be encouraged to stimulate their children to be physically active on days when they are not participating in these sports and not rely solely on the sports to provide all their away-from-school physical activity. This should include participation in physical activities with the entire family. Communities designed with green spaces and biking trails help provide families the means to enjoy such active lifestyles.

During late childhood and adolescence, strength training may be additionally beneficial. Youth taking part in this type of exercise may gain strength, improve sport performance, and derive long-term health benefits.[44] Obese children often prefer strength training because it does not require agility or aerobic ability, and the benefits become apparent within as little as 2 to 3 weeks. Because of their added body mass, overweight participants also tend to be stronger than their peers, giving them a relative psychological advantage. Recent studies have shown that obese students are more compliant and increase their free fat mass when weight training is added to aerobic exercise or a standardized energy-reduction diet.[45,46]

Recommended physical activity levels for children and youth vary somewhat in different countries. The Centers for Disease Control and Prevention and the United Kingdom Health Education Authority recommend that children and youth accumulate at least 60 minutes daily of moderate to vigorous physical activity in a variety of enjoyable individual and group activities.[47,48] Health Canada guidelines recommend increasing physical activity above the current level by at least 30 minutes (10 minutes vigorous) and reducing sedentary activity by the same amount per day. Each month, physical activity should be increased and sedentary behavior should be decreased by 15 minutes until at least 90 minutes more active time and 90 minutes less inactive time are accumulated (www.paguide.com). The Canadian Paediatric Society has endorsed these recommendations and emphasizes a wide variety of activities as part of recreation, transportation, chores, work, and planned exercise to encourage lifestyle changes that may last a lifetime.[49]

Age-Appropriate Recommendations for Physical Activity

Clinicians should encourage parents to limit sedentary activity and make physical activity and sport recommendations to parents and caregivers that are consistent with the developmental level of the child.[50] The following are guidelines from the AAP for different age groups.

Infants and Toddlers

There is insufficient evidence to recommend exercise programs or classes for infants and toddlers as a means of promoting increased physical activity or preventing obesity in later years. The AAP has recommended that children younger than 2 years not watch any television. The AAP suggests that parents be encouraged to provide a safe, nurturing, and minimally structured play environment for their infant.[51] Infants and toddlers should also be allowed to develop enjoyment of outdoor physical activity and unstructured exploration under the supervision of a responsible adult caregiver. Such activities include walking in the neighborhood, unorganized free play outdoors, and walking through a park or zoo.

Preschool-Aged Children (4–6 Years)

Free play should be encouraged with emphasis on fun, playfulness, exploration, and experimentation while being mindful of safety and proper supervision. Preschool-aged children should take part in unorganized play, preferably on flat surfaces with few variables and instruction limited to a show-and-tell format. Appropriate activities might include running, swimming, tumbling, throwing, and catching. Preschoolers should also begin walking tolerable distances with family members. In addition, parents should reduce sedentary transportation by car and stroller and, as applies to all age groups, limit screen time to <2 hours per day.

Elementary School-Aged Children (6–9 Years)

In this age group, children improve their motor skills, visual tracking, and balance. Parents should continue to encourage free play involving more sophisticated movement patterns with emphasis on fundamental skill acquisition. These children should be encouraged to walk, dance, or jump rope and may enjoy playing miniature golf. There is little difference between the sexes in weight, height, endurance, and motor skill development at this age; thus, co-ed participation is not contraindicated. Organized sports (soccer, baseball) may be initiated, but they should have flexible rules and short instruction time, allow free time in practices, and focus on enjoyment rather than competition. These children have a limited ability to learn team strategy.

Middle School–Aged Children (10–12 Years)

Preferred physical activities that focus on enjoyment with family members and friends should be encouraged as with previous groups. Emphasis on skill development and increasing focus on tactics and strategy as well as factors promoting continued participation are needed. Fully developed visual tracking, balance, and motor skills are typical in late childhood. Middle school–aged children are better able to process verbal instruction and integrate information from multiple sources so that participation in complex sports (football, basketball, ice hockey) is more feasible. Puberty may begin at different rates, making some individuals bigger and stronger than others. Basing placement in contact and collision sports on maturity rather than chronologic age may result in less risk of injury and enhanced chance of success, especially for those at lower Tanner stages. Weight training may be initiated, provided that the program is well supervised, that small free weights are used with high repetitions (15–20), that proper technique is demonstrated, and that shorter sets using heavier weights and maximum lifts (squat lifts, clean and jerk, dead lifts) are avoided.[44]

Adolescents

Adolescents are highly social and influenced by their peers. Identifying activities that are of interest to the adolescent, especially those that are fun and include friends, is crucial for long-term participation. Physical activities may include personal fitness preferences (eg, dance, yoga, running), active transportation (walking, cycling), household chores, and competitive and non-competitive sports. Ideally, enrollment in competitive contact and collision sports should be based on size and ability instead of chronologic age. Weight training may continue, and as the individual reaches physical maturity (Tanner stage 5), longer sets using heavier weights and fewer repetitions may be safely pursued while continuing to stress the importance of proper technique.

Office-Based Physical Activity Assessment

An accurate assessment of an individual child's physical activity level by history or questionnaire is difficult and fraught with methodologic problems. It may be easier for parents to recall the number of times per week their child plays outside for at least 30 minutes than to estimate the average daily minutes spent in physical activity. In addition, asking parents about the number of hours per day their child spends in front of a television, video game, or computer screen may be simpler to quantify and track than time spent in active play. Pedometers may also be helpful, because they provide a simple and more objective method of measuring activity, are inexpensive, and have a "gadget appeal" among youngsters. It has been recommend that adults accumulate 10 000 steps per day to follow a healthy lifestyle.[52] Requirements are less clearly defined in children, but guidelines range from 11 000 to 12 000 steps per day for girls and 13 000 to 15 000 steps per day for boys.[53,54]

CONCLUSIONS

The prevalence of pediatric obesity has reached epidemic proportions. It is unlikely that the medical profession alone will be able to solve this serious health problem. The promotion of decreased caloric intake and increased energy expenditure will need to take place within all aspects of society. Among the most difficult but most important challenges for society are making exercise alternatives as attractive, exciting, and enjoyable as video games for children, convincing school boards that PE and other school-based physical activity opportunities are as important to long-term productivity as are academics, changing both supplier and consumer attitudes about food selection and portion sizes, and reengineering living environments to promote physical activity.

RECOMMENDATIONS

Research has shown the importance of social, physical, and cultural environments in determining the extent to which people are able to be active in all facets of daily life, including work, education, family life, and leisure.[55] Creating active school communities is an ideal way to ensure that children and youth adopt active, healthy lifestyles. These communities require a collaborative framework between families, schools, community recreation leaders, and health care professionals. Physicians can be instrumental in the development of active school communities by advocating for policy changes at the community, state, and national levels that support healthy nutrition, reducing sedentary time, and increasing physical activity levels while providing education and health supervision about regular physical activity and reduced sedentary time to families in their practices.

ADVOCACY

In addition to promoting healthy nutrition recommendations suggested by the AAP Committee on Nutrition, physicians and health care professionals and their national organizations should advocate for:

- Social marketing that promotes increased physical activity.
- The appropriate allocation of funding for quality research in the prevention of childhood obesity.
- The development and implementation of a school wellness counsel on which local physician representation is encouraged.
- A school curriculum that teaches children and youth the health benefits of regular physical activity.

- Comprehensive community sport and recreation programs that allow for community and school facilities to be open after hours and make physical activities available to all children and youth at reasonable costs; access to recreation facilities should be equally available to both sexes.

- The reinstatement of compulsory, quality, daily PE classes in all schools (kindergarten through grade 12) taught by qualified, trained educators. The curricula should emphasize enjoyable participation in physical activity that helps students develop the knowledge, attitudes, motor skills, behavioral skills, and confidence required to adopt and maintain healthy active lifestyles. These classes should allow participation by all children regardless of ability, illness, injury, and developmental disability, including those with obesity and those who are disinterested in traditional competitive team sports. Commitment of adequate resources for program funding, trained PE personnel, safe equipment, and facilities is also recommended.

- The provision of a variety of physical activity opportunities in addition to PE, including the protection of children's recess time and the requirement of extracurricular physical activity programs and nonstructured physical activity before, during, and after school hours, that address the needs and interests of all students.

- The reduction of environmental barriers to an active lifestyle through the construction of safe recreational facilities, parks, playgrounds, bicycle paths, sidewalks, and crosswalks.

PROMOTING A HEALTHY LIFESTYLE

Physicians and health care professionals should promote active healthy living within each family unit by:

- Serving as role models through the adoption of an active lifestyle.

- Inquiring about nutritional intake, calculating and plotting BMI, identifying obesity-related comorbidities, and promoting healthy eating as suggested by the AAP Committee on Nutrition.

- Documenting the number of hours per day spent on sedentary activities and limiting screen (television, video game, and computer) time according to AAP guidelines.

- Determining physical activity levels of the child and family members at regular health care visits.

- Tabulating the amount of physical activity the child or youth does each day at home, school, or child care as part of transportation, work, recreation, and unorganized sports, which should include determining the actual minutes of PE and recess-related physical activity achieved at school each week. In addition, the number of times per week spent in outdoor play for at least 30 minutes and/or the number of daily steps achieved (monitored by using a pedometer) should be documented. Specific involvement in organized sports and dance also should be noted.

- Encouraging children and adolescents to be physically active for at least 60 minutes per day, which does not need to be acquired in a continuous fashion but rather may be accumulated by using smaller increments. Events should be of moderate intensity and include a wide variety of activities as part of sports, recreation, transportation, chores, work, planned exercise, and school-based PE classes. These activities should be primarily unstructured and fun if they are to achieve best compliance.

- Identifying any barriers the child, youth, or parent might have against increasing physical activity, which might include lack of time, competing interests, perceived lack of motor skills, and fear of injury on the part of the child. Parents might be additionally concerned about financial and safety issues. Efforts must then be made to work with the family to educate them regarding the importance of lifelong physical activity and to identify potential strategies to overcome some of their barriers.

- Recommending that parents become good role models by increasing their own level of physical activity. Parents should also incorporate physical activities that family members of all ages and abilities can do together. They should encourage children to play outside as much as possible. Safety should be promoted by the use of appropriate protective equipment (bicycle helmets, life jackets, etc).

- Advising parents to support their children and youth in developmentally and age-appropriate sports and recreational activities. The child's favorite types of physical activity should be a priority. These might best occur in the school setting during extracurricular activities, in which parents/grandparents can take part as leaders and coaches.

- Suggesting that overweight children partake in activities that take advantage of their tall stature and muscle strength, such as water-based sports and strength training, rather than those that require weight bearing (eg, jumping, jogging).

- Recommending that parents of overweight children and youth play a supporting, accepting, and encouraging role in returning them to healthier lifestyles to increase self-esteem.

- Encouraging youth to promote physical activities for their peers and become role models and leaders for younger students.

COUNCIL ON SPORTS MEDICINE AND FITNESS, 2005–2006
Teri M. McCambridge, MD, Chairperson
David T. Bernhardt, MD
Joel S. Brenner, MD, MPH
Joseph A. Congeni, MD
*Jorge E. Gomez, MD
Andrew J.M. Gregory, MD
Douglas B. Gregory, MD
Bernard A. Griesemer, MD
Frederick E. Reed, MD
Stephen G. Rice, MD, PhD
Eric W. Small, MD
Paul R. Stricker, MD

LIAISONS
*Claire LeBlanc, MD
    Canadian Paediatric Society
James Raynor, MS, ATC
    National Athletic Trainers Association

STAFF
Jeanne Christensen Lindros, MPH

COUNCIL ON SCHOOL HEALTH, 2005–2006
Barbara L. Frankowski, MD, MPH, Chairperson
Rani S. Gereige, MD, MPH
Linda M. Grant, MD, MPH
Daniel Hyman, MD
Harold Magalnick, MD
Cynthia J. Mears, DO
George J. Monteverdi, MD
*Robert D. Murray, MD
Evan G. Pattishall III, MD
Michele M. Roland, MD
Thomas L. Young, MD

LIAISONS
Nancy LaCursia, PhD
    American School Health Association
Mary Vernon-Smiley, MD, MPH
    Centers for Disease Control and Prevention
Donna Mazyck, MS, RN
    National Association of School Nurses
Robin Wallace, MD
    Independent School Health Association

STAFF
Su Li, MPA

*Lead authors

REFERENCES
1. World Health Organization. *Obesity: Preventing and Managing the Global Epidemic. Report of a WHO Consultation on Obesity, 3–5 June 1997, Geneva*. Geneva, Switzerland: World Health Organization; 2001. WHO/NUT/NCD 98.1
2. Ogden CL, Carroll MD, Flegal KM. Epidemiologic trends in overweight and obesity. *Endocrinol Metab Clin North Am.* 2003; 32:741–760, vii

3. Rosenbloom AL. Increasing incidence of type 2 diabetes in children and adolescents: treatment considerations. *Paediatr Drugs.* 2002;4:209–221

4. Sorof JM, Lai D, Turner J, Poffenbarger T, Portman RJ. Overweight, ethnicity, and the prevalence of hypertension in school-aged children. *Pediatrics.* 2004;113:475–482

5. Wing YK, Hui SH, Pak WM, et al. A controlled study of sleep related disordered breathing in obese children. *Arch Dis Child.* 2003;88:1043–1047

6. Rashid M, Roberts EA. Nonalcoholic steatohepatitis in children. *J Pediatr Gastroenterol Nutr.* 2000;30:48–53

7. Schwimmer JB, Burwinkle TM, Varni JW. Health-related quality of life of severely obese children and adolescents. *JAMA.* 2003;289:1813–1819

8. Whitaker RC, Wright JA, Pepe MS, Seidel KD, Dietz WH. Predicting obesity in young adulthood from childhood and parental obesity. *N Engl J Med.* 1997;337:869–873

9. Guo SS, Chumlea WC. Tracking of body mass index in children in relation to overweight in adulthood. *Am J Clin Nutr.* 1999;70(1 pt 2):145S–148S

10. Belay B, Belamarich P, Racine AD. Pediatric precursors of adult atherosclerosis. *Pediatr Rev.* 2004;25:4–16

11. Lobstein T, Baur L, Uauy R. Obesity in children and young people: a crisis in public health. *Obesity Rev.* 2004;5(suppl 1):4–104

12. Kuczmarski RJ, Ogden CL, Grummer-Strawn LM, et al. CDC growth charts: United States. *Adv Data.* 2000;(314):1–28

13. Himes JH, Dietz WH. Guidelines for overweight in adolescent preventive services: recommendations from an expert committee. The Expert Committee on Clinical Guidelines for Overweight in Adolescent Preventive Services. *Am J Clin Nutr.* 1994;59:307–316

14. Sardinha LB, Going SB, Teixeira PJ, Lohman TG. Receiver operating characteristic analysis of body mass index, triceps skinfold thickness, and arm girth for obesity screening in children and adolescents. *Am J Clin Nutr.* 1999;70:1090–1095

15. Krebs NF, Jacobson MS; American Academy of Pediatrics, Committee on Nutrition. Prevention of pediatric overweight and obesity. *Pediatrics.* 2003;112:424–430

16. American Academy of Pediatrics, Committee on School Health. Soft drinks in schools. *Pediatrics.* 2004;113:152–154

17. Andersen RE, Crespo CJ, Bartlett SJ, Cheskin LJ, Pratt M. Relationship of physical activity and television watching with body weight and level of fatness among children: results from the Third National Health and Nutrition Examination Survey. *JAMA.* 1998;279:938–942

18. Centers for Disease Control and Prevention. Physical activity levels among children aged 9–13 years: United States, 2002. *MMWR Morb Mortal Wkly Rep.* 2003;52:785–788

19. US Department of Health and Human Services. *Healthy People 2010: Understanding and Improving Health.* 2nd ed. Washington, DC: US Department of Health and Human Services; 2001

20. Raine KD. *Overweights and Obesity in Canada: A Population Health Perspective.* Ottawa, Ontario, Canada: Canadian Institute for Health Information; 2004. Available at: http://secure.cihi.ca/cihiweb/products/CPHIOverweightandObesityAugust2004.e.pdf. Accessed March 30, 2005

21. Sallis JF. Epidemiology of physical activity and fitness in children and adolescents. *Crit Rev Food Sci Nutr.* 1993;33:403–408

22. Burgeson CR, Wechsler H, Brener ND, Young JC, Spain CG. Physical education and activity: results from the School Health Policies and Programs Study 2000. *J Sch Health.* 2001;71:279–293

23. National Association of State Boards of Education. *Fit, Healthy, and Ready to Learn: A School Health Policy Guide.* Alexandria, VA: National Association of State Boards of Education; 2000

24. Nader PR. Frequency and intensity of activity of third-grade children in physical education. National Institute of Child Health and Human Development Study of Early Child Care and Youth Development Network. *Arch Pediatr Adolesc Med.* 2003;157:185–190

25. Grunbaum JA, Kann L, Kinchen S, et al. Youth risk behavior surveillance: United States, 2003 [published corrections appear in *MMWR Morb Mortal Wkly Rep.* 2004;53(24):536 and *MMWR Morb Mortal Wkly Rep.* 2005;54(24):608]. *MMWR Surveill Summ.* 2004;53(2):1–96

26. Summerbell CD, Ashton V, Campbell KJ, Edmonds L, Kelly S, Waters E. Interventions for treating obesity in children. *Cochrane Database Syst Rev.* 2003;(3):CD001872

27. Epstein LH. Methodological issues and ten-year outcomes for obese children. *Ann N Y Acad Sci.* 1993;699:237–249

28. Robinson TN. Reducing children's television viewing to prevent obesity: a randomized controlled trial. *JAMA.* 1999;282:1561–1567

29. American Academy of Pediatrics, Committee on Public Education. Children, adolescents, and television. *Pediatrics.* 2001;107:423–426

30. Epstein LH, Wing RR, Koeske R, Valoski A. A comparison of lifestyle exercise, aerobic exercise, and calisthenics on weight loss in obese children. *Behav Ther.* 1985;16:345–356

31. American Diabetes Association. Type 2 diabetes in children and adolescents. *Pediatrics.* 2000;105:671–680

32. Hansen HS, Froberg K, Hyldebrandt N, Nielsen JR. A controlled study of eight months of physical training and reduction of blood pressure in children: the Odense schoolchild study. *BMJ.* 1991;303:682–685

33. Hagberg JM, Ehsani AA, Goldring D, Hernandez A, Sinacore DR, Holloszy JO. Effect of weight training on blood pressure and hemodynamics in hypertensive adolescents. *J Pediatr.* 1984;104:147–151

34. Roberts EA. Nonalcoholic steatohepatitis in children. *Curr Gastroenterol Rep.* 2003;5:253–259

35. Calfas KJ, Taylor WC. Effects of physical activity on psychological variables in adolescents. *Pediatr Exerc Sci.* 1994;6:406–423

36. Campbell K, Waters E, O'Meara S, Kelly S, Summerbell C. Interventions for preventing obesity in children. *Cochrane Database Syst Rev.* 2002;(2):CD001871

37. Robinson TN, Sirard JR. Preventing childhood obesity: a solution-oriented research paradigm. *Am J Prev Med.* 2005;28(2 suppl 2):194–201

38. Centers for Disease Control and Prevention. Youth risk behavior surveillance. National College Health Risk Behavior Survey—United States, 1995. *MMWR CDC Surveill Summ.* 1997;46(6):1–56

39. Datar A, Sturm R. Physical education in elementary school and body mass index: evidence from the Early Childhood Longitudinal Study. *Am J Public Health.* 2004;94:1501–1506

40. Sallis JF, McKenzie TL, Kolody B, Lewis M, Marshall S, Rosengard P. Effects of health-related physical education on academic achievement: project SPARK. *Res Q Exerc Sport.* 1999;70:127–134

41. Taras H. Physical activity and student performance at school. *J Sch Health.* 2005;75:214–218

42. Donnelly JE, Jacobsen DJ, Whatley JE, et al. Nutrition and physical activity program to attenuate obesity and promote physical and metabolic fitness in elementary school children. *Obes Res.* 1996;4:229–243

43. Pangrazi RP, Beighle A, Vehige T, Vack C. Impact of Promoting Lifestyle Activity for Youth (PLAY) on children's physical activity. *J Sch Health.* 2003;73:317–321

44. Bernhardt DT, Gomez J, Johnson MD, et al. Strength training by children and adolescents. *Pediatrics.* 2001;107:1470–1472

45. Sothern MS, Loftin JM, Udall JN, et al. Safety, feasibility, and

efficacy of a resistance training program in preadolescent obese children. *Am J Med Sci.* 2000;319:370–375

46. Schwingshandl J, Sudi K, Eibl B, Wallner S, Borkenstein M. Effect of an individualised training programme during weight reduction on body composition: a randomised trial. *Arch Dis Child.* 1999;81:426–428

47. Strong WB, Malina RM, Blimkie CJ, et al. Evidence based physical activity for school-age youth. *J Pediatr.* 2005;146:732–737

48. Biddle S, Sallis J, Cavill N. Policy framework for young people and health-enhancing physical activity. In: Biddle S, Sallis J, Cavill N, eds. *Young and Active: Young People and Physical Activity.* London, England: Health Education Authority; 1998:3–16

49. Canadian Paediatric Society, Healthy Active Living Committee. Healthy active living for children and youth. *Paediatr Child Health.* 2002;7:339–345

50. Harris SS. Readiness to participate in sports. In: Sullivan JA, Anderson SJ, eds. *Care of the Young Athlete.* Rosemont, IL:

American Academy of Orthopaedic Surgeons/American Academy of Pediatrics; 2000:19–24

51. American Academy of Pediatrics, Committee on Sports Medicine and Fitness. Infant exercise programs. *Pediatrics.* 1988;82: 800

52. Hatano Y. Use of the pedometer for promoting daily walking exercise. *Int Council Health Phys Ed Rec.* 1993;29:4–8

53. Vincent SD, Pangrazi RP. An examination of the activity patterns of elementary school children. *Pediatr Exerc Sci.* 2002;14: 432–441

54. Tudor-Locke C, Pangrazi RP, Corbin CB, et al. BMI-referenced standards for recommended pedometer-determined steps/day in children. *Prev Med.* 2004;38:857–864

55. Health Canada, Population and Public Health Branch, Policy Directorate. *The Population Health Template: Key Elements and Actions That Define a Population Health Approach.* Ottawa, Ontario, Canada: Health Canada; 2001

AMERICAN ACADEMY OF PEDIATRICS

Committee on Public Education

Children, Adolescents, and Television

ABSTRACT. This statement describes the possible negative health effects of television viewing on children and adolescents, such as violent or aggressive behavior, substance use, sexual activity, obesity, poor body image, and decreased school performance. In addition to the television ratings system and the v-chip (electronic device to block programming), media education is an effective approach to mitigating these potential problems. The American Academy of Pediatrics offers a list of recommendations on this issue for pediatricians and for parents, the federal government, and the entertainment industry.

ABBREVIATIONS. AAP, American Academy of Pediatrics; MTV, Music Television; E/I, educational/informational.

For the past 15 years, the American Academy of Pediatrics (AAP) has expressed its concerns about the amount of time children and adolescents spend viewing television and the content of what they view.[1] According to recent Nielsen Media Research data, the average child or adolescent watches an average of nearly 3 hours of television per day.[2] This figure does not include time spent watching videotapes or playing video games[3] (a 1999 study found that children spend an average of 6 hours 32 minutes per day with various media combined).[4] By the time the average person reaches age 70, he or she will have spent the equivalent of 7 to 10 years watching television.[5] One recent study found that 32% of 2- to 7-year-olds and 65% of 8- to 18-year-olds have television sets in their bedrooms.[4] Time spent with various media may displace other more active and meaningful pursuits, such as reading, exercising, or playing with friends.

Although there are potential benefits from viewing some television shows, such as the promotion of positive aspects of social behavior (eg, sharing, manners, and cooperation), many negative health effects also can result. Children and adolescents are particularly vulnerable to the messages conveyed through television, which influence their perceptions and behaviors.[6] Many younger children cannot discriminate between what they see and what is real. Research has shown primary negative health effects on violence and aggressive behavior[7–12]; sexuality[7,13–15]; academic performance[16]; body concept and self-im-

age[17–19]; nutrition, dieting, and obesity[17,20,21]; and substance use and abuse patterns.[7]

In the scientific literature on media violence, the connection of media violence to real-life aggressive behavior and violence has been substantiated.[8–12] As much as 10% to 20% of real-life violence may be attributable to media violence.[22] The recently completed 3-year National Television Violence Study found the following: 1) nearly two thirds of all programming contains violence; 2) children's shows contain the most violence; 3) portrayals of violence are usually glamorized; and 4) perpetrators often go unpunished.[23] A recent comprehensive analysis of music videos found that nearly one fourth of all Music Television (MTV) videos portray overt violence and depict weapon carrying.[24] Research has shown that even television news can traumatize children or lead to nightmares.[25] In a random survey of parents with children in kindergarten through sixth grade, 37% reported that their child had been frightened or upset by a television story in the preceding year.[26]

According to a recent content analysis, mainstream television programming contains large numbers of references to cigarettes, alcohol, and illicit drugs.[27] One fourth of all MTV videos contain alcohol or tobacco use.[28] A longitudinal study found a positive correlation between television and music video viewing and alcohol consumption among teens.[29] Finally, content analyses show that children and teenagers continue to be bombarded with sexual imagery and innuendoes in programming and advertising.[14,30,31] To date, there are no data available to substantiate the behavioral impact of this exposure.[31]

The new television ratings system and the v-chip are tools that can help protect children from potentially harmful content. All new television sets with screens measuring 13 inches or greater contain a v-chip that enables parents to program televisions to block out any shows that they deem inappropriate for their children.[32] To block out television shows, parents must use the television ratings system, which has age and content descriptors for violence, sexual situations, suggestive dialogue, and adult language. Although the ratings system and the v-chip can assist parents, ongoing evaluation is necessary to ensure that these tools are as effective as possible.[33–35] For example, the ratings should be applied uniformly and listed in television guides, newspapers, and journals so parents know what they mean.

Besides the v-chip, there are other means of protecting children from what is on television. Evidence now shows that media education can help mitigate the harmful effects of media violence[36-40] and alcohol advertising[41,42] on children and adolescents. Media education programs have been included in the school curricula beginning in early elementary school in many states across the United States.[43]

Furthermore, continued support of the Children's Television Act of 1990[44] and additional regulations made in 1996[45] will help to ensure the airing of television programs specifically designated for children. The act requires broadcasters to air educational and informational programming for children at least 3 hours per week and to limit the amount of advertising time allowed during children's programming. The shows must be labeled E/I (for educational and informational) on the television screen.

RECOMMENDATIONS

The following recommendations are given for pediatricians and other health care professionals:

1. Remain knowledgeable about the effects of television, including violent and aggressive behavior, obesity, poor body concept and self-image, substance use, and early sexual activity, by becoming involved in the AAP *Media Matters* campaign.[46] Educate patients and their parents about these effects.
2. Use the AAP *Media History* form[46] to help parents recognize the extent of their children's media consumption.
3. Work with local schools to implement comprehensive media-education programs that deal with important public health issues.[36]
4. Serve as good role models by using television appropriately and by implementing reading programs using volunteer readers in waiting rooms and hospital inpatient units.
5. Become involved in the AAP's Media Resource Team (contact the Division of Public Education), and learn how to work effectively with writers, directors, and producers to make media more appropriate for children and adolescents. Contact networks and producers of television programs with concerns about the content of specific shows and episodes.
6. Ensure that appropriate entertainment options are available for hospitalized children and adolescents. Work with child life staff to assemble a screening committee that selects programs for closed circuit broadcast or a video library. Develop institution-specific, formal guidelines based on the established ratings system (which takes profanity, sex, and violence into account), and screen for content containing ethnic and sex role stereotyping. Considerations should also be made to avoid themes hospitalized children might find upsetting, and efforts should be made to enforce the ratings system in the hospital setting.
7. Support the Children's Television Act of 1990 and its 1996 rules by working to ensure that local television stations are in compliance with the act and by urging local newspapers to list ratings and E/I denotations of programs.

8. Monitor the television ratings system for appropriateness and advocate for substantive, content-based ratings in the future.

Pediatricians should recommend the following guidelines for parents:

1. Limit children's total media time (with entertainment media) to no more than 1 to 2 hours of quality programming per day.
2. Remove television sets from children's bedrooms.
3. Discourage television viewing for children younger than 2 years, and encourage more interactive activities that will promote proper brain development, such as talking, playing, singing, and reading together.
4. Monitor the shows children and adolescents are viewing. Most programs should be informational, educational, and nonviolent.
5. View television programs along with children, and discuss the content. Two recent surveys involving a total of nearly 1500 parents found that less than half of parents reported always watching television with their children.[5,47]
6. Use controversial programming as a stepping-off point to initiate discussions about family values, violence, sex and sexuality, and drugs.
7. Use the videocassette recorder wisely to show or record high-quality, educational programming for children.
8. Support efforts to establish comprehensive media-education programs in schools.
9. Encourage alternative entertainment for children, including reading, athletics, hobbies, and creative play.

Pediatricians should lead efforts in their communities to do the following:

1. Form coalitions including libraries, religious organizations, and other community groups to broaden media education beyond the schools.
2. Organize activities promoting media education, such as letter-writing campaigns to local television stations to advocate for better programming for children, and developing local TV turnoff week projects.[48]

Pediatricians should work with the Academy and local chapters to challenge the federal government to do the following:

1. Initiate legislation and rules that would ban alcohol advertising from television.
2. Fund ongoing annual research, such as the National Television Violence Study, and fund more research on the effects of television on children and adolescents, particularly in the area of sex and sexuality.
3. Assemble a *National Institutes of Health Comprehensive Report on Children, Adolescents, and Media* that would bring together all of the current relevant research.
4. Work with the US Department of Education to support the creation and implementation of media-education curricula for school children.

Pediatricians should work with the Academy and local chapters to challenge the entertainment industry to do the following:

1. Take responsibility for the programming it produces.
2. Adhere to the current television ratings system, and label programs conscientiously.
3. Collaborate with other public health advocates to convene a series of seminars with writers, directors, and producers to discuss ways to make media more appropriate for children and adolescents.
4. Produce more educational programming for children and adolescents, and ensure that the programming it produces is of higher quality, with less content that is gratuitously violent, sexually suggestive, or drug oriented.

COMMITTEE ON PUBLIC EDUCATION, 2000–2001
Miriam E. Bar-on, MD, Chairperson
Daniel D. Broughton, MD
Susan Buttross, MD
Suzanne Corrigan, MD
Alberto Gedissman, MD
M. Rosario González de Rivas, MD
Michael Rich, MD, MPH
Donald L. Shifrin, MD

LIAISONS
Michael Brody, MD
    American Academy of Child and Adolescent
    Psychiatry
Brian Wilcox, PhD
    American Psychological Association

CONSULTANTS
Marjorie Hogan, MD
H. James Holroyd, MD
Linda Reid, MD
S. Norman Sherry, MD
Victor Strasburger, MD

STAFF
Jennifer Stone

REFERENCES

1. American Academy of Pediatrics, Task Force on Children, and Television. Children, adolescents and television. *News and Comment.* December 1984;35:8
2. 1998 Report on Television. New York, NY. Nielsen Media Research; 1998.
3. Mares ML. Children's use of VCRs. *Ann Am Acad Pol Soc Science.* 1998;557:120–131
4. Roberts DF, Foehr UG, Rideout VJ, Brodie, M. *Kids and Media at the New Millennium: A Comprehensive National Analysis of Children's Media Use.* Menlo Park, CA: The Henry J Kaiser Family Foundation Report; 1999
5. Strasburger VC. Children, adolescents, and the media: five crucial issues. *Adolesc Med.* 1993;4:479–493
6. Gerbner G, Gross L, Morgan M, Signorielli N. Growing up with television: the cultivation perspective. In: Bryant J, Zillmann D, eds. *Media Effects: Advances in Theory and Research.* Hillsdale, NJ: Lawrence Erlbaum; 1994:17–41
7. Strasburger VC. "Sex, drugs, rock'n'roll," and the media: are the media responsible for adolescent behavior? *Adolesc Med.* 1997;8:403–414
8. Strasburger VC. *Adolescents and the Media: Medical and Psychological Impact.* Thousand Oaks, CA: Sage; 1995
9. Huston AC, Donnerstein E, Fairchild H, et al. *Big World, Small Screen: The Role of Television in American Society.* Lincoln, NE: University of Nebraska Press; 1992
10. Donnerstein E, Linz D. The mass media: a role in injury causation and prevention. *Adolesc Med.* 1995;6:271–284
11. Eron LR. Media violence. *Pediatr Ann.* 1995;24:84–87
12. Willis E, Strasburger VC. Media violence. *Pediatr Clin North Am.* 1998; 45:319–331
13. Kunkel D, Cope KM, Farinola WJM, Biely E, Rollin E, Donnerstein E. *Sex on TV: Content and Context.* Menlo Park, CA: The Henry J Kaiser Family Foundation; 1999
14. Huston AC, Wartella E, Donnerstein E. *Measuring, the Effects of Sexual Content in the Media.* Menlo Park, CA: The Henry J Kaiser Family Foundation Report; 1998
15. Brown JD, Greenberg BS, Buerkel-Rothfuss NL. Mass media, sex and sexuality. *Adolesc Med.* 1993;4:511–525
16. Morgan M. Television and school performance. *Adolesc Med.* 1993;4: 607–622
17. Harrison K, Cantor J. The relationship between media consumption and eating disorders. *J Commun.* 1997;47:40–67
18. Signorielli N. Sex roles and stereotyping on television. *Adolesc Med.* 1993;4:551–561
19. A Different World. *Children's Perceptions of Race and Class in the Media.* Oakland, CA: Children Now; 1998
20. Andersen RE, Crespo CJ, Bartlett SJ, Cheskin LJ, Pratt M. Relationship of physical activity and television watching with body weight and level of fatness among children: results from the Third National Health and Nutrition Examination Study. *JAMA.* 1998;279:938–942
21. Jeffrey RW, French SA. Epidemic obesity in the United States: are fast foods and television viewing contributing? *Am J Public Health.* 1998;88: 277–280
22. Comstock GC, Strasburger VC. Media violence: Q & A. *Adolesc Med.* 1993;4:495–509
23. Federman J, ed. *National Television Violence Study.* Vol 3. Thousand Oaks, CA: Sage; 1998
24. DuRant RH, Rich M, Emans SJ, Rome ES, Allred E, Woods ER. Violence and weapon carrying in music videos: a content analysis. *Arch Pediatr Adolesc Med.* 1997;151:443–448
25. Cantor J. *"Mommy, I'm Scared": How TV and Movies Frighten Children and What We Can Do to Protect Them.* New York, NY: Harcourt Brace; 1998
26. Cantor J, Nathanson AI. Children's fright reactions to television news. *J Commun.* 1996;46:139–152
27. Gerbner G, Ozyegin N. *Alcohol, Tobacco, and Illicit Drugs in Entertainment Television, Commercials, News, "Reality Shows," Movies, and Music Channels.* Princeton, NJ: Robert Wood Johnson Foundation; 1997
28. DuRant RH, Rome ES, Rich M, Allred E, Emans SJ, Woods ER. Tobacco and alcohol use behaviors portrayed in music videos: a content analysis. *Am J Public Health.* 1997;87:1131–1135
29. Robinson TN, Chen HL, Killen JD. Television and music video exposure and risk of adolescent alcohol use. *Pediatrics* [serial online]. 1998;102:e54. Available at: http://www.pediatrics.org/cgi/content/full/102/5/e54. Accessed May 2, 2000.
30. Brown JD, Steele, JR. *Sex and the Mass Media.* Menlo Park, CA: The Henry J Kaiser Family Foundation; 1995
31. Kunkel D, Cope KM, Colvin C. *Sexual Messages on Family Hour Television: Content and Context.* Menlo Park, CA: Henry J Kaiser Family Foundation; 1996
32. Telecommunications Act of., Pub L No. 104–104, 1996.
33. Cantor J. Ratings for program content: the role of research findings. *Ann Am Acad Pol Soc Science.* 1998;557:54–69
34. Kunkel D, Farinola WJM, Cope KM, Donnerstein E et al. *Rating, the TV Ratings: One Year Out. An Assessment of the Television Industry's Use of V-Chip Ratings.* Menlo Park, CA: Henry J Kaiser Family Foundation; 1998
35. *Parents Rate the TV Ratings.* Minneapolis, MN: National Institute on Media and the Family; 1998
36. Potter WJ. *Media Literacy.* Thousand Oaks, CA: Sage; 1998
37. Huesmann LR, Eron LD, Klein R, Brice P, Fischer P. Mitigating, the imitation of aggressive behaviors by changing children's attitudes about media violence. *J Pers Soc Psychol.* 1983;44:899–910
38. Gunter B. The question of media violence. In: Bryant J, Zillmann D, eds. *Media Effects: Advances in Theory and Research.* Hillsdale, NJ: Lawrence Erlbaum; 1994:163–211
39. Kubey RW. Television dependence, diagnosis, and prevention. In: MacBeth TM, ed. *Tuning in to Young Viewers: Social Science Perspectives on Television.* Thousand Oaks, CA: Sage; 1996:221–260
40. Singer DG, Singer JL. Developing critical viewing skills and media literacy in children. In: Jordan AB, Jamieson KH, eds. Children and television. *Ann Am Acad Pol Soc Science.* 1998;557:164–179

41. Austin EW, Johnson KK. Effects of general and alcohol-specific media literacy training on children's decision making about alcohol. *J Health Commun.* 1997;2:17–42

42. Austin EW, Pinkleton BE, Fujioka Y. The role of interpretation processes and parental discussion in the media's effects on adolescents' use of alcohol. *Pediatrics.* 2000;105:343–349

43. Kubey R, Baker F. Has media literacy found a curricular foothold? *Education Week.* 1999;19:38,56

44. Children's Television Act. 47 USC §303a, 303b, 394

45. Revision of Programming Policies for Television Broadcast Stations. Washington, DC. Federal Communications Commission; August 8, 1996. FCC 96–335 (MM Docket 93–48)

46. American Academy of Pediatrics. *Media Matters: A National Media Education Campaign.* Elk Grove Village, IL: American Academy of Pediatrics; 1997

47. Valerio M, Amodio P, Dal Zio M, Vianello A, Zacchello GP. The use of television in 2- to 8-year-old children and the attitude of parents about such use. *Arch Pediatr Adolesc Med.* 1997;151:22–26

48. TV Turnoff Network Web site. Available at: http://www.tvturnoff.org. Accessed December 27, 2000

AMERICAN ACADEMY OF PEDIATRICS

POLICY STATEMENT

Organizational Principles to Guide and Define the Child Health Care System and/or Improve the Health of All Children

Committee on Adolescence

Identifying and Treating Eating Disorders

ABSTRACT. Pediatricians are called on to become involved in the identification and management of eating disorders in several settings and at several critical points in the illness. In the primary care pediatrician's practice, early detection, initial evaluation, and ongoing management can play a significant role in preventing the illness from progressing to a more severe or chronic state. In the subspecialty setting, management of medical complications, provision of nutritional rehabilitation, and coordination with the psychosocial and psychiatric aspects of care are often handled by pediatricians, especially those who have experience or expertise in the care of adolescents with eating disorders. In hospital and day program settings, pediatricians are involved in program development, determining appropriate admission and discharge criteria, and provision and coordination of care. Lastly, primary care pediatricians need to be involved at local, state, and national levels in preventive efforts and in providing advocacy for patients and families. The roles of pediatricians in the management of eating disorders in the pediatric practice, subspecialty, hospital, day program, and community settings are reviewed in this statement.

ABBREVIATIONS. DSM-IV, *Diagnostic and Statistical Manual of Mental Disorders, Fourth Edition*; BMI, body mass index; DSM-PC, *Diagnostic and Statistic Manual for Primary Care.*

INTRODUCTION

Increases in the incidence and prevalence of anorexia and bulimia nervosa in children and adolescents have made it increasingly important that pediatricians be familiar with the early detection and appropriate management of eating disorders. Epidemiologic studies document that the numbers of children and adolescents with eating disorders increased steadily from the 1950s onward.[1–4] During the past decade, the prevalence of obesity in children and adolescents has increased significantly,[5,6] accompanied by an unhealthy emphasis on dieting and weight loss among children and adolescents, especially in suburban settings[7–10]; increasing concerns with weight-related issues in children at progressively younger ages[11,12]; growing awareness of the presence of eating disorders in males[13,14]; increases in the prevalence of eating disorders among minority populations in the United States[15–18]; and the identi-

PEDIATRICS (ISSN 0031 4005). Copyright © 2003 by the American Academy of Pediatrics.

fication of eating disorders in countries that had not previously been experiencing those problems.[3,4,19,20] It is estimated that 0.5% of adolescent females in the United States have anorexia nervosa, that 1% to 5% meet criteria for bulimia nervosa, and that up to 5% to 10% of all cases of eating disorders occur in males. There are also a large number of individuals with milder cases who do not meet all of the criteria in the *Diagnostic and Statistical Manual of Mental Disorders, Fourth Edition (DSM-IV)* for anorexia or bulimia nervosa but who nonetheless experience the physical and psychologic consequences of having an eating disorder.[21–25] Long-term follow-up for these patients can help reduce sequelae of the diseases; *Healthy People 2010* includes an objective (#18.5) seeking to reduce the relapse rates for persons with eating disorders including anorexia nervosa and bulimia nervosa.[26]

THE ROLE OF THE PEDIATRICIAN IN THE IDENTIFICATION AND EVALUATION OF EATING DISORDERS

Primary care pediatricians are in a unique position to detect the onset of eating disorders and stop their progression at the earliest stages of the illness. Primary and secondary prevention is accomplished by screening for eating disorders as part of routine annual health care, providing ongoing monitoring of weight and height, and paying careful attention to the signs and symptoms of an incipient eating disorder. Early detection and management of an eating disorder may prevent the physical and psychologic consequences of malnutrition that allow for progression to a later stage.[23,24]

Screening questions about eating patterns and satisfaction with body appearance should be asked of all preteens and adolescents as part of routine pediatric health care. Weight and height need to be determined regularly (preferably in a hospital gown, because objects may be hidden in clothing to falsely elevate weight). Ongoing measurements of weight and height should be plotted on pediatric growth charts to evaluate for decreases in both that can occur as a result of restricted nutritional intake.[27] Body mass index (BMI), which compares weight with height, can be a helpful measurement in tracking concerns; BMI is calculated as:

weight in pounds × 700/(height in inches squared)

or
weight in kilograms/(height in meters squared).
Newly developed growth charts are available for
plotting changes in weight, height, and BMI over
time and for comparing individual measurements
with age-appropriate population norms.[27] Any evidence of inappropriate dieting, excessive concern
with weight, or a weight loss pattern requires further
attention, as does a failure to achieve appropriate
increases in weight or height in growing children. In
each of these situations, careful assessment for the
possibility of an eating disorder and close monitoring at intervals as frequent as every 1 to 2 weeks may
be needed until the situation becomes clear.

A number of studies have shown that most adolescent females express concerns about being overweight, and many may diet inappropriately.[7–10]
Most of these children and adolescents do not have
an eating disorder. On the other hand, it is known
that patients with eating disorders may try to hide
their illness, and usually no specific signs or symptoms are detected, so a simple denial by the adolescent does not negate the possibility of an eating
disorder. It is wise, therefore, for the pediatrician to
be cautious by following weight and nutrition patterns very closely or referring to a specialist experienced in the treatment of eating disorders when suspected. In addition, taking a history from a parent
may help identify abnormal eating attitudes or behaviors, although parents may at times be in denial
as well. Failure to detect an eating disorder at this
early stage can result in an increase in severity of the
illness, either further weight loss in cases of anorexia
nervosa or increases in bingeing and purging behaviors in cases of bulimia nervosa, which can then
make the eating disorder much more difficult to
treat. In situations in which an adolescent is referred
to the pediatrician because of concerns by parents,
friends, or school personnel that he or she is displaying evidence of an eating disorder, it is most likely
that the adolescent does have an eating disorder,
either incipient or fully established. Pediatricians
must, therefore, take these situations very seriously
and not be lulled into a false sense of security if the
adolescent denies all symptoms. Table 1 outlines
questions useful in eliciting a history of eating disorders, and Table 2 delineates possible physical findings in children and adolescents with eating disorders.

Initial evaluation of the child or adolescent with a
suspected eating disorder includes establishment of
the diagnosis; determination of severity, including
evaluation of medical and nutritional status; and
performance of an initial psychosocial evaluation.
Each of these initial steps can be performed in the
pediatric primary care setting. The American Psychiatric Association has established DSM-IV criteria for
the diagnosis of anorexia and bulimia nervosa (Table
3).[24] These criteria focus on the weight loss, attitudes
and behaviors, and amenorrhea displayed by patients with eating disorders. Of note, studies have
shown that more than half of all children and adolescents with eating disorders may not fully meet all
DSM-IV criteria for anorexia or bulimia nervosa

TABLE 1. Specific Screening Questions to Identify the Child,
Adolescent, or Young Adult With an Eating Disorder

What is the most you ever weighed? How tall were you then?
   When was that?
What is the least you ever weighed in the past year? How tall
   were you then? When was that?
What do you think you ought to weigh?
Exercise: how much, how often, level of intensity? How stressed
   are you if you miss a workout?
Current dietary practices: ask for specifics—amounts, food
   groups, fluids, restrictions?
 • 24-h diet history?
 • Calorie counting, fat gram counting? Taboo foods (foods
   you avoid)?
 • Any binge eating? Frequency, amount, triggers?
 • Purging history?
 • Use of diuretics, laxatives, diet pills, ipecac? Ask about
   elimination pattern, constipation, diarrhea.
 • Any vomiting? Frequency, how long after meals?
Any previous therapy? What kind and how long? What was
   and was not helpful?
Family history: obesity, eating disorders, depression, other
   mental illness, substance abuse by parents or other family
   members?
Menstrual history: age at menarche? Regularity of cycles? Last
   menstrual period?
Use of cigarettes, drugs, alcohol? Sexual history? History of
   physical or sexual abuse?
Review of symptoms:
 • Dizziness, syncope, weakness, fatigue?
 • Pallor, easy bruising or bleeding?
 • Cold intolerance?
 • Hair loss, lanugo, dry skin?
 • Vomiting, diarrhea, constipation?
 • Fullness, bloating, abdominal pain, epigastric burning?
 • Muscle cramps, joint paints, palpitations, chest pain?
 • Menstrual irregularities?
 • Symptoms of hyperthyroidism, diabetes, malignancy,
   infection, inflammatory bowel disease?

while still experiencing the same medical and psychologic consequences of these disorders[28]; these patients are included in another DSM-IV diagnosis,
referred to as eating disorder-not otherwise specified.[24] The pediatrician needs to be aware that patients with eating disorders not otherwise specified
require the same careful attention as those who meet
criteria for anorexia or bulimia nervosa. A patient
who has lost weight rapidly but who does not meet
full criteria because weight is not yet 15% below that
which is expected for height may be more physically
and psychologically compromised than may a patient of lower weight. Also, in growing children, it is
failure to make appropriate gains in weight and
height, not necessarily weight loss per se, that indicates the severity of the malnutrition. It is also common for adolescents to have significant purging behaviors without episodes of binge eating; although
these patients do not meet the full DSM-IV criteria
for bulimia nervosa, they may become severely medically compromised. These issues are addressed in
the Diagnostic and Statistical Manual for Primary Care
(DSM-PC) Child and Adolescent Version, which provides diagnostic codes and criteria for purging and
bingeing, dieting, and body image problems that do
not meet DSM-IV criteria.[29] In general, determination of total weight loss and weight status (calculated
as percent below ideal body weight and/or as BMI),
along with types and frequency of purging behaviors

TABLE 2.   Possible Findings on Physical Examination in Children and Adolescents With Eating Disorders

Anorexia Nervosa	Bulimia Nervosa
Bradycardia	Sinus bradycardia
Orthostatic by pulse or blood pressure	Orthostatic by pulse or blood pressure
Hypothermia	Hypothermia
Cardiac murmur (one third with mitral valve prolapse)	Cardiac murmur (mitral valve prolapse)
Dull, thinning scalp hair	Hair without shine
Sunken cheeks, sallow skin	Dry skin
Lanugo	Parotitis
Atrophic breasts (postpubertal)	Russell's sign (callous on knuckles from self-induced emesis)
Atrophic vaginitis (postpubertal)	Mouth sores
Pitting edema of extremities	Palatal scratches
Emaciated, may wear oversized clothes	Dental enamel erosions
Flat affect	May look entirely normal
Cold extremities, acrocyanosis	Other cardiac arrhythmias

TABLE 3.   Diagnosis of Anorexia Nervosa, Bulimia Nervosa, and Eating Disorders Not Otherwise Specified, From *DSM-IV*[25]

Anorexia Nervosa
1. Intense fear of becoming fat or gaining weight, even though underweight.
2. Refusal to maintain body weight at or above a minimally normal weight for age and height (ie, weight loss leading to maintenance of body weight <85% of that expected, or failure to make expected weight gain during period of growth, leading to body weight <85% of that expected).
3. Disturbed body image, undue influence of shape or weight on self-evaluation, or denial of the seriousness of the current low body weight.
4. Amenorrhea or absence of at least 3 consecutive menstrual cycles (those with periods only inducible after estrogen therapy are considered amenorrheic).
   Types:
   Restricting—no regular bingeing or purging (self-induced vomiting or use of laxatives and diuretics).
   Binge eating/purging—regular bingeing and purging in a patient who also meets the above criteria for anorexia nervosa.
Bulimia Nervosa
1. Recurrent episodes of binge eating, characterized by:
   a. Eating a substantially larger amount of food in a discrete period of time (ie, in 2 h) than would be eaten by most people in similar circumstances during that same time period.
   b. A sense of lack of control over eating during the binge.
2. Recurrent inappropriate compensatory behavior to prevent weight gain; ie, self-induced vomiting, use of laxatives, diuretics, fasting, or hyperexercising.
3. Binges or inappropriate compensatory behaviors occurring, on average, at least twice weekly for at least 3 mo.
4. Self-evaluation unduly influenced by body shape or weight.
5. The disturbance does not occur exclusively during episodes of anorexia nervosa
   Types:
   Purging—regularly engages in self-induced vomiting or use of laxatives or diuretics.
   Nonpurging—uses other inappropriate compensatory behaviors; ie, fasting or hyperexercising, without regular use of vomiting or medications to purge.
Eating Disorder Not Otherwise Specified (those who do not meet criteria for anorexia nervosa or bulimia nervosa, per *DSM-IV*
1. All criteria for anorexia nervosa, except has regular menses.
2. All criteria for anorexia nervosa, except weight still in normal range.
3. All criteria for bulimia nervosa, except binges <twice a wk or <3 times a mo.
4. A patient with normal body weight who regularly engages in inappropriate compensatory behavior after eating small amounts of food (ie, self-induced vomiting after eating 2 cookies).
5. A patient who repeatedly chews and spits out large amounts of food without swallowing.
6. Binge eating disorder: recurrent binges but does not engage in the inappropriate compensatory behaviors of bulimia nervosa.

(including vomiting and use of laxatives, diuretics, ipecac, and over-the-counter or prescription diet pills as well as use of starvation and/or exercise) serve to establish an initial index of severity for the child or adolescent with an eating disorder.

The medical complications associated with eating disorders are listed in Table 4, and details of these complications have been described in several reviews.[23,24,30–34] It is uncommon for the pediatrician to encounter most of these complications in a patient with a newly diagnosed eating disorder. However, it is recommended that an initial laboratory assessment be performed and that this include complete blood cell count, electrolyte measurement, liver function tests, urinalysis, and a thyroid-stimulating hormone test. Additional tests (urine pregnancy, luteinizing and follicle-stimulating hormone, prolactin, and estradiol tests) may need to be performed in patients

who are amenorrheic to rule out other causes for amenorrhea, including pregnancy, ovarian failure, or prolactinoma. Other tests, including an erythrocyte sedimentation rate and radiographic studies (such as computed tomography or magnetic resonance imaging of the brain or upper or lower gastrointestinal system studies), should be performed if there are uncertainties about the diagnosis. An electrocardiogram should be performed on any patient with bradycardia or electrolyte abnormalities. Bone densitometry should be considered in those amenorrheic for more than 6 to 12 months. It should be noted, however, that most test results will be normal in most patients with eating disorders, and normal laboratory test results do not exclude serious illness or medical instability in these patients.

The initial psychosocial assessment should include an evaluation of the patient's degree of obsession

TABLE 4. Medical Complications Resulting From Eating Disorders

Medical Complications Resulting From Purging
1. Fluid and electrolyte imbalance; hypokalemia; hyponatremia; hypochloremic alkalosis.
2. Use of ipecac: irreversible myocardial damage and a diffuse myositis.
3. Chronic vomiting: esophagitis; dental erosions; Mallory-Weiss tears; rare esophageal or gastric rupture; rare aspiration pneumonia.
4. Use of laxatives: depletion of potassium bicarbonate, causing metabolic acidosis; increased blood urea nitrogen concentration and predisposition to renal stones from dehydration; hyperuricemia; hypocalcemia; hypomagnesemia; chronic dehydration. With laxative withdrawal, may get fluid retention (may gain up to 10 lb in 24 h).
5. Amenorrhea (can be seen in normal or overweight individuals with bulimia nervosa), menstrual irregularities, osteopenia.

Medical Complications From Caloric Restriction
1. Cardiovascular
   Electrocardiographic abnormalities: low voltage; sinus bradycardia (from malnutrition); T wave inversions; ST segment depression (from electrolyte imbalances). Prolonged corrected QT interval is uncommon but may predispose patient to sudden death. Dysrhythmias include supraventricular beats and ventricular tachycardia, with or without exercise. Pericardial effusions can occur in those severely malnourished. All cardiac abnormalities except those secondary to emetine (ipecac) toxicity are completely reversible with weight gain.
2. Gastrointestinal system: delayed gastric emptying; slowed gastrointestinal motility; constipation; bloating; fullness; hypercholesterolemia (from abnormal lipoprotein metabolism); abnormal liver function test results (probably from fatty infiltration of the liver). All reversible with weight gain.
3. Renal: increased blood urea nitrogen concentration (from dehydration, decreased glomerular filtration rate) with increased risk of renal stones; polyuria (from abnormal vasopressin secretion, rare partial diabetes insipidus). Total body sodium and potassium depletion caused by starvation; with refeeding, 25% can get peripheral edema attributable to increased renal sensitivity to aldosterone and increased insulin secretion (affects renal tubules).
4. Hematologic: leukopenia; anemia; iron deficiency; thrombocytopenia.
5. Endocrine: euthyroid sick syndrome; amenorrhea; osteopenia.
6. Neurologic: cortical atrophy; seizures.

with food and weight, understanding of the diagnosis, and willingness to receive help; an assessment of the patient's functioning at home, in school, and with friends; and a determination of other psychiatric diagnoses (such as depression, anxiety, and obsessive-compulsive disorder), which may be comorbid with or may be a cause or consequence of the eating disorder. Suicidal ideation and history of physical or sexual abuse or violence should also be assessed. The parents' reaction to the illness should be assessed, because denial of the problem or parental differences in how to approach treatment and recovery may exacerbate the patient's illness. The pediatrician who feels competent and comfortable in performing the full initial evaluation is encouraged to do so. Others should refer to appropriate medical subspecialists and mental health personnel to ensure that a complete evaluation is performed. A differential diagnosis for the adolescent with symptoms of an eating disorder can be found in Table 5.

Several treatment decisions follow the initial evaluation, including the questions of where and by whom the patient will be treated. Patients who have minimal nutritional, medical, and psychosocial issues and show a quick reversal of their condition may be treated in the pediatrician's office, usually in conjunction with a registered dietitian and a mental health practitioner. Pediatricians who do not feel comfortable with issues of medical and psychosocial

TABLE 5. Differential Diagnosis of Eating Disorders

- Malignancy, central nervous system tumor
- Gastrointestinal system: inflammatory bowel disease, malabsorption, celiac disease
- Endocrine: diabetes mellitus, hyperthyroidism, hypopituitarism, Addison disease
- Depression, obsessive-compulsive disorder, psychiatric diagnosis
- Other chronic disease or chronic infections
- Superior mesenteric artery syndrome (can also be a consequence of an eating disorder)

management can refer these patients at this early stage. Pediatricians can choose to stay involved even after referral to the team of specialists, as the family often appreciates the comfort of the relationship with their long-term care provider. Pediatricians comfortable with the ongoing care and secondary prevention of medical complications in patients with eating disorders may choose to continue care themselves. More severe cases require the involvement of a multidisciplinary specialty team working in outpatient, inpatient, or day program settings.

THE PEDIATRICIAN'S ROLE IN THE TREATMENT OF EATING DISORDERS IN OUTPATIENT SETTINGS

Pediatricians have several important roles to play in the management of patients with diagnosed eating disorders. These aspects of care include medical and nutritional management and coordination with mental health personnel in provision of the psychosocial and psychiatric aspects of care. Most patients will have much of their ongoing treatment performed in outpatient settings. Although some pediatricians in primary care practice may perform these roles for some patients in outpatient settings on the basis of their levels of interest and expertise, many general pediatricians do not feel comfortable treating patients with eating disorders and prefer to refer patients with anorexia or bulimia nervosa for care by those with special expertise.[35] A number of pediatricians specializing in adolescent medicine have developed this skill set, with an increasing number involved in the management of eating disorders as part of multidisciplinary teams.[23,36] Other than the most severely affected patients, most children and adolescents with eating disorders will be managed in an outpatient setting by a multidisciplinary team coordinated by a pediatrician or subspecialist with appropriate expertise in the care of children and adolescents with eating disorders. Pediatricians

• •

generally work with nursing, nutrition, and mental health colleagues in the provision of medical, nutrition, and mental health care required by these patients.

As listed in Table 4, medical complications of eating disorders can occur in all organ systems. Pediatricians need to be aware of several complications that can occur in the outpatient setting. Although most patients do not have electrolyte abnormalities, the pediatrician must be alert to the possibility of development of hypokalemic, hypochloremic alkalosis resulting from purging behaviors (including vomiting and laxative or diuretic use) and hyponatremia or hypernatremia resulting from drinking too much or too little fluid as part of weight manipulation. Endocrine abnormalities, including hypothyroidism, hypercortisolism, and hypogonadotropic hypogonadism, are common, with amenorrhea leading to the potentially long-term complication of osteopenia and, ultimately, osteoporosis.[37–40] Gastrointestinal symptoms caused by abnormalities in intestinal motility resulting from malnutrition, laxative abuse, or refeeding are common but are rarely dangerous and may require symptomatic relief. Constipation during refeeding is common and should be treated with dietary manipulation and reassurance; the use of laxatives in this situation should be avoided.

The components of nutritional rehabilitation required in the outpatient management of patients with eating disorders are presented in several reviews.[23,24,41–44] These reviews highlight the dietary stabilization that is required as part of the management of bulimia nervosa and the weight gain regimens that are required as the hallmark of treatment of anorexia nervosa. The reintroduction or improvement of meals and snacks in those with anorexia nervosa is generally done in a stepwise manner, leading in most cases to an eventual intake of 2000 to 3000 kcal per day and a weight gain of 0.5 to 2 lb per week. Changes in meals are made to ensure ingestion of 2 to 3 servings of protein per day (with 1 serving equal to 3 oz of cheese, chicken, meat, or other protein sources). Daily fat intake should be slowly shifted toward a goal of 30 to 50 g per day. Treatment goal weights should be individualized and based on age, height, stage of puberty, premorbid weight, and previous growth charts. In postmenarchal girls, resumption of menses provides an objective measure of return to biological health, and weight at resumption of menses can be used to determine treatment goal weight. A weight approximately 90% of standard body weight is the average weight at which menses resume and can be used as an initial treatment goal weight, because 86% of patients who achieve this weight resume menses within 6 months.[45] For a growing child or adolescent, goal weight should be reevaluated at 3- to 6-month intervals on the basis of changing age and height. Behavioral interventions are often required to encourage otherwise reluctant (and often resistant) patients to accomplish necessary caloric intake and weight gain goals. Although some pediatric specialists, pediatric nurses, or dietitians may be able to handle this aspect of care alone, a combined medical and nutritional

team is usually required, especially for more difficult patients.[46]

Similarly, the pediatrician must work with mental health experts to provide the necessary psychologic, social, and psychiatric care.[47–49] The model used by many interdisciplinary teams, especially those based in settings experienced in the care of adolescents, is to establish a division of labor such that the medical and nutritional clinicians work on the issues described in the preceding paragraph and the mental health clinicians provide such modalities as individual, family, and group therapy. It is generally accepted that medical stabilization and nutritional rehabilitation are the most crucial determinants of short-term and intermediate-term outcome. Individual and family therapy, the latter being especially important in working with younger children and adolescents, are crucial determinants of the long-term prognosis.[50–53] It is also recognized that correction of malnutrition is required for the mental health aspects of care to be effective. Psychotropic medications have been shown to be helpful in the treatment of bulimia nervosa and prevention of relapse in anorexia nervosa in adults.[54–56] These medications are also used for many adolescent patients and may be prescribed by the pediatrician or the psychiatrist, depending on the delegation of roles within the team.

THE ROLE OF THE PEDIATRICIAN IN HOSPITAL AND DAY PROGRAM SETTINGS

Criteria for the hospitalization of children and adolescents with eating disorders have been established by the Society for Adolescent Medicine[23] (Table 6). These criteria, in keeping with those published by the American Psychiatric Association,[24] acknowledge that hospitalization may be required because of medical or psychiatric needs or because of failure of outpatient treatment to accomplish needed medical, nutritional, or psychiatric progress. Unfortunately, many insurance companies do not use similar crite-

TABLE 6.   Criteria for Hospital Admission for Children, Adolescents, and Young Adults With Eating Disorders

Anorexia Nervosa
- <75% ideal body weight, or ongoing weight loss despite intensive management
- Refusal to eat
- Body fat <10%
- Heart rate <50 beats per minute daytime; <45 beats per min nighttime
- Systolic pressure <90
- Orthostatic changes in pulse (>20 beats per min) or blood pressure (>10 mm Hg)
- Temperature <96°F
- Arrhythmia

Bulimia Nervosa
- Syncope
- Serum potassium concentration <3.2 mmol/L
- Serum chloride concentration <88 mmol/L
- Esophageal tears
- Cardiac arrhythmias including prolonged QTc
- Hypothermia
- Suicide risk
- Intractable vomiting
- Hematemesis
- Failure to respond to outpatient treatment

ria, thus making it difficult for some children and adolescents with eating disorders to receive an appropriate level of care.[57-59] Children and adolescents have the best prognosis if their disease is treated rapidly and aggressively[36] (an approach that may not be as effective in adults with a more long-term, protracted course). Hospitalization, which allows for adequate weight gain in addition to medical stabilization and the establishment of safe and healthy eating habits, improves the prognosis in children and adolescents.[60]

The pediatrician involved in the treatment of hospitalized patients must be prepared to provide nutrition via a nasogastric tube or occasionally intravenously when necessary. Some programs use this approach frequently, and others apply it more sparingly. Also, because these patients are generally more malnourished than those treated as outpatients, more severe complications may need to be treated. These include the possible metabolic, cardiac, and neurologic complications listed in Table 2. Of particular concern is the refeeding syndrome that can occur in severely malnourished patients who receive nutritional replenishment too rapidly.[61] The refeeding syndrome consists of cardiovascular, neurologic, and hematologic complications that occur because of shifts in phosphate from extracellular to intracellular spaces in individuals who have total body phosphorus depletion as a result of malnutrition. Recent studies have shown that this syndrome can result from use of oral, parenteral, or enteral nutrition.[62-64] Slow refeeding, with the possible addition of phosphorus supplementation, is required to prevent development of the refeeding syndrome in severely malnourished children and adolescents.

Day treatment (partial hospitalization) programs have been developed to provide an intermediate level of care for patients with eating disorders who require more than outpatient care but less than 24-hour hospitalization.[65-68] In some cases, these programs have been used in an attempt to prevent the need for hospitalization; more often, they are used as a transition from inpatient to outpatient care. Day treatment programs generally provide care (including meals, therapy, groups, and other activities) 4 to 5 days per week from 8 or 9 AM until 5 or 6 PM. An additional level of care, referred to as an "intensive outpatient" program, has also been developed for these patients and generally provides care 2 to 4 afternoons or evenings per week. It is recommended that intensive outpatient and day programs that include children and adolescents should incorporate pediatric care into the management of the developmental and medical needs of their patients. Pediatricians can play an active role in the development of objective, evidence-based criteria for the transition from one level of care to the next. Additional research can also help clarify other questions, such as the use of enteral versus parenteral nutrition during refeeding, to serve as the foundation for evidence-based guidelines.

THE ROLE OF THE PEDIATRICIAN IN PREVENTION AND ADVOCACY

Prevention of eating disorders can take place in the practice and community setting. Primary care pediatricians can help families and children learn to apply the principles of proper nutrition and physical activity and to avoid an unhealthy emphasis on weight and dieting. In addition, pediatricians can implement screening strategies (as described earlier) to detect the early onset of an eating disorder and be careful to avoid seemingly innocuous statements (such as "you're just a little above the average weight") that can sometimes serve as the precipitant for the onset of an eating disorder. At the community level, there is general agreement that changes in the cultural approaches to weight and dieting issues will be required to decrease the growing numbers of children and adolescents with eating disorders. School curricula have been developed to try to accomplish these goals. Initial evaluations of these curricula show some success in changing attitudes and behaviors, but questions about their effectiveness remain, and single-episode programs (eg, 1 visit to a classroom) are clearly not effective and may do more harm than good.[69-74] Additional curricula are being developed and additional evaluations are taking place in this field.[75] Some work has also been done with the media, in an attempt to change the ways in which weight and dieting issues are portrayed in magazines, television shows, and movies.[76] Pediatricians can work in their local communities, regionally, and nationally to support the efforts that are attempting to change the cultural norms being experienced by children and adolescents.

Pediatricians can also help support advocacy efforts that are attempting to ensure that children and adolescents with eating disorders are able to receive necessary care. Length of stay, adequacy of mental health services, and appropriate level of care have been a source of contention between those who treat eating disorders on a regular basis and the insurance industry.

Work is being done with insurance companies and on legislative and judicial levels to secure appropriate coverage for the treatment of mental health conditions, including eating disorders.[77,78] Parent groups, along with some in the mental health professions, have been leading this battle. Support by pediatrics in general, and pediatricians in particular, is required to help this effort.

RECOMMENDATIONS

1. Pediatricians need to be knowledgeable about the early signs and symptoms of disordered eating and other related behaviors.
2. Pediatricians should be aware of the careful balance that needs to be in place to decrease the growing prevalence of eating disorders in children and adolescents. When counseling children on risk of obesity and healthy eating, care needs to be taken not to foster overaggressive dieting and to help children and adolescents build self-esteem while still addressing weight concerns.

3. Pediatricians should be familiar with the screening and counseling guidelines for disordered eating and other related behaviors.

4. Pediatricians should know when and how to monitor and/or refer patients with eating disorders to best address their medical and nutritional needs, serving as an integral part of the multidisciplinary team.

5. Pediatricians should be encouraged to calculate and plot weight, height, and BMI using age- and gender-appropriate graphs at routine annual pediatric visits.

6. Pediatricians can play a role in primary prevention through office visits and community- or school-based interventions with a focus on screening, education, and advocacy.

7. Pediatricians can work locally, nationally, and internationally to help change cultural norms conducive to eating disorders and proactively to change media messages.

8. Pediatricians need to be aware of the resources in their communities so they can coordinate care of various treating professionals, helping to create a seamless system between inpatient and outpatient management in their communities.

9. Pediatricians should help advocate for parity of mental health benefits to ensure continuity of care for the patients with eating disorders.

10. Pediatricians need to advocate for legislation and regulations that secure appropriate coverage for medical, nutritional, and mental health treatment in settings appropriate to the severity of the illness (inpatient, day hospital, intensive outpatient, and outpatient).

11. Pediatricians are encouraged to participate in the development of objective criteria for the optimal treatment of eating disorders, including the use of specific treatment modalities and the transition from one level of care to another.

Committee on Adolescence, 2002–2003
David W. Kaplan, MD, MPH, Chairperson
Margaret Blythe, MD
Angela Diaz, MD
Ronald A. Feinstein, MD
*Martin M. Fisher, MD
Jonathan D. Klein, MD, MPH
W. Samuel Yancy, MD

Consultant
*Ellen S. Rome, MD, MPH

Liaisons
S. Paige Hertweck, MD
    American College of Obstetricians and
    Gynecologists
Miriam Kaufman, RN, MD
    Canadian Paediatric Society
Glen Pearson, MD
    American Academy of Child and Adolescent
    Psychiatry

Staff
Tammy Piazza Hurley

*Lead authors

REFERENCES

1. Whitaker AH. An epidemiological study of anorectic and bulimic symptoms in adolescent girls: implications for pediatricians. *Pediatr Ann.* 1992;21:752–759

2. Lucas AR, Beard CM, O'Fallon WM, Kurland LT. 50-year trends in the incidence of anorexia nervosa in Rochester, Minn.: a population-based study. *Am J Psychiatry.* 1991;148:917–922

3. Hsu LK. Epidemiology of the eating disorders. *Psychiatry Clin North Am.* 1996;19:681–700

4. Dorian BJ, Garfinkel PE. The contributions of epidemiologic studies to the etiology and treatment of the eating disorders. *Psychiatry Ann.* 1999;29:187–192

5. Troiano RP, Flegal KM, Kuczmarski RJ, Campbell SM, Johnson CL. Overweight prevalence and trends for children and adolescents: the National Health and Nutrition Examination Surveys, 1963 to 1991. *Arch Pediatr Adolesc Med.* 1995;149:1085–1091

6. Troiano RP, Flegal KM. Overweight children and adolescents: description, epidemiology, and demographics. *Pediatrics.* 1998;101(suppl): 497–504

7. Strauss RS. Self-reported weight status and dieting in a cross-sectional sample of young adolescents: National Health and Nutrition Examination Survey III. *Arch Pediatr Adolesc Med.* 1999;153:741–747

8. Fisher M, Schneider M, Pegler C, Napolitano B. Eating attitudes, health risk behaviors, self-esteem, and anxiety among adolescent females in a suburban high school. *J Adolesc Health.* 1991;12:377–384

9. Stein D, Meged S, Bar-Hanin T, Blank S, Elizur A, Weizman A. Partial eating disorders in a community sample of female adolescents. *J Am Acad Child Adolesc Psychiatry.* 1997;36:1116–1123

10. Patton GC, Carlin JB, Shao Q, et al. Adolescent dieting: healthy weight control or borderline eating disorder? *J Child Psychol Psychiatry.* 1997; 38:299–306

11. Krowchuk DP, Kreiter SR, Woods CR, Sinal SH, DuRant RH. Problem dieting behaviors among young adolescents. *Arch Pediatr Adolesc Med.* 1998;152:884–888

12. Field AE, Camargo CA Jr, Taylor CB, et al. Overweight, weight concerns, and bulimic behaviors among girls and boys. *J Am Acad Child Adolesc Psychiatry.* 1999;38:754–760

13. Andersen AE. Eating disorders in males. In: Brownell KD, Fairburn CG, eds. *Eating Disorders and Obesity: A Comprehensive Handbook.* New York, NY: Guilford Press; 1995:177–187

14. Carlat DJ, Camargo CA Jr, Herzog DB. Eating disorders in males: a report on 135 patients. *Am J Psychiatry.* 1997;154:1127–1132

15. Robinson TN, Killen JD, Litt IF, et al. Ethnicity and body dissatisfaction: are Hispanic and Asian girls at increased risk for eating disorders? *J Adolesc Health.* 1996;19:384–393

16. Crago M, Shisslak CM, Estes LS. Eating disturbances among American minority groups: a review. *Int J Eat Disord.* 1996;19:239–248

17. Gard MC, Freeman CP. The dismantling of a myth: a review of eating disorders and socioeconomic status. *Int J Eat Disord.* 1996;20:1–12

18. Pike KM, Walsh BT. Ethnicity and eating disorders: implications for incidence and treatment. *Psychopharmacol Bull.* 1996;32:265–274

19. Lai KY. Anorexia nervosa in Chinese adolescents—does culture make a difference? *J Adolesc.* 2000;23:561–568

20. le Grange D, Telch CF, Tibbs J. Eating attitudes and behaviors in 1435 South African Caucasian and non-Caucasian college students. *Am J Psychiatry.* 1998;155:250–254

21. Becker AE, Grinspoon SK, Klibanski A, Herzog DB. Eating disorders. *N Engl J Med.* 1999;340:1092–1098

22. Steiner H, Lock J. Anorexia nervosa and bulimia nervosa in children and adolescents: a review of the past 10 years. *J Am Acad Child Adolesc Psychiatry.* 1998;37:352–359

23. Fisher M, Golden NH, Katzman DK, et al. Eating disorders in adolescents: a background paper. *J Adolesc Health.* 1995;16:420–437

24. American Psychiatric Association, Work Group on Eating Disorders. Practice guideline for the treatment of patients with eating disorders (revision). *Am J Psychiatry.* 2000;157(1 suppl):1–39

25. American Psychiatric Association. *Diagnostic and Statistical Manual of Mental Disorders, 4th ed (DSM-IV).* Washington, DC: American Psychiatric Association; 1994

26. US Department of Health and Human Services. *Mental health and mental disorders.* In: *Healthy People 2010.* Vol II. Washington, DC: US Public Health Service, US Department of Health and Human Services; 2000. Available at: http://www.health.gov/healthypeople/document/html/volume2/18mental.htm. Accessed September 4, 2002

27. Kuczmarski RJ, Ogden CL, Grummer-Strawn LM, et al. *CDC Growth Charts: United States.* Hyattsville, MD: National Center for Health

Statistics; 2000. Available at: http://www.cdc.gov/growthcharts/. Accessed February 26, 2002

28. Bunnell DW, Shenker IR, Nussbaum MP, et al. Subclinical versus formal eating disorders: differentiating psychological features. *Int J Eat Disord.* 1990;9:357–362

29. Wolraich ML, Felice ME, Drotar D, eds. *The Classification of Child and Adolescent Mental Diagnoses in Primary Care: Diagnostic and Statistical Manual for Primary Care (DSM-PC) Child and Adolescent Version.* Elk Grove Village, IL: American Academy of Pediatrics; 1996

30. Palla B, Litt IF. Medical complications of eating disorders in adolescents. *Pediatrics.* 1988;81:613–623

31. Fisher M. Medical complications of anorexia and bulimia nervosa. *Adolesc Med.* 1992;3:487–502

32. Rome ES. Eating disorders in adolescents and young adults: what's a primary care clinician to do? *Cleveland Clin J Med.* 1996;63:387–395

33. Mehler PS, Gray MC, Schulte M. Medical complications of anorexia nervosa. *J Womens Health.* 1997;6:533–541

34. Nicholls D, Stanhope R. Medical complications of anorexia nervosa in children and young adolescents. *Eur Eat Disord Rev.* 2000;8:170–180

35. Fisher M, Golden NH, Bergeson R, et al. Update on adolescent health care in pediatric practice. *J Adolesc Health.* 1996;19:394–400

36. Kreipe RE, Golden NH, Katzman DK, et al. Eating disorders in adolescents. A position paper of the Society for Adolescent Medicine. *J Adolesc Health.* 1995;16:476–479

37. Wong JCH, Lewindon P, Mortimer R, Shepherd R. Bone mineral density in adolescent females with recently diagnosed anorexia nervosa. *Int J Eat Disord.* 2001;29:11–16

38. Grinspoon S, Thomas E, Pitts S, et al. Prevalence and predictive factors for regional osteopenia in women with anorexia nervosa. *Ann Intern Med.* 2000;133:790–794

39. Castro J, Lazaro L, Pons F, Halperin I, Toro J. Predictors of bone mineral density reduction in adolescents with anorexia nervosa. *J Am Acad Child Adolesc Psychiatry.* 2000;39:1365–1370

40. Golden NH, Shenker IR. Amenorrhea in anorexia nervosa: etiology and implications. *Adolesc Med.* 1992;3:503–518

41. Schebendach J, Nussbaum MP. Nutrition management in adolescents with eating disorders. *Adolesc Med.* 1992;3:541–558

42. Rock CL, Curran-Celentano J. Nutritional disorder of anorexia nervosa: a review. *Int J Eat Disord.* 1994;15:187–203

43. Rock CL, Curran-Celentano J. Nutritional management of eating disorders. *Psychiatry Clin North Am.* 1996;19:701–713

44. Rome ES, Vazquez IM, Emans SJ. Nutritional problems in adolescence: anorexia nervosa/bulimia nervosa for young athletes. In: Walker WA, Watkins JB, eds. *Nutrition in Pediatrics: Basic Science and Clinical Applications.* 2nd ed. Hamilton, Ontario: BC Decker Inc; 1997:691–704

45. Golden NH, Jacobson MS, Schebendach J, Solanto MV, Hertz SM, Shenker IR. Resumption of menses in anorexia nervosa. *Arch Pediatr Adolesc Med.* 1997;151:16–21

46. Kreipe R, Uphoff M. Treatment and outcome of adolescents with anorexia nervosa. *Adolesc Med.* 1992;3:519–540

47. Yager J. Psychosocial treatments for eating disorders. *Psychiatry.* 1994; 57:153–164

48. Powers PS. Initial assessment and early treatment options for anorexia nervosa and bulimia nervosa. *Psychiatry Clin North Am.* 1996;19:639–655

49. Robin AL, Gilroy M, Dennis AB. Treatment of eating disorders in children and adolescents. *Clin Psychol Rev.* 1998;18:421–446

50. Russell GF, Szmukler GI, Dare C, Eisler I. An evaluation of family therapy in anorexia nervosa and bulimia nervosa. *Arch Gen Psychiatry.* 1987;44:1047–1056

51. Eisler I, Dare C, Russell GF, Szmukler G, le Grange D, Dodge E. Family and individual therapy in anorexia nervosa: a 5-year follow-up. *Arch Gen Psychiatry.* 1997;54:1025–1030

52. North C, Gowers S, Byram V. Family functioning in adolescent anorexia nervosa. *Br J Psychiatry.* 1995;167:673–678

53. Geist R, Heinmaa M, Stephens D, Davis R, Katzman DK. Comparison of family therapy and family group psychoeducation in adolescents with anorexia nervosa. *Can J Psychiatry.* 2000;45:173–178

54. Jimerson DC, Wolfe BE, Brotman AW, Metzger ED. Medications in the treatment of eating disorders. *Psychiatry Clin North Am.* 1996;19:739–754

55. Walsh BT, Wilson GT, Loeb KL, et al. Medication and psychotherapy in the treatment of bulimia nervosa. *Am J Psychiatry.* 1997;154:523–531

56. Strober M, Freeman R, De Antonio M, Lampert C, Diamond J. Does adjunctive fluoxetine influence the post-hospital course of restrictor-type anorexia nervosa? A 24-month prospective, longitudinal follow up and comparison with historical controls. *Psychopharmacol Bull.* 1997;33: 425–431

57. Silber TJ, Delaney D, Samuels J Anorexia nervosa. Hospitalization on adolescent medicine units and third-party payments. *J Adolesc Health.* 1989;10:122–125

58. Silber TJ. Eating disorders and health insurance. *Arch Pediatr Adolesc Med.* 1994;148:785–788

59. Sigman G. How has the care of eating disorder patients been altered and upset by payment and insurance issues? Let me count the ways [letter]. *J Adolesc Health.* 1996;19:317–318

60. Baran SA, Weltzin TE, Kaye WH. Low discharge weight and outcome in anorexia nervosa. *Am J Psychiatry.* 1995;152:1070–1072

61. Solomon SM, Kirby DF. The refeeding syndrome: a review. *JPEN J Parenter Enteral Nutr.* 1990;14:900–97

62. Birmingham CL, Alothman AF, Goldner EM. Anorexia nervosa: refeeding and hypophosphatemia. *Int J Eat Disord.* 1996;20:211–213

63. Kohn MR, Golden NH, Shenker IR. Cardiac arrest and delirium: presentations of the refeeding syndrome in severely malnourished adolescents with anorexia nervosa. *J Adolesc Health.* 1998;22:239–243

64. Fisher M, Simpser E, Schneider M. Hypophosphatemia secondary to oral refeeding in anorexia nervosa. *Int J Eat Disord.* 2000;28:181–187

65. Kaye WH, Kaplan AS, Zucker ML. Treating eating-disorder patients in a managed care environment. Contemporary American issues and Canadian response. *Psychiatry Clin North Am.* 1996;19:793–810

66. Kaplan AS, Olmstead MP. Partial hospitalization. In: Garner DM, Garfinkel PE, eds. *Handbook of Treatment for Eating Disorders.* 2nd ed. New York, NY: Guilford Press; 1997:354–360

67. Kaplan AS, Olmstead MP, Molleken L. Day treatment of eating disorders. In: Jimerson D, Kaye WH, eds. *Bailliere's Clinical Psychiatry, Eating Disorders.* Philadelphia, PA: Bailliere Tindall; 1997:275–289

68. Howard WT, Evans KK, Quintero-Howard CV, Bowers WA, Andersen AE. Predictors of success or failure of transition to day hospital treatment for inpatients with anorexia nervosa. *Am J Psychiatry.* 1999;156: 1697–1702

69. Killen JD, Taylor CB, Hammer LD, et al. An attempt to modify unhealthful eating attitudes and weight regulation practices of young adolescent girls. *Int J Eat Disord.* 1993;13:369–384

70. Neumark-Sztainer D, Butler R, Palti H. Eating disturbances among adolescent girls: evaluation of a school-based primary prevention program. *J Nutr Educ.* 1995;27:24–31

71. Neumark-Sztainer D. School-based programs for preventing eating disturbances. *J Sch Health.* 1996;66:64–71

72. Carter JC, Stewart DA, Dunn VJ, Fairburn CG. Primary prevention of eating disorders: might it do more harm than good? *Int J Eat Disord.* 1997;22:167–172

73. Martz DM, Bazzini DG. Eating disorder prevention programs may be failing: evaluation of 2 one-shot programs. *J Coll Stud Dev.* 1999;40: 32–42

74. Hartley P. Does health education promote eating disorders? *Eur Eat Disord Rev.* 1996;4:3–11

75. Story M, Neumark-Sztainer D. Promoting healthy eating and physical activity in adolescents. *Adolesc Med.* 1999;10:109–123

76. Becker AE, Hamburg P. Culture, the media, and eating disorders. *Harv Rev Psychiatry.* 1996;4:163–167

77. Andersen AE. Third-party payment for inpatient treatment of anorexia nervosa. *Eat Disord Rev.* 1997;7:1, 4–5

78. Stein MK. House bill aims to raise eating disorder awareness. *Eat Disord Rev.* 2000;11:1–2

All policy statements from the American Academy of Pediatrics automatically expire 5 years after publication unless reaffirmed, revised, or retired at or before that time.

AMERICAN ACADEMY OF PEDIATRICS

POLICY STATEMENT
Organizational Principles to Guide and Define the Child Health Care System and/or Improve the Health of All Children

Committee on Nutrition

Prevention of Pediatric Overweight and Obesity

ABSTRACT. The dramatic increase in the prevalence of childhood overweight and its resultant comorbidities are associated with significant health and financial burdens, warranting strong and comprehensive prevention efforts. This statement proposes strategies for early identification of excessive weight gain by using body mass index, for dietary and physical activity interventions during health supervision encounters, and for advocacy and research.

ABBREVIATION. BMI, body mass index.

INTRODUCTION

Prevention is one of the hallmarks of pediatric practice and includes such diverse activities as newborn screenings, immunizations, and promotion of car safety seats and bicycle helmets. Documented trends in increasing prevalence of overweight and inactivity mean that pediatricians must focus preventive efforts on childhood obesity, with its associated comorbid conditions in childhood and likelihood of persistence into adulthood. These trends pose an unprecedented burden in terms of children's health as well as present and future health care costs. A number of statements have been published that address the scope of the problem and treatment strategies.[1-6]

The intent of this statement is to propose strategies to foster prevention and early identification of overweight and obesity in children. Evidence to support the recommendations for prevention is presented when available, but unfortunately, too few studies on prevention have been performed. The enormity of the epidemic, however, necessitates this call to action for pediatricians using the best information available.

DEFINITIONS AND DESCRIPTION OF THE PROBLEM

Body mass index (BMI) is the ratio of weight in kilograms to the square of height in meters. BMI is widely used to define overweight and obesity, because it correlates well with more accurate measures of body fatness and is derived from commonly available data—weight and height.[7] It has also been correlated with obesity-related comorbid conditions in

PEDIATRICS (ISSN 0031 4005). Copyright © 2003 by the American Academy of Pediatrics.

adults and children. Clinical judgment must be used in applying these criteria to a patient, because obesity refers to excess adiposity rather than excess weight, and BMI is a surrogate for adiposity. The pediatric growth charts for the US population now include BMI for age and gender, are readily available online (http://www.cdc.gov/growthcharts), and allow longitudinal tracking of BMI.[8]

BMI between 85th and 95th percentile for age and sex is considered at risk of overweight, and BMI at or above the 95th percentile is considered overweight or obese.[9,10] The prevalence of childhood overweight and obesity is increasing at an alarming rate in the United States as well as in other developed and developing countries. Prevalence among children and adolescents has doubled in the past 2 decades in the United States. Currently, 15.3% of 6- to 11-year-olds and 15.5% of 12- to 19-year-olds are at or above the 95th percentile for BMI on standard growth charts based on reference data from the 1970s, with even higher rates among subpopulations of minority and economically disadvantaged children.[10,11] Recent data from the Centers for Disease Control and Prevention also indicate that children younger than 5 years across all ethnic groups have had significant increases in the prevalence of overweight and obesity.[12,13] American children and adolescents today are less physically active as a group than were previous generations, and less active children are more likely to be overweight and to have higher blood pressure, insulin and cholesterol concentrations and more abnormal lipid profiles.[14,15]

Obesity is associated with significant health problems in the pediatric age group and is an important early risk factor for much of adult morbidity and mortality.[15,16] Medical problems are common in obese children and adolescents and can affect cardiovascular health (hypercholesterolemia and dyslipidemia, hypertension),[14,17-19] the endocrine system (hyperinsulinism, insulin resistance, impaired glucose tolerance, type 2 diabetes mellitus, menstrual irregularity),[20-22] and mental health (depression, low self-esteem).[23,24] Because of the increasing incidence of type 2 diabetes mellitus among obese adolescents and because diabetes-related morbidities may worsen if diagnosis is delayed, the clinician should be alert to the possibility of type 2 diabetes mellitus in all obese adolescents, especially those with a family history of early-onset (younger than 40 years) type 2 diabetes mellitus.[25] The psychologic stress of social stigmatization imposed on obese children may be just as damaging as the medical morbidities. The negative images of obesity are so strong that growth failure and pubertal delay have been reported in children practicing self-imposed caloric restriction because of fears of becoming obese.[26] Other important complications and associations include pulmonary (asthma, obstructive sleep apnea syndrome, pickwickian syndrome),[27-32] orthopedic (genu varum, slipped capital femoral epiphysis),[33,34] and gastrointestinal/hepatic (nonalcoholic steatohepatitis)[35] complications. All these disturbances are seen at an increased rate in obese individuals and have become more common in the pediatric population. The probability of childhood obesity persisting into adulthood is estimated to increase from approximately 20% at 4 years of age to approximately 80% by adolescence.[36] In addition, it is probable that comorbidities will persist into adulthood.[16,37] Thus, the potential future health care costs associated with pediatric obesity and its comorbidities are staggering, prompting the surgeon general to predict that preventable morbidity and mortality associated with obesity may exceed those associated with cigarette smoking.[10,38]

Although treatment approaches for pediatric obesity may be effective in the short term,[39-44] long-term outcome data for successful treatment approaches are limited.[45,46] The intractable nature of adult obesity is well known. Therefore, it is incumbent on the pediatric community to take a leadership role in prevention and early recognition of pediatric obesity.

RISK FACTORS

Development of effective prevention strategies mandates that physicians recognize populations and individuals at risk. Interactions between genetic, biological, psychologic, sociocultural, and environmental factors clearly are evident in childhood obesity. Elucidation of hormonal and neurochemical mechanisms that promote the energy imbalance that generates obesity has come from molecular genetics and neurochemistry. Knowledge of the genetic basis of differences in the complex of hormones and neurotransmitters (including growth hormone, leptin, ghrelin, neuropeptide Y, melanocortin, and others) that are responsible for regulating satiety, hunger, lipogenesis, and lipolysis as well as growth and reproductive development will eventually refine our understanding of risk of childhood overweight and obesity and may lead to more effective therapies.[47,48]

Genetic conditions known to be associated with propensity for obesity include Prader-Willi syndrome, Bardet-Biedl syndrome, and Cohen syndrome. In these conditions, early diagnosis allows collaboration with subspecialists, such as geneticists, endocrinologists, behavioralists, and nutritionists, to optimize growth and development while promoting healthy eating and activity patterns from a young age. For example, data suggest that growth hormone may improve some of the signs of Prader-Willi syndrome.[49-51]

It has long been recognized that obesity "runs in families"—high birth weight, maternal diabetes, and obesity in family members all are factors—but there are likely to be multiple genes and a strong interaction between genetics and environment that influence the degree of adiposity.[47,48,52,53] For young children, if 1 parent is obese, the odds ratio is approximately 3 for obesity in adulthood, but if both parents are obese, the odds ratio increases to more than 10. Before 3 years of age, parental obesity is a stronger predictor of obesity in adulthood than the child's weight status.[54] Such observations have important implications for recognition of risk and routine anticipatory guidance that is directed toward healthy eating and activity patterns in families.

There are critical periods of development for excessive weight gain. Extent and duration of breastfeeding have been found to be inversely associated with risk of obesity in later childhood, possibly mediated by physiologic factors in human milk as well as by the feeding and parenting patterns associated with nursing.[55-58] Investigations of dietary factors in infancy, such as high protein intake or the timing of introduction of complementary foods, have not consistently revealed effects on childhood obesity. It has been known for decades that adolescence is another critical period for development of obesity.[59] The normal tendency during early puberty for insulin resistance may be a natural cofactor for excessive weight gain as well as various comorbidities of obesity.[60] Early menarche is clearly associated with degree of overweight, with a twofold increase in rate of early menarche associated with BMI greater than the 85th percentile.[61] The risk of obesity persisting into adulthood is higher among obese adolescents than among younger children.[54] The roles of leptin, adiponectin, ghrelin, fat mass, and puberty on development of adolescent obesity are being actively investigated. Data suggest that adolescents who engage in highrisk behaviors, such as smoking, ethanol use, and early sexual experimentation also may be at greater risk of poor dietary and exercise habits.[62]

Environmental risk factors for overweight and obesity, including family and parental dynamics, are numerous and complicated. Although clinical interventions cannot change these factors directly, they can influence parents' adaptations to them, and the physician can advocate for change at the community level. Food insecurity may contribute to the inverse relation of obesity prevalence with socioeconomic status, but the relationship is a complex one.[63] Other barriers low-income families may face are lack of safe places for physical activity and lack of consistent access to healthful food choices, particularly fruits and vegetables. Low cognitive stimulation in the home, low socioeconomic status, and maternal obesity all predict development of obesity.[64] In research settings, there is accumulating evidence for the detrimental effects of overcontrolling parental behavior on children's ability to self-regulate energy intake. For example, maternal-child feeding practices, maternal perception of daughter's risk of overweight,[65] maternal restraint, verbal prompting to eat at mealtime, attentiveness to noneating behavior, and close parental monitoring[66] all may promote undesired consequences for children's eating behaviors. Parental food choices influence child food preferences,[67] and degree of parental adiposity is a marker for children's fat preferences.[68] Children and adolescents of lower socioeconomic status have been reported to be less likely to eat fruits and vegetables and to have a higher intake of total and saturated fat.[69–71] Absence of family meals is associated with lower fruit and vegetable consumption as well as consumption of more fried food and carbonated beverages. Although our understanding of the development of eating behaviors is improving, there are not yet good trials to demonstrate effective translation of this knowledge base into clinical practices to prevent obesity. At a minimum, however, pediatricians need to proactively discuss and promote healthy eating behaviors for children at an early age and empower parents to promote children's ability to self-regulate energy intake while providing appropriate structure and boundaries around eating.

Widespread and profound societal changes during the last several decades have affected child rearing, which in turn has affected childhood patterns of physical activity as well as diet. National survey data indicate that children are currently less active than they have been in previous surveys. Leisure activity is increasingly sedentary, with wide availability of entertainment such as television, videos, and computer games. In addition, with increasing urbanization, there has been a decrease in frequency and duration of physical activities of daily living for children, such as walking to school and doing household chores. Changes in availability and requirements of school physical education programs have also generally decreased children's routine physical activity, with the possible exception of children specifically enrolled in athletic programs. All these factors play a potential part in the epidemic of overweight.[72]

National survey data indicate that 20% of US children 8 to 16 years of age reported 2 or fewer bouts of vigorous physical activity per week, and more than 25% watched at least 4 hours of television per day.[73] Children who watched 4 or more hours of television per day had significantly greater BMI, compared with those watching fewer than 2 hours per day.[73] Furthermore, having a television in the bedroom has been reported to be a strong predictor of being overweight, even in preschool-aged children.[74] Some cross-sectional data have found significant correlation between obesity prevalence and television viewing,[75–77] but others have not.[78,79] The results of a randomized trial to decrease television viewing for school-aged children has provided the strongest evidence to support the role of limiting television in prevention of obesity. In this study, decreasing "media use" without specifically promoting more active behaviors in the intervention group resulted in a significantly lower increase in BMI at the 1-year follow-up, compared with the control group.[80] Additional support for the importance of decreasing television viewing comes from controlled investigations that demonstrated that obese children who were reinforced for decreasing sedentary activity (and following an energy-restricted diet) had significantly

greater weight loss than those who were reinforced for increasing physical activity.[42] These findings have important implications for anticipatory guidance and provide additional support for recommendations to limit television exposure for young children.[2]

EARLY RECOGNITION

Routine assessments of eating and activity patterns in children and recognition of excessive weight gain relative to linear growth are essential throughout childhood. At any age, an excessive rate of weight gain relative to linear growth should be recognized, and underlying predisposing factors should be addressed with parents and other caregivers. The Centers for Disease Control and Prevention percentile grids for BMI are important tools for anticipatory guidance and discussion of longitudinal tracking of a child's BMI. Significant changes on growth patterns (eg, upward crossing of weight for age or BMI percentiles) can be recognized and addressed before children are severely overweight.[81] An increase in BMI percentiles should be discussed with parents, some of whom may be overly concerned and some of whom may not recognize or accept potential risk.[82]

Although data are extremely limited, it is likely that anticipatory guidance or treatment intervention before obesity has become severe will be more successful. Discussions to raise parental awareness should be conducted in a nonjudgmental, blame-free manner so that unintended negative impact on the child's self-concept is avoided.[24] Data from adult patient surveys indicate that those who were asked by their physician about diet were more likely to report positive changes.[83] Similarly, the efficacy of physicians discussing physical activity,[84] breastfeeding,[85] and smoking prevention[86] is well documented. Thus, pediatricians are strongly encouraged to incorporate assessment and anticipatory guidance about diet, weight, and physical activity into routine clinical practice, being careful to discuss habits rather than focusing on habitus to avoid stigmatizing the child, adolescent, or family.

ADVOCACY

Abundant opportunities exist for pediatricians to take a leadership role in this critical area of child health, including action in the following areas: opportunities for physical activity, the food supply, research, and third-party reimbursement. Change is desperately needed in opportunities for physical activity in child care centers, schools, after-school programs, and other community settings. As leaders in their communities, pediatricians can be effective advocates for health- and fitness-promoting programs and policies. Foods that are nutrient rich and palatable yet low in excess energy from added sugars and fat need to be readily available to parents, school and child care food services, and others responsible for feeding children. Potential affordable sources include community gardens and farmers' market projects. Advertising and promotion of energy-dense, nutrient-poor food products to children may need to be regulated or curtailed. The increase in carbonated beverage intake has been linked to obesity[87]; therefore, the sale of such beverages should not be promoted at school. Pediatricians are encouraged to work with school administrators and others in the community on ways to decrease the availability of foods and beverages with little nutritional value and to decrease the dependence on vending machines, snack bars, and school stores for school revenue. Regarding physical activity, advocacy is sorely needed for physical education programs that emphasize and model learning of daily activities for personal fitness (as opposed to physical education limited to a few team sports).

New initiatives for pilot projects to test prevention strategies have been funded by the National Institutes of Health and other organizations, but a long-term commitment of substantial funds from many sources and to many disciplines will be needed to attack this serious, widespread, and potentially intractable problem. Support for development and testing of primary prevention strategies for the primary care setting will be critical. Likewise, investment of substantial resources will be required for development of effective treatment approaches for normalizing or improving body weight and fitness and for determining long-term effects of weight loss on comorbidities of childhood obesity. Collaboration and coalitions with nutrition, behavioral health, physical therapy, and exercise physiology professionals will be needed. Working with communities and schools to develop needed counseling services, physical activity opportunities, and strategies to reinforce the gains made in clinical management is also important.

Pediatric referral centers will need to develop specialized programs for treatment of complex and difficult cases, and for research into etiology and new methods of prevention and treatment. Efforts are needed to ensure adequate health care coverage for preventive and treatment services. Even when serious comorbidities are documented, insurance reimbursement is limited.[88] Lack of reimbursement is a disincentive for physicians to develop prevention and treatment programs and presents a significant barrier to families seeking professional care.

SUMMARY/CONCLUSIONS

1. Prevalence of overweight and its significant comorbidities in pediatric populations has rapidly increased and reached epidemic proportions.
2. Prevention of overweight is critical, because long-term outcome data for successful treatment approaches are limited.
3. Genetic, environmental, or combinations of risk factors predisposing children to obesity can and should be identified.
4. Early recognition of excessive weight gain relative to linear growth should become routine in pediatric ambulatory care settings. BMI (kg/m^2 [see http://www.cdc.gov/growthcharts]) should be calculated and plotted periodically.
5. Families should be educated and empowered through anticipatory guidance to recognize the impact they have on their children's development

of lifelong habits of physical activity and nutritious eating.
6. Dietary practices should be fostered that encourage moderation rather than overconsumption, emphasizing healthful choices rather than restrictive eating patterns.
7. Regular physical activity should be consciously promoted, prioritized, and protected within families, schools, and communities.
8. Optimal approaches to prevention need to combine dietary and physical activity interventions.
9. Advocacy is needed in the areas of physical activity and food policy for children; research into pathophysiology, risk factors, and early recognition and management of overweight and obesity; and improved insurance coverage and third-party reimbursement for obesity care.

RECOMMENDATIONS

1. Health supervision
   a. Identify and track patients at risk by virtue of family history, birth weight, or socioeconomic, ethnic, cultural, or environmental factors.
   b. Calculate and plot BMI once a year in all children and adolescents.
   c. Use change in BMI to identify rate of excessive weight gain relative to linear growth.
   d. Encourage, support, and protect breastfeeding.
   e. Encourage parents and caregivers to promote healthy eating patterns by offering nutritious snacks, such as vegetables and fruits, low-fat dairy foods, and whole grains; encouraging children's autonomy in self-regulation of food intake and setting appropriate limits on choices; and modeling healthy food choices.
   f. Routinely promote physical activity, including unstructured play at home, in school, in child care settings, and throughout the community.
   g. Recommend limitation of television and video time to a maximum of 2 hours per day.
   h. Recognize and monitor changes in obesity-associated risk factors for adult chronic disease, such as hypertension, dyslipidemia, hyperinsulinemia, impaired glucose tolerance, and symptoms of obstructive sleep apnea syndrome.
2. Advocacy
   a. Help parents, teachers, coaches, and others who influence youth to discuss health habits, not body habitus, as part of their efforts to control overweight and obesity.
   b. Enlist policy makers from local, state, and national organizations and schools to support a healthful lifestyle for all children, including proper diet and adequate opportunity for regular physical activity.
   c. Encourage organizations that are responsible for health care and health care financing to provide coverage for effective obesity prevention and treatment strategies.
   d. Encourage public and private sources to direct funding toward research into effective strategies to prevent overweight and obesity and to maximize limited family and community re-

• •

sources to achieve healthful outcomes for youth.
  e. Support and advocate for social marketing intended to promote healthful food choices and increased physical activity.

COMMITTEE ON NUTRITION, 2002–2003
*Nancy F. Krebs, MD, Chairperson
Robert D. Baker, Jr, MD, PhD
Frank R. Greer, MD
Melvin B. Heyman, MD
Tom Jaksic, MD, PhD
Fima Lifshitz, MD

*Marc S. Jacobson, MD
  Past Committee Member

LIAISONS
Donna Blum-Kemelor, MS, RD
  US Department of Agriculture
Margaret P. Boland, MD
  Canadian Paediatric Society
William Dietz, MD, PhD
  Centers for Disease Control and Prevention
Van S. Hubbard, MD, PhD
  National Institute of Diabetes and Digestive and Kidney Diseases
Elizabeth Yetley, PhD
  US Food and Drug Administration

STAFF
Pamela Kanda, MPH

*Lead authors

REFERENCES

1. American Academy of Pediatrics, Committee on Sports Medicine and Fitness. Promotion of healthy weight-control practices in young athletes. *Pediatrics*. 1996;97:752–753
2. American Academy of Pediatrics, Committee on Public Education. Children, adolescents, and television. *Pediatrics*. 2001;107:423–426
3. American Dietetic Association. Position of the American Dietetic Association. Dietary guidance for healthy children aged 2 to 11 years. *J Am Diet Assoc*. 1999;99:93–101
4. Gidding SS, Leibel RL, Daniels S, Rosenbaum M, Van Horn L, Marx GR. Understanding obesity in youth. A statement for healthcare professionals from the Committee on Atherosclerosis and Hypertension in the Young of the Committee on Cardiovascular Disease in the Young and Nutrition Committee, American Heart Association. *Circulation*. 1996;94: 3383–3387
5. American Medical Association, Council on Scientific Affairs. *Obesity as a Major Public Health Problem*. Chicago, IL: American Medical Association; 1999. Available at: http://www.ama-assn.org/meetings/public/annual99/reports/csa/rtf/csa6.rtf. Accessed September 4, 2002
6. Barlow SE, Dietz WH. Obesity evaluation and treatment: expert committee recommendations. The Maternal and Child Health Bureau, Health Resources and Services Administration and the Department of Health and Human Services. *Pediatrics*. 1998;102(3). Available at: http://www.pediatrics.org/cgi/content/full/102/3/e29
7. Pietrobelli A, Faith MS, Allison DB, Gallagher D, Chiumello G, Heymsfield SB. Body mass index as a measure of adiposity among children and adolescents: a validation study. *J Pediatr*. 1998;132:204–210
8. Kuczmarski RJ, Ogden CL, Grummer-Strawn LM, et al. CDC growth charts: United States. *Adv Data*. 2000 Jun 8;(314):1–27
9. Himes JH, Dietz WH. Guidelines for overweight in adolescent preventive services: recommendations from an expert committee. *Am J Clin Nutr*. 1994;59:307–316
10. US Dept Health and Human Services. *The Surgeon General's Call to Action to Prevent and Decrease Overweight and Obesity*. Rockville, MD: US Department of Health and Human Services, Public Health Service, Office of the Surgeon General; 2001
11. Ogden CL, Flegal KM, Carroll MD, Johnson CL. Prevalence and trends in overweight among US children and adolescents, 1999–2000. *JAMA*. 2002;288:1728–1732

12. Mei Z, Scanlon KS, Grummer-Strawn LM, Freedman DS, Yip R, Trowbridge FL. Increasing prevalence of overweight among US low-income preschool children: The Centers for Disease Control and Prevention Pediatric Nutrition Surveillance, 1983 to 1995. *Pediatrics*. 1998;101(1). Available at: http://www.pediatrics.org/cgi/content/full/101/1/e12
13. Ogden CL, Troiano RP, Breifel RR, Kuczmarski RJ, Flegal KM, Johnson CL. Prevalence of overweight among preschool children in the United States, 1971 through 1994. *Pediatrics*. 1997;99(4). Available at: http://www.pediatrics.org/cgi/content/full/99/4/e1
14. Gidding SS, Bao W, Srinivasan SR, Berenson GW. Effects of secular trends in obesity on coronary risk factors in children: the Bogalusa Heart Study. *J Pediatr*. 1995;127:868–874
15. Freedman DS, Dietz WH, Srinivasan SR, Berenson GS. The relation of overweight to cardiovascular risk factors among children and adolescents: the Bogalusa heart study. *Pediatrics*. 1999;103:1175–1182
16. Must A, Jacques PF, Dallal GE, Bajema CJ, Dietz WH. Long-term morbidity and mortality of overweight adolescents. A follow-up of the Harvard Growth Study of 1922 to 1935. *N Engl J Med*. 1992;327: 1350–1355
17. Clarke WR, Woolson RF, Lauer RM. Changes in ponderosity and blood pressure in childhood: the Muscatine Study. *Am J Epidemiol*. 1986;124: 195–206
18. Johnson AL, Cornoni JC, Cassel JC, Tyroler HA, Heyden S, Hames CG. Influence of race, sex and weight on blood pressure behavior in young adults. *Am J Cardiol*. 1975;35:523–530
19. Morrison JA, Laskerzewski PM, Rauh JL, et al. Lipids, lipoproteins, and sexual maturation during adolescence: the Princeton Maturation Study. *Metabolism*. 1979;28:641–649
20. Shinha R, Fisch G, Teague B, et al. Prevalence of impaired glucose tolerance among children and adolescents with marked obesity. *N Engl J Med*. 2002;346:802–810
21. Pinhas-Hamiel O, Dolan LM, Daniels SR, Standiford D, Khoury PR, Zeitler P. Increased incidence of non-insulin-dependent diabetes mellitus among adolescents. *J Pediatr*. 1996;128:608–615
22. Richards GE, Cavallo A, Meyer WJ III, et al. Obesity, acanthosis nigricans, insulin resistance, and hyperandrogenemia: pediatric perspective and natural history. *J Pediatr*. 1985;107:893–897
23. Strauss RS. Childhood obesity and self-esteem. *Pediatrics*. 2000;105(1). Available at: http://www.pediatrics.org/cgi/content/full/105/1/e15
24. Davison KK, Birch LL. Weight status, parent reaction, and self-concept in five-year-old girls. *Pediatrics*. 2001;107:46–53
25. Mitchell BD, Kammerer CM, Reinhart LJ, Stern MP. NIDDM in Mexican-American families. Heterogeneity by age of onset. *Diabetes Care*. 1994;17:567–573
26. Pugliese MT, Lifshitz F, Grad G, Fort P, Marks-Katz M. Fear of obesity. A cause of short stature and delayed puberty. *N Engl J Med*. 1983;309: 513–518
27. American Academy of Pediatrics, Section on Pediatric Pulmonology, Subcommittee on Obstructive Sleep Apnea Syndrome. Clinical practice guideline: diagnosis and management of childhood obstructive sleep apnea syndrome. *Pediatrics*. 2002;109:704–712
28. Rodriguez MA, Winkleby MA, Ahn D, Sundquist J, Kraemer HC. Identification of population subgroups of children and adolescents with high asthma prevalence: findings from the Third National Health and Nutrition Examination Survey. *Arch Pediatr Adolesc Med*. 2002;156: 269–275
29. Riley DJ, Santiago TV, Edelman NH. Complications of obesity-hypoventilation syndrome in childhood. *Am J Dis Child*. 1976;130: 671–674
30. Boxer GH, Bauer AM, Miller BD. Obesity-hypoventilation in childhood. *J Am Acad Child Adolesc Psychiatry*. 1988;27:552–558
31. Mallory GB Jr, Fiser DH, Jackson R. Sleep-associated breathing disorders in obese children and adolescents. *J Pediatr*. 1989;115:892–897
32. Silvestri JM, Weese-Mayer DE, Bass MT, Kenny AS, Hauptman SA, Pearsall SM. Polysomnography in obese children with a history of sleep-associated breathing disorders. *Pediatr Pulmonol*. 1993;16:124–129
33. Dietz WH, Gross WL, Kirkpatrick JA Jr. Blount disease (tibia vara): another skeletal disorder associated with childhood obesity. *J Pediatr*. 1982;101:735–737
34. Loder RT, Aronson DD, Greenfield ML. The epidemiology of bilateral slipped capital femoral epiphysis. A study of children in Michigan. *J Bone Joint Surg*. 1993;75:1141–1147
35. Rashid M, Roberts EA. Nonalcoholic steatohepatitis in children. *J Pediatr Gastroenterol Nutr*. 2000;30:48–53
36. Guo SS, Chumlea WC. Tracking of body mass index in children in relation to overweight into adulthood. *Am J Clin Nutr*. 1999;70(suppl): 145S–148S
37. Wisemandle W, Maynard LM, Guo SS, Siervogel RM. Childhood

weight, stature, and body mass index among never overweight, early-onset overweight and late-onset overweight groups. *Pediatrics*. 2000; 106(1). Available at: http://www.pediatrics.org/cgi/content/full/106/1/e14

38. Wolf AM, Colditz GA. Current estimates of the economic cost of obesity in the United States. *Obes Res*. 1998;6:97–106
39. Becque MD, Katch VL, Rocchini AP, Marks CR, Moorehead C. Coronary risk incidence of obese adolescents: reduction by exercise plus diet intervention. *Pediatrics*. 1988;81:605–612
40. Sothern MS, von Almen TK, Schumacher H, et al. An effective multidisciplinary approach to weight reduction in youth. *Ann N Y Acad Sci*. 1993;699:292–294
41. Jacobson MS, Copperman N, Haas T, Shenker IR. Adolescent obesity and cardiovascular risk: a rational approach to management. *Ann N Y Acad Sci*. 1993;699:220–229
42. Epstein LH, Myers MD, Raynor HA, Saelens BE. Treatment of pediatric obesity. *Pediatrics*. 1998;101(suppl):554–570
43. Harrell JS, Gansky SA, McMurray RG, Bangdiwala SI, Frauman AC, Bradley CB. School-based interventions improve heart health in children with multiple cardiovascular disease risk factors. *Pediatrics*. 1998; 102:371–380
44. Willi SM, Oexamm MJ, Wright NM, Collup NA, Key LL Jr. The effects of a high protein, low-fat, ketogenic diet on adolescents with morbid obesity: body composition, blood chemistries, and sleep abnormalities. *Pediatrics*. 1998;101:61–67
45. Epstein LH, Valoski A, Wing RR, McCurley J. Ten-year follow-up of behavioral family-based treatment for obese children. *JAMA*. 1990;264: 2519–2523
46. Wadden TA, Foster GD, Letizia KA. One-year behavioral treatment of obesity: comparison of moderate and severe caloric restriction and the effects of weight maintenance therapy. *J Consult Clin Psychol*. 1994;62: 165–171
47. Rosenbaum M, Leibel RL, Hirsch J. Obesity. *N Engl J Med*. 1997;337: 396–407
48. Rosenbaum M, Leibel RL. The physiology of body weight regulation: relevance to the etiology of obesity in children. *Pediatrics*. 1998; 101(suppl):525–539
49. Ritzen EM, Lindgren AC, Hagenas L, Marcus C, Muller J, Blichfeldt S. Growth hormone treatment of patients with Prader-Willi syndrome. Swedish Growth Hormone Advisory Group. *J Pediatr Endocrinol Metab*. 1999 Apr;12(suppl 1):345–349
50. Whitman BY, Myers S, Carrel A, Allen D. The behavioral impact of growth hormone treatment for children and adolescents with Prader-Willi syndrome: a 2-year, controlled study. *Pediatrics*. 2002;109(2). Available at: http://www.pediatrics.org/cgi/content/full/109/2/e35
51. Carrel AL, Myers SE, Whitman BY, Allen DB. Sustained benefits of growth hormone on body composition, fat utilization, physical strength and agility, and growth in Prader-Willi syndrome are dose-dependent. *J Pediatr Endocrinol Metab*. 2002;15:1549–1554
52. Stunkard AJ, Harris JR, Pedersen NL, McClearn GE. The body mass index of twins who have been reared apart. *N Engl J Med*. 1990;322: 1483–1487
53. Bouchard C, Tremblay A, Despres JP, et al. The response to long-term overfeeding in identical twins. *N Engl J Med*. 1990;322:1477–1482
54. Whitaker RC, Wright JA, Pepe MS, Seidel KD, Dietz WH. Predicting obesity in young adulthood from childhood and parental obesity. *N Engl J Med*. 1997;337:869–873
55. Agras SW, Kraemer HC, Berkowitz RI, Hammer LD. Influence of early feeding style on adiposity at 6 years of age. *J Pediatr*. 1990;116:805–809
56. von Kries R, Koletzko B, Sauerwald T, et al. Breast feeding and obesity: cross sectional study. *BMJ*. 1999;319:147–150
57. Gilman MW, Rifas-Shiman SL, Camargo CA Jr, et al. Risk of overweight among adolescents who were breastfed as infants. *JAMA*. 2001;285: 2461–2467
58. Hediger ML, Overpeck MD, Kuczmarski RJ, Ruan WJ. Association between infant breastfeeding and overweight in young children. *JAMA*. 2001;285:2453–2460
59. Heald FP. Natural history and physiological basis of adolescent obesity. *Fed Proc*. 1966;25:1–3
60. Travers SH, Jeffers BW, Bloch CA, Hill JO, Eckel RH. Gender and Tanner stage differences in body composition and insulin sensitivity in early pubertal children. *J Clin Endocrinol Metab*. 1995;80:172–178
61. Adair LS, Gordon-Larsen P. Maturational timing and overweight prevalence in US adolescents. *Am J Public Health*. 2001;91:642–644
62. Irwin CE Jr, Igra V, Eyre S, Millstein S. Risk-taking behavior in adolescents: the paradigm. *Ann N Y Acad Sci*. 1997;817:1–35
63. Alaimo K, Olson CM, Frongillo EA Jr. Low family income and food

insufficiency in relation to overweight in US children: is there a paradox? *Arch Pediatr Adolesc Med*. 2001;155:1161–1167
64. Strauss RS, Knight J. Influence of the home environment on the development of obesity in children. *Pediatrics*. 1999;103(6). Available at: http://www.pediatrics.org/cgi/content/full/103/6/e85
65. Birch LL, Fisher JO. Mothers' child-feeding practices influence daughters' eating and weight. *Am J Clin Nutr*. 2000;71:1054–1061
66. Klesges RC, Stein RJ, Eck LH, Isbell TR, Klesges LM. Parental influence on food selection in young children and its relationships to childhood obesity. *Am J Clin Nutr*. 1991;53:859–864
67. Ray JW, Klesges RC. Influences on the eating behavior of children. *Ann N Y Acad Sci*. 1993;699:57–69
68. Fisher JO, Birch LL. Fat preferences and fat consumption of 3- to 5-year-old children are related to parental adiposity. *J Am Diet Assoc*. 1995;95:759–764
69. Neumark-Sztainer D, Story M, Resnick MD, Blum RW. Correlates of inadequate fruit and vegetable consumption among adolescents. *Prev Med*. 1996;25:497–505
70. Krebs-Smith SM, Cook A, Subar AF, Cleveland L, Friday J, Kahle LL. Fruit and vegetable intakes of children and adolescents in the United States. *Arch Pediatr Adolesc Med*. 1996;150:81–86
71. Kennedy E, Powell R. Changing eating patterns of American children: a view from 1996. *J Am Coll Nutr*. 1997;16:524–529
72. Berkey CS, Rockett HR, Field AE, et al. Activity dietary intake, and weight changes in a longitudinal study of preadolescent and adolescent boys and girls. *Pediatrics*. 2000;105(4). Available at: http://www.pediatrics.org/cgi/content/full/105/4/e56
73. Anderson RE, Crespo CJ, Bartlett SJ, Cheskin LJ, Pratt M. Relationship of physical activity and television watching with body weight and level of fatness among children: results from the Third National Health and Nutrition Examination Survey. *JAMA*. 1998;279:938–942
74. Dennison BA, Erb TA, Jenkins PL. Television viewing and television in bedroom associated with overweight risk among low-income preschool children. *Pediatrics*. 2002;109:1028–1035
75. Pate RR, Ross JG. The National Children and Youth Fitness Study II: factors associated with health-related fitness. *J Physical Educ Recreation Dance*. 1987;58:93–96
76. Dietz WH Jr, Gortmaker SL. Do we fatten our children at the TV set? Obesity and television viewing in children and adolescents. *Pediatrics*. 1985;75:807–812
77. Gortmaker SL, Must A, Sobol AM, Peterson K, Colditz GA, Dietz WH. Television viewing as a cause of increasing obesity among children in the United States, 1986–1990. *Arch Pediatr Adolesc Med*. 1996;150:356–362
78. Tucker LA. The relationship of television viewing to physical fitness and obesity. *Adolescence*. 1986;21:797–806
79. Robinson TN, Hammer LD, Killen JD, et al. Does television viewing increase obesity and reduce physical activity? Cross-sectional and longitudinal analyses among adolescent girls. *Pediatrics*. 1993;91:273–280
80. Robinson T. Reducing children's television viewing to prevent obesity: a randomized controlled trial. *JAMA*. 1999;282:1561–1567
81. Miller LA, Grunwald G, Johnson SL, Krebs NF. Disease severity at time of referral for pediatric failure to thrive and obesity: time for a paradigm shift? *J Pediatr*. 2002;141:121–124
82. Jain A, Sherman SN, Chamberlin DL, Carter Y, Powers SW, Whitaker RC. Why don't low-income mothers worry about their preschoolers being overweight? *Pediatrics*. 2001;107:1138–1146
83. Nawaz H, Adams ML, Katz DL. Physician-patient interactions regarding diet, exercise, and smoking. *Prev Med*. 2000;31:652–657
84. Calfas KJ, Long BJ, Sallis JF, Wooten WJ, Pratt M, Patrick K. A controlled trial of physician counseling to promote the adoption of physical activity. *Prev Med*. 1996;25:225–233
85. Lu MC, Lange L, Slusser W, Hamilton J, Halfon N. Provider encouragement of breast-feeding: evidence from a national survey. *Obstet Gynecol*. 2001;97:290–295
86. Epps RP, Manley MW. The clinician's role in preventing smoking initiation. *Med Clin North Am*. 1992;76:439–449
87. Ludwig DS, Peterson KE, Gortmaker SL. Relation between consumption of sugar-sweetened drinks and childhood obesity: a prospective, observational analysis. *Lancet*. 2001;357:505–508
88. Tershakovec AM, Watson MH, Wenner WJ Jr, Marx AL. Insurance reimbursement for the treatment of obesity in children. *J Pediatr*. 1999; 134:573–578

ADDITIONAL RESOURCES

American Academy of Pediatrics, Committee on Nutrition. Cholesterol in childhood. *Pediatrics*. 1998;101:141–147
American Academy of Pediatrics, Committee on Sports Medicine and Fit-

ness and Committee on School Health. Physical fitness and activity in schools. *Pediatrics.* 2000;105:1156–1157

Centers for Disease Control and Prevention. *2000 CDC Growth Charts: United States.* Atlanta, GA: Centers for Disease Control and Prevention; 2000. Available at: http://www.cdc.gov/growthcharts

Jacobson MS, Rees J, Golden NH, Irwin C. Adolescent nutritional disorders. *Ann N Y Acad Sci.* 1997;817

National Association for Sports and Physical Activity Web site. Available at: http://www.aahperd.org

National Institutes of Health, National Heart, Lung, and Blood Institute. *The Practical Guide: Identification, Evaluation, and Treatment of Overweight and Obesity in Adults.* Rockville, MD: National Heart, Lung, and Blood Institute; 2000. NIH Publ. No. 00-4084

Story M, Holt K, Sofka D, eds. *Bright Futures in Practice: Nutrition.* Arlington, VA: National Center for Education in Maternal and Child Health; 2000

US Department of Health and Human Services, Office of Public Health and Science, Office of Disease Prevention and Health Promotion, Public Health Foundation. *Healthy People 2010 Toolkit: A Field Guide to Health Planning.* Washington, DC: Public Health Foundation; 2002. Available at: http://www.health.gov/healthypeople/state/toolkit or by calling toll-free 877/252–1200 (Item RM-005)

Weight-control Information Network Web site. Available at: http://www.niddk.nih.gov/health/nutrit/win.htm

All policy statements from the American Academy of Pediatrics automatically expire 5 years after publication unless reaffirmed, revised, or retired at or before that time.

AMERICAN ACADEMY OF PEDIATRICS

POLICY STATEMENT

Organizational Principles to Guide and Define the Child Health Care System and/or Improve the Health of All Children

Committee on School Health

Soft Drinks in Schools

ABSTRACT. This statement is intended to inform pediatricians and other health care professionals, parents, superintendents, and school board members about nutritional concerns regarding soft drink consumption in schools. Potential health problems associated with high intake of sweetened drinks are 1) overweight or obesity attributable to additional calories in the diet; 2) displacement of milk consumption, resulting in calcium deficiency with an attendant risk of osteoporosis and fractures; and 3) dental caries and potential enamel erosion. Contracts with school districts for exclusive soft drink rights encourage consumption directly and indirectly. School officials and parents need to become well informed about the health implications of vended drinks in school before making a decision about student access to them. A clearly defined, district-wide policy that restricts the sale of soft drinks will safeguard against health problems as a result of overconsumption.

BACKGROUND AND INFORMATION

Overweight

Overweight is now the most common medical condition of childhood, with the prevalence having doubled over the past 20 years. Nearly 1 of every 3 children is at risk of overweight (defined as body mass index [BMI] between the 85th and 95th percentiles for age and sex), and 1 of every 6 is overweight (defined as BMI at or above the 95th percentile).[1] Complications of the obesity epidemic include high cholesterol, high blood pressure, type 2 diabetes mellitus, coronary plaque formation, and serious psychosocial implications.[2-6] Annually, obesity-related diseases in adults and children account for more than 300 000 deaths and more than $100 billion per year in treatment costs.[7-9]

Soft Drinks and Fruit Drinks

In the United States, children's daily food selections are excessively high in discretionary, or added, fat and sugar.[10-15] This category of fats and sugars accounts for 40% of children's daily energy intake.[10] Soft drink consumers have a higher daily energy intake than nonconsumers at all ages.[16] Sweetened drinks (fruitades, fruit drinks, soft drinks, etc) constitute the primary source of added sugar in the daily diet of children.[17] High-fructose corn syrup, the principle nutrient in sweetened drinks, is not a problem

food when consumed in smaller amounts, but each 12-oz serving of a carbonated, sweetened soft drink contains the equivalent of 10 teaspoons of sugar and 150 kcal. Soft drink consumption increased by 300% in 20 years,[12] and serving sizes have increased from 6.5 oz in the 1950s to 12 oz in the 1960s and 20 oz by the late 1990s. Between 56% and 85% of children in school consume at least 1 soft drink daily, with the highest amounts ingested by adolescent males. Of this group, 20% consume 4 or more servings daily.[16]

Each 12-oz sugared soft drink consumed daily has been associated with a 0.18-point increase in a child's BMI and a 60% increase in risk of obesity, associations not found with "diet" (sugar-free) soft drinks.[18] Sugar-free soft drinks constitute only 14% of the adolescent soft drink market.[19] Sweetened drinks are associated with obesity, probably because overconsumption is a particular problem when energy is ingested in liquid form[20] and because these drinks represent energy added to, not displacing, other dietary intake.[21-23] In addition to the caloric load, soft drinks pose a risk of dental caries because of their high sugar content and enamel erosion because of their acidity.[24]

Calcium

Milk consumption decreases as soft drinks become a favorite choice for children, a transition that occurs between the third and eighth grades.[12,15] Milk is the principle source of calcium in the typical American diet.[11] Dairy products contain substantial amounts of several nutrients, including 72% of calcium, 32% of phosphorus, 26% of riboflavin, 22% of vitamin B_{12}, 19% of protein, and 15% of vitamin A in the US food supply.[25] The percent daily value for milk is considered either "good" or "excellent" for 9 essential nutrients depending on age and gender. Intake of protein and micronutrients is decreased in diets low in dairy products.[19,26] The resulting diminished calcium intake jeopardizes the accrual of maximal peak bone mass at a critical time in life, adolescence.[27] Nearly 100% of the calcium in the body resides in bone.[27] Nearly 40% of peak bone mass is accumulated during adolescence. Studies suggest that a 5% to 10% deficit in peak bone mass may result in a 50% greater lifetime prevalence of hip fracture,[28] a problem certain to worsen if steps are not taken to improve calcium intake among adolescents.[29]

STATEMENT OF PROBLEM

Soft drinks and fruit drinks are sold in vending machines, in school stores, at school sporting events, and at school fund drives. "Exclusive pouring rights" contracts, in which the school agrees to promote one brand exclusively in exchange for money, are being signed in an increasing number of school districts across the country,[30] often with bonus incentives tied to sales.[31] Although they are a new phenomenon, such contracts already have provided schools with more than $200 million in unrestricted revenue.

Some superintendents, school board members, and principals claim that the financial gain from soft drink contracts is an unquestioned "win" for students, schools, communities, and taxpayers.[31,32] Parents and school authorities generally are uninformed about the potential risk to the health of their children that may be associated with the unrestricted consumption of soft drinks. The decision regarding which foods will be sold in schools more often is made by school district business officers alone rather than with input from local health care professionals.

Subsidized school lunch programs are associated with a high intake of dietary protein, complex carbohydrates, dairy products, fruits, and vegetables.[16] The US Department of Agriculture, which oversees the National School Lunch Program, is concerned that foods with high sugar content (especially foods of minimal nutritional value, such as soft drinks) are displacing nutrients within the school lunch program, and there is evidence to support this.[26]

There are precedents for using optimal nutrition standards to create a model district-wide school nutrition policy,[33] but this is not yet a routine practice in most states. The discussion engendered by the creation of such a policy would be an important first step in establishing an ideal nutritional environment for students.

RECOMMENDATIONS

1. Pediatricians should work to eliminate sweetened drinks in schools. This entails educating school authorities, patients, and patients' parents about the health ramifications of soft drink consumption. Offerings such as real fruit and vegetable juices, water, and low-fat white or flavored milk provide students at all grade levels with healthful alternatives. Pediatricians should emphasize the notion that every school in every district shares a responsibility for the nutritional health of its student body.

2. Pediatricians should advocate for the creation of a school nutrition advisory council comprising parents, community and school officials, food service representatives, physicians, school nurses, dietitians, dentists, and other health care professionals. This group could be one component of a school district's health advisory council. Pediatricians should ensure that the health and nutritional interests of students form the foundation of nutritional policies in schools.

3. School districts should invite public discussion before making any decision to create a vended food or drink contract.

4. If a school district already has a soft drink contract in place, it should be tempered such that it does not promote overconsumption by students.
   - Soft drinks should not be sold as part of or in competition with the school lunch program, as stated in regulations of the US Department of Agriculture.[34]
   - Vending machines should not be placed within the cafeteria space where lunch is sold. Their location in the school should be chosen by the school district, not the vending company.
   - Vending machines with foods of minimal nutritional value, including soft drinks, should be turned off during lunch hours and ideally during school hours.
   - Vended soft drinks and fruit-flavored drinks should be eliminated in all elementary schools.
   - Incentives based on the amount of soft drinks sold per student should not be included as part of exclusive contracts.
   - Within the contract, the number of machines vending sweetened drinks should be limited. Schools should insist that the alternative beverages listed in recommendation 1 be provided in preference over sweetened drinks in school vending machines.
   - Schools should preferentially vend drinks that are sugar-free or low in sugar to lessen the risk of overweight.

5. Consumption or advertising of sweetened soft drinks within the classroom should be eliminated.

COMMITTEE ON SCHOOL HEALTH, 2002–2003
Howard L. Taras, MD, Chairperson
Barbara L. Frankowski, MD, MPH
Jane W. McGrath, MD
Cynthia J. Mears, DO
*Robert D. Murray, MD
Thomas L. Young, MD

LIAISONS
Janis Hootman, RN, PhD
  National Association of School Nurses
Janet Long, MEd
  American School Health Association
Jerald L. Newberry, MEd
  National Education Association, Health Information
Mary Vernon-Smiley, MD, MPH
  Centers for Disease Control and Prevention

STAFF
Su Li, MPA

*Lead author

REFERENCES

1. American Academy of Pediatrics, Committee on Nutrition. Prevention of pediatric overweight and obesity. *Pediatrics.* 2003;112:424–430
2. Freedman DS, Dietz WH, Srinivasan SR, Berenson GS. The relation of overweight to cardiovascular risk factors among children and adolescents: the Bogalusa Heart Study. *Pediatrics.* 1999;103:1175–1182
3. Pinhas-Hamiel O, Dolan LM, Daniels SR, Standiford D, Khoury PR, Zeitler P. Increased incidence of non-insulin-dependent diabetes mellitus among adolescents. *J Pediatr.* 1996;128:608–615
4. Ludwig DS, Ebbeling CB. Type 2 diabetes mellitus in children: primary care and public health considerations. *JAMA.* 2001;286:1427–1430

5. Dietz W. Health consequences of obesity in youth: childhood predictors of adult disease. *Pediatrics.* 1998;101:518–525

6. Davison KK, Birch LL. Weight status, parent reaction, and self-concept in five-year-old girls. *Pediatrics.* 2001;107:46–53

7. Allison DB, Fontaine KR, Manson JE, Stevens J, VanItallie TB. Annual deaths attributable to obesity in the United States. *JAMA.* 1999;282: 1530–1538

8. Must A, Spadano J, Coakley EH, Field AE, Colditz G, Dietz WH. The disease burden associated with overweight and obesity. *JAMA.* 1999; 282:1523–1529

9. Blumenthal D. Controlling health care expenditures. *N Engl J Med.* 2001;344:766–769

10. Muñoz KA, Krebs-Smith SM, Ballard-Barbash R, Cleveland LE. Food intakes of US children and adolescents compared with recommendations. *Pediatrics.* 1997;100:323–329

11. Subar AF, Krebs-Smith SM, Cook A, Kahle LL. Dietary sources of nutrients among US children, 1989–1991. *Pediatrics.* 1998;102:913–923

12. Calvadini C, Siega-Riz AM, Popkin BM. US adolescent food intake trends from 1965 to 1996. *Arch Dis Child.* 2000;83:18–24

13. Borrud LG, Enns CW, Mickle S. What we eat in America: USDA surveys food consumption changes. *Food Rev.* 1996;19:14–19. Available at: http://www.ers.usda.gov/publications/foodreview/sep1996/ sept96d.pdf. Accessed February 12, 2003

14. Borrud LG, Mickle S, Nowverl A, Tippett K. *Eating Out in America: Impact on Food Choices and Nutrient Profiles.* Beltsville, MD: Food Surveys Research Group, US Department of Agriculture; 1998. Available at: http://www.barc.usda.gov/bhnrc/foodsurvey/Eatout95.html. Accessed February 12, 2003

15. Lytle LA, Seifert S, Greenstein J, McGovern P. How do children's eating patterns and food choices change over time? Results from a cohort study. *Am J Health Promot.* 2000;14:222–228

16. Gleason P, Suitor C. *Children's Diets in the Mid-1990s: Dietary Intake and Its Relationship with School Meal Participation.* Alexandria, VA: US Department of Agriculture, Food and Nutrition Service, Office of Analysis, Nutrition and Evaluation; 2001. Available at: http://www.fns.usda. gov/oane/menu/published/cnp/files/childiet.pdf. Accessed February 12, 2003

17. Guthrie JF, Morton JF. Food sources of added sweeteners in the diets of Americans. *J Am Diet Assoc.* 2000;100:43–51

18. Ludwig DS, Peterson KE, Gortmaker SL. Relation between consumption of sugar-sweetened drinks and childhood obesity: a prospective observational analysis. *Lancet.* 2001;357:505–508

19. Harnack L, Stang J, Story M. Soft drink consumption among US children and adolescents: nutritional consequences. *J Am Diet Assoc.* 1999; 99:436–441

20. Mattes RD. Dietary compensation by humans for supplemental energy provided as ethanol or carbohydrates in fluids. *Physiol Behav.* 1996;59: 179–187

21. Bellisle F, Rolland-Cachera M-F. How sugar-containing drinks might increase adiposity in children. *Lancet.* 2001;357:490–491

22. Tordoff MG, Alleva AM. Effect of drinking soda sweetened with aspartame or high-fructose corn syrup on food intake and body weight. *Am J Clin Nutr.* 1990;51:963–969

23. De Castro JM, Orozco S. Moderate alcohol intake and spontaneous eating patterns of humans: evidence of unregulated supplementation. *Am J Clin Nutr.* 1990;52:246–253

24. Heller K, Burt BA, Eklund SA. Sugared soda consumption and dental caries in the United States. *J Dent Res.* 2001;80:1949–1953

25. Gerrior S, Bente L. *Nutrient Content of the US Food Supply, 1909–97.* Home Economics Research Report No. 54. Washington, DC: Center for Nutrition Policy and Promotion, US Department of Agriculture; 2001. Available at: http://www.usda.gov/cnpp/Pubs/Food%20Supply/ foodsupplyrpt.pdf. Accessed February 12, 2003

26. Johnson RK, Panely C, Wang MQ. The association between noon beverage consumption and the diet quality of school-age children. *J Child Nutr Manage.* 1998;22:95–100

27. American Academy of Pediatrics, Committee on Nutrition. Calcium requirements of infants, children, and adolescents. *Pediatrics.* 1999;104: 1152–1157

28. Wyshak G. Teenaged girls, carbonated beverage consumption, and bone fractures. *Arch Pediatr Adolesc Med.* 2000;154:610–613

29. NIH Consensus Development Panel on Osteoporosis Prevention, Diagnosis, and Therapy. Osteoporosis: prevention, diagnosis, and therapy. *JAMA.* 2001;285:785–795

30. Henry T. Coca-cola rethinks school contracts. Bottlers asked to fall in line. *USA Today.* March 14, 2001:A01

31. Nestle M. Soft drink "pouring rights": marketing empty calories to children. *Public Health Rep.* 2000;115:308–319

32. Zorn RL. The great cola wars: how one district profits from the competition for vending machines. *Am Sch Board J.* 1999;186:31–33

33. Stuhldreher WL, Koehler AN, Harrison MK, Deel H. The West Virginia Standards for School Nutrition. *J Child Nutr Manage.* 1998;22:79–86

34. National School Lunch Program Regulations. 7 CFR §210.11 (2002). Competitive food services

All policy statements from the American Academy of Pediatrics automatically expire 5 years after publication unless reaffirmed, revised, or retired at or before that time.

AMERICAN ACADEMY OF PEDIATRICS

Committee on Nutrition

The Use and Misuse of Fruit Juice in Pediatrics

ABSTRACT. Historically, fruit juice was recommended by pediatricians as a source of vitamin C and an extra source of water for healthy infants and young children as their diets expanded to include solid foods with higher renal solute. Fruit juice is marketed as a healthy, natural source of vitamins and, in some instances, calcium. Because juice tastes good, children readily accept it. Although juice consumption has some benefits, it also has potential detrimental effects. Pediatricians need to be knowledgeable about juice to inform parents and patients on its appropriate uses.

ABBREVIATIONS. FDA, Food and Drug Administration; AAP, American Academy of Pediatrics.

INTRODUCTION

In 1997, US consumers spent almost $5 billion on refrigerated and bottled juice.[1] Mean juice consumption in America is more than 2 billion gal/y or 9.2 gal/y per person.[2] Children are the single largest group of juice consumers. Children younger than 12 years account for only about 18% of the total population but consume 28% of all juice and juice drinks.[3] By 1 year of age, almost 90% of infants consume juice. The mean daily juice consumption by infants is approximately 2 oz/d, but 2% consume more than 16 oz/d, and 1% of infants consume more than 21 oz/d.[2,4,5] Toddlers consume a mean of approximately 6 oz/d.[2] Ten percent of children 2 to 3 years old and 8% of children 4 to 5 years old drink on average more than 12 oz/d.[2] Adolescents consume the least, accounting for only 10% of juice consumption.

DEFINITIONS

To be labeled as a fruit juice, the Food and Drug Administration (FDA) mandates that a product be 100% fruit juice. For juices reconstituted from concentrate, the label must state that the product is reconstituted from concentrate. Any beverage that is less than 100% fruit juice must list the percentage of the product that is fruit juice, and the beverage must include a descriptive term, such as "drink," "beverage," or "cocktail." In general, juice drinks contain between 10% and 99% juice and added sweeteners, flavors, and sometimes fortifiers, such as vitamin C or calcium. These ingredients must be listed on the label, according to FDA regulations.

The recommendations in this statement do not indicate an exclusive course of treatment or serve as a standard of medical care. Variations, taking into account individual circumstances, may be appropriate.
PEDIATRICS (ISSN 0031 4005). Copyright © 2001 by the American Academy of Pediatrics.

COMPOSITION OF FRUIT JUICE

Water is the predominant component of fruit juice. Carbohydrates, including sucrose, fructose, glucose, and sorbitol, are the next most prevalent nutrient in juice. The carbohydrate concentration varies from 11 g/100 mL (0.44 kcal/mL) to more than 16 g/100 mL (0.64 kcal/mL). Human milk and standard infant formulas have a carbohydrate concentration of 7 g/100 mL.

Juice contains a small amount of protein and minerals. Juices fortified with calcium have approximately the same calcium content as milk but lack other nutrients present in milk. Some juices have high contents of potassium, vitamin A, and vitamin C. In addition, some juices and juice drinks are fortified with vitamin C. The vitamin C and flavonoids in juice may have beneficial long-term health effects, such as decreasing the risk of cancer and heart disease.[6,7] Drinks that contain ascorbic acid consumed simultaneously with food can increase iron absorption by twofold.[8,9] This may be important for children who consume diets with low iron bioavailability.

Juice contains no fat or cholesterol, and unless the pulp is included, it contains no fiber. The fluoride concentration of juice and juice drinks varies. One study found fluoride ion concentrations ranged from 0.02 to 2.8 parts per million.[10] The fluoride content of concentrated juice varies with the fluoride content of the water used to reconstitute the juice.

Grapefruit juice contains substances that suppress a cytochrome P-450 enzyme in the small bowel wall. This results in altered absorption of some drugs, such as cisapride, calcium antagonists, and cyclosporin.[11–13] Grapefruit juice should not be consumed when these drugs are used.

Some manufacturers specifically produce juice for infants. These juices do not contain sulfites or added sugars and are more expensive than regular fruit juice.

ABSORPTION OF CARBOHYDRATE FROM JUICE

The 4 major sugars in juice are sucrose, glucose, fructose, and sorbitol. Sucrose is a disaccharide that is hydrolyzed into 2 component monosaccharides, glucose and fructose, by sucrase present in the small bowel epithelium. Glucose is then absorbed rapidly via an active-carrier–mediated process in the brush border of the small bowel. Fructose is absorbed by a facilitated transport mechanism via a carrier but not against a concentration gradient. In addition, fructose may be absorbed by a disaccharidase-related transport system, because the absorption of fructose is more efficient in the presence of glucose, with maximal absorption occurring when fructose and glucose are present in equimolar concentrations.[14] Clinical studies have demonstrated this, with more apparent malabsorption when fructose concentration exceeds that of glucose (eg, apple and pear juice) than when the 2 sugars are present in equal concentrations (eg, white grape juice).[15,16] However, when provided in appropriate amounts (10 mL/kg of body weight), these different juices are absorbed equally as well.[17] Sorbitol is absorbed via passive diffusion at slow rates, resulting in much of the ingested sorbitol being unabsorbed.[18]

Carbohydrate that is not absorbed in the small intestine is fermented by bacteria in the colon. This bacterial fermentation results in the production of hydrogen, carbon dioxide, methane, and the short-chain fatty acids—acetic, propionic, and butyric. Some of these gases and fatty acids are reabsorbed through the colonic epithelium, and in this way, a portion of the malabsorbed carbohydrate can be scavenged.[19] Nonabsorbed carbohydrate presents an osmotic load to the gastrointestinal tract, which causes diarrhea.[20]

Malabsorption of carbohydrate in juice, especially when consumed in excessive amounts, can result in chronic diarrhea, flatulence, bloating, and abdominal pain.[21–27] Fructose and sorbitol have been implicated most commonly,[15,16,28–30] but the ratios of specific carbohydrates may also be important.[31] The malabsorption of carbohydrate that can result from large intakes of juice is the basis for some health care providers to recommend juice for the treatment of constipation.[32]

JUICE IN THE FOOD GUIDE PYRAMID

Fruit is 1 of the 5 major food groups in the Food Guide Pyramid.[33] It is recommended that children consuming approximately 1600 kcal/d (depending on size, 1–4 years old) should have 2 fruit servings and those consuming 2800 kcal/d (depending on size, 10–18 years old) should consume 4 fruit servings. Half of these servings can be provided in the form of fruit juice (not fruit drinks). A 6-oz glass of fruit juice equals 1 fruit serving. Fruit juice offers no nutritional advantage over whole fruit. In fact, fruit juice lacks the fiber of whole fruit. Kilocalorie for kilocalorie, fruit juice can be consumed more quickly than whole fruit. Reliance on fruit juice instead of whole fruit to meet the recommended daily intake of fruits does not promote eating behaviors associated with consumption of whole fruits.

MICROBIAL SAFETY OF JUICE

Only pasteurized juice is safe for infants, children, and adolescents. Pasteurized fruit juices are free of microorganisms. Unpasteurized juice may contain pathogens, such as *Escherichia coli* and *Salmonella* and *Cryptosporidium* organisms.[34] These organisms can cause serious disease, such as hemolytic-uremic syndrome, and should never be given to infants and children. Unpasteurized juice must contain a warning on the label that the product may contain harmful bacteria.[35]

INFANTS

The American Academy of Pediatrics (AAP) recommends that breast milk be the only nutrient fed to infants until 4 to 6 months of age.[36] For mothers who cannot breastfeed or choose not to breastfeed, a prepared infant formula can be used and is a complete source of nutrition. No additional nutrients are needed. There is no nutritional indication to feed juice to infants younger than 6 months. Offering juice before solid foods are introduced into the diet could risk having juice replace breast milk or infant formula in the diet. This can result in reduced intake of protein, fat, vitamins, and minerals such as iron, calcium, and zinc.[37] Malnutrition and short stature in children have been associated with excessive consumption of juice.[4,38]

After approximately 4 to 6 months of age, solid foods can be introduced into the diets of infants. The AAP recommends that single-ingredient foods be chosen and introduced 1 at a time at weekly intervals. Iron-fortified infant cereals or pureed meats are good choices for first weaning foods. Because foods high in iron are recommended as weaning foods, beverages that contain vitamin C do not offer a nutritional advantage for iron-sufficient individuals.

It is prudent to give juice only to infants who can drink from a cup (approximately 6 months or older). Teeth begin to erupt at approximately 6 months of age. Dental caries have also been associated with juice consumption.[39] Prolonged exposure of the teeth to the sugars in juice is a major contributing factor to dental caries. The AAP and the American Academy of Pedodontics recommendations state that juice should be offered to infants in a cup, not a bottle, and that infants not be put to bed with a bottle in their mouth.[40] The practice of allowing children to carry a bottle, cup, or box of juice around throughout the day leads to excessive exposure of the teeth to carbohydrate, which promotes development of dental caries.

Fruit juice should be used as part of a meal or snack. It should not be sipped throughout the day or used as a means to pacify an unhappy infant or child. Because infants consume fewer than 1600 kcal/d, 4 to 6 oz of juice per day, representing 1 food serving of fruit, is more than adequate. Infants can be encouraged to consume whole fruits that are mashed or pureed.

The AAP practice guideline on the management of acute gastroenteritis in young children recommends that only oral electrolyte solutions be used to rehydrate infants and young children and that a normal diet be continued throughout an episode of gastroenteritis.[41] Surveys show that many health care providers do not follow the recommended procedures for management of diarrhea.[42] The high carbohydrate content of juice (11–16 g %), compared with oral electrolyte solutions (2.5–3 g %), may exceed the intestine's ability to absorb carbohydrate, resulting in carbohydrate malabsorption. Carbohydrate malabsorption causes osmotic diarrhea, increasing the severity of the diarrhea already present.[43] Fruit juice is low in electrolytes. The sodium concentration is 1

• •

to 3 mEq/L. Stool sodium concentration in children with acute diarrhea is 20 to 40 mEq/L. Oral electrolyte solutions contain 40 to 45 mEq/L of sodium. As a replacement for fluid losses, juice may predispose infants to development of hyponatremia.

In the past, there was concern that infants who were fed orange juice were likely to develop an allergy to it. The development of a perioral rash in some infants after being fed freshly squeezed citrus juice is most likely a contact dermatitis attributable to peel oils.[44] Diarrhea and other gastrointestinal symptoms observed in some infants were most likely attributable to carbohydrate malabsorption. Although allergies to fruit may develop early in life, they are uncommon.[45]

TODDLERS AND YOUNG CHILDREN

Most issues relevant to juice intake for infants are also are relevant for toddlers and young children. Fruit juice and fruit drinks are easily overconsumed by toddlers and young children because they taste good. In addition, they are conveniently packaged or can be placed in a bottle and carried around during the day. Because juice is viewed as nutritious, limits on consumption are not usually set by parents. Like soda, it can contribute to energy imbalance. High intakes of juice can contribute to diarrhea, overnutrition or undernutrition, and development of dental caries.

OLDER CHILDREN AND ADOLESCENTS

Juice consumption presents fewer nutritional issues for older children and adolescents, because they consume less of these beverages. Nevertheless, it seems prudent to limit juice intake to two 6-oz servings, or half of the recommended fruit servings each day. It is important to encourage consumption of the whole fruit for the benefit of fiber intake and a longer time to consume the same kilocalories.

Excessive juice consumption and the resultant increase in energy intake may contribute to the development of obesity. One study found a link between juice intake in excess of 12 oz/d and obesity.[4] Other studies, however, found that children who consumed greater amounts of juice were taller and had lower body mass index than those who consumed less juice[46] or found no relationship between juice intake and growth parameters.[47] More research is needed to better define this relationship.

CONCLUSIONS

1. Fruit juice offers no nutritional benefit for infants younger than 6 months.
2. Fruit juice offers no nutritional benefits over whole fruit for infants older than 6 months and children.
3. One hundred percent fruit juice or reconstituted juice can be a healthy part of the diet when consumed as part of a well-balanced diet. Fruit drinks, however, are not nutritionally equivalent to fruit juice.
4. Juice is not appropriate in the treatment of dehydration or management of diarrhea.

5. Excessive juice consumption may be associated with malnutrition (overnutrition and undernutrition).
6. Excessive juice consumption may be associated with diarrhea, flatulence, abdominal distention, and tooth decay.
7. Unpasteurized juice may contain pathogens that can cause serious illnesses.
8. A variety of fruit juices, provided in appropriate amounts for a child's age, are not likely to cause any significant clinical symptoms.
9. Calcium-fortified juices provide a bioavailable source of calcium but lack other nutrients present in breast milk, formula, or cow's milk.

RECOMMENDATIONS

1. Juice should not be introduced into the diet of infants before 6 months of age.
2. Infants should not be given juice from bottles or easily transportable covered cups that allow them to consume juice easily throughout the day. Infants should not be given juice at bedtime.
3. Intake of fruit juice should be limited to 4 to 6 oz/d for children 1 to 6 years old. For children 7 to 18 years old, juice intake should be limited to 8 to 12 oz or 2 servings per day.
4. Children should be encouraged to eat whole fruits to meet their recommended daily fruit intake.
5. Infants, children, and adolescents should not consume unpasteurized juice.
6. In the evaluation of children with malnutrition (overnutrition and undernutrition), the health care provider should determine the amount of juice being consumed.
7. In the evaluation of children with chronic diarrhea, excessive flatulence, abdominal pain, and bloating, the health care provider should determine the amount of juice being consumed.
8. In the evaluation of dental caries, the amount and means of juice consumption should be determined.
9. Pediatricians should routinely discuss the use of fruit juice and fruit drinks and should educate parents about differences between the two.

COMMITTEE ON NUTRITION, 1999–2000
Susan S. Baker, MD, PhD, Chairperson
William J. Cochran, MD
Frank R. Greer, MD
Melvin B. Heyman, MD
Marc S. Jacobson, MD
Tom Jaksic, MD, PhD
Nancy F. Krebs, MD

LIAISONS
Donna Blum-Kemelor, MS, RD
    US Department of Agriculture
William Dietz, MD, PhD
    Centers for Disease Control and Prevention
Gilman Grave, MD
    National Institute of Child Health and Human Development
Suzanne S. Harris, PhD
    International Life Sciences Institute

Van S. Hubbard, MD, PhD
  National Institute of Diabetes and Digestive
  and Kidney Diseases
Ann Prendergast, RD, MPH
  Maternal and Child Health Bureau
Alice E. Smith, MS, RD
  American Dietetic Association
Elizabeth Yetley, PhD
  Food and Drug Administration
Doris E. Yuen, MD, PhD
  Canadian Paediatric Society

SECTION LIAISONS
Scott C. Denne, MD
  Section on Perinatal Pediatrics
Ronald M. Lauer, MD
  Section on Cardiology

STAFF
Pamela Kanda, MPH

REFERENCES

1. Food Marketing Institute Information Service. *Food Institute Report.* Washington, DC: Food Marketing Institute Information Service; 1998
2. Agriculture Research Service. *Food and Nutrient Intakes by Individuals in the United States by Sex and Age, 1994–96.* Washington, DC: US Department of Agriculture; 1998. NFS Report No. 96-2
3. National Family Opinion Research. Share of Intake Panel [database]. Greenwich, CT: National Family Opinion Research. Cited by: Clydesdale FM, Kolasa KM, Ikeda JP. All you want to know about fruit juice. *Nutrition Today.* 1994;March/April:14–28
4. Dennison BA, Rockwell HL, Baker SL. Excess fruit juice consumption by preschool-aged children is associated with short stature and obesity. *Pediatrics.* 1997;99:15–22
5. Dennison BA. Fruit juice consumption by infants and children: a review. *J Am Coll Nutr.* 1996;15(suppl 5):4S–11S
6. Ames BN. Micronutrients prevent cancer and delay aging. *Toxicol Lett.* 1998;102–103:5–18
7. Hollman PC, Hertog MG, Katan MB. Role of dietary flavonoids in protection against cancer and coronary heart disease. *Biochem Soc Trans.* 1996;24:785–789
8. Fairweather-Tait S, Fox T, Wharf SG, Eagles J. The bioavailability of iron in different weaning foods and the enhancing effect of a fruit drink containing ascorbic acid. *Pediatr Res.* 1995;37:389–394
9. Abrams SA, O'Brien KO, Wen J, Liang LK, Stuff JE. Absorption by 1-year old children of an iron supplement given with cow's milk or juice. *Pediatr Res.* 1996;39:171–175
10. Kiritsy MC, Levy SM, Warren JJ, Guha-Chowdhury N, Heilman JR, Marshall T. Assessing fluoride concentrations of juices and juice-flavored drinks. *J Am Dent Assoc.* 1996;127:895–902
11. Bailey DG, Malcolm J, Arnold O, Spence JD. Grapefruit juice-drug interactions. *Br J Clin Pharmacol.* 1998;46:101–110
12. Gross AS, Goh YD, Addison RS, Shenfield GM. Influence of grapefruit juice on cisapride pharmacokinetics. *Clin Pharmacol Ther.* 1999;65: 395–401
13. Fuhr U. Drug interactions with grapefruit juice. Extent, probable mechanism and clinical relevance. *Drug Saf.* 1998;18:251–272
14. Riby JE, Fujisawa T, Kretchmer N. Fructose absorption. *Am J Clin Nutr.* 1993;58(suppl 5):748S–753S
15. Smith MM, Davis M, Chasalow FI, Lifshitz F. Carbohydrate absorption from fruit juice in young children. *Pediatrics.* 1995;95:340–344
16. Nobigrot T, Chasalow FI, Lifshitz F. Carbohydrate absorption from one serving of fruit juice in young children: age and carbohydrate composition effects. *J Am Coll Nutr.* 1997;16:152–158
17. Lifshitz CH. Carbohydrate absorption from fruit juices in infants. *Pediatrics.* 2000;105(1). URL: http://www.pediatrics.org/cgi/content/full/105/1/e4
18. Southgate DA. Digestion and metabolism of sugar. *Am J Clin Nutr.* 1995;62(suppl 1):203S–211S
19. Lifshitz CH. Role of colonic scavengers of unabsorbed carbohydrate in infants and children. *J Am Coll Nutr.* 1996;15(suppl 5):30S–34S
20. Gryboski JD. Diarrhea from dietetic candies. *N Engl J Med.* 1966;275:718
21. Hyams JS, Leichtner AM. Apple juice: an unappreciated cause of chronic diarrhea. *Am J Dis Child.* 1985;139:503–505
22. Hyams JS, Etienne NL, Leichtner AM, Theuer RC. Carbohydrate malabsorption following fruit juice ingestion in young children. *Pediatrics.* 1988;82:64–68
23. Rumessen JJ, Gudmand-Hoyer E. Functional bowel disease: malabsorption and abdominal distress after ingestion of fructose, sorbitol, and fructose-sorbitol mixtures. *Gastroenterology.* 1988;95:694–700
24. Hoekstra JH, van den Aker JHL, Ghoos YF, Hartemink R, Kneepkens CM. Fluid intake and industrial processing in apple juice induced chronic non-specific diarrhea. *Arch Dis Child.* 1995;73:126–130
25. Ament ME. Malabsorption of apple juice and pear nectar in infants and children: clinical implications. *J Am Coll Nutr.* 1996;15(suppl 5):26S–29S
26. Davidson M, Wasserman R. The irritable colon of childhood (chronic non-specific diarrhea syndrome). *J Pediatr.* 1996;69:1027–1038
27. Lifshitz F, Ament ME, Kleinman RE, et al. Role of juice carbohydrate malabsorption in chronic nonspecific diarrhea in children. *J Pediatr.* 1992;120:825–829
28. Hoekstra JH, van Kempen AA, Kneepkens C. Apple juice malabsorption: fructose or sorbitol? *J Pediatr Gastroenterol Nutr.* 1993;16:39–42
29. Kneepkens CM, Jakobs C, Douwes AC. Apple juice, fructose and chronic nonspecific diarrhoea. *Eur J Pediatr.* 1989;148:571–573
30. Hoekstra JH, van den Aker JH, Hartemink R, Kneepkens CM. Fruit juice malabsorption: not only fructose. *Acta Paediatr.* 1995;84:1241–1244
31. Fujisawa T, Riby J, Kretchmer N. Intestinal absorption of fructose in the rat. *Gastroenterology.* 1991;101:360–367
32. Baker SS, Liptak GS, Colletti RB, et al. Constipation in infants and children: evaluation and treatment. *J Pediatr Gastroenterol Nutr.* 1999;29: 612–626
33. US Department of Agriculture, Human Nutrition Information Service. *The Food Guide Pyramid.* Washington, DC: US Government Printing Office; 1992. Home and Garden Bull No. 252
34. Parish ME. Public health and nonpasteurized fruit juices. *Crit Rev Microbiol.* 1997;23:109–119
35. Food Labeling. Warning and Notice Statement: Labeling of Juice Products; Final Rule. 63 *Federal Register* 37029–37056 (1998) (codified at 21 CFR §101, 120)
36. American Academy of Pediatrics, Committee on Nutrition. Supplemental foods for infants. In: Kleinman RE, ed. *Pediatric Nutrition Handbook.* 4th ed. Elk Grove Village, IL: American Academy of Pediatrics; 1998: 43–53
37. Gibson SA. Non-milk extrinsic sugars in the diets of pre-school children: association with intakes of micronutrients, energy, fat and NSP. *Br J Nutr.* 1997;78:367–378
38. Smith MM, Lifshitz F. Excess fruit juice consumption as a contributing factor in nonorganic failure to thrive. *Pediatrics.* 1994;93:438–443
39. Konig KG, Navia JM. Nutritional role of sugars in oral health. *Am J Clin Nutr.* 1995;62(suppl 1):275S–283S
40. American Academy of Pediatrics and American Academy of Pedodontics. Juice in ready-to-use bottles and nursing bottle caries. *AAP News and Comment.* 1978;29(1):11
41. American Academy of Pediatrics, Provisional Committee on Quality Improvement, Subcommittee on Acute Gastroenteritis. Practice parameter: the management of acute gastroenteritis in young children. *Pediatrics.* 1996;97:424–433
42. Bezerra JA, Stathos TH, Duncan B, Gaines JA, Udall JN Jr. Treatment of infants with acute diarrhea: what's recommended and what's practiced. *Pediatrics.* 1992;90:1–4
43. Cochran WJ, Klish WJ. Treating acute gastroenteritis in infants. *Drug Prot.* 1987;2:88–93
44. Ratner B, Untracht S, Malone J, Retsina M. Allergenicity of modified and processed food stuffs: IV. Orange: allergenicity of orange studied in man. *J Pediatr.* 1953;43:421–428
45. Blanco Quiros A, Sanchez Villares E. Pathogenic basis of food allergy treatment. In: Reinhardt D, Schmidt E, eds. *Food Allergy.* New York, NY: Raven Press; 1988:265–270
46. Alexy U, Sichert Hellert W, Kersting M, Manz F, Schoch G. Fruit juice consumption and the prevalence of obesity and short stature in German preschool children: results of the DONALD study. *J Pediatr Gastroenterol Nutr.* 1999;29:343–349
47. Skinner JD, Carruth BR, Moran J III, Houck K, Coletta F. Fruit juice intake is not related to children's growth. *Pediatrics.* 1999;103:58–64

Index